Minimally Invasive and Robotic Thyroid and Parathyroid Surgery

David J. Terris • Michael C. Singer
Editors

Minimally Invasive and Robotic Thyroid and Parathyroid Surgery

Springer

Editors
David J. Terris, MD, FACS
Department of Otolaryngology – Head and Neck Surgery
GRU Thyroid Center
Georgia Regents University
Augusta, GA
USA

Michael C. Singer, MD
Division of Thyroid and Parathyroid Surgery
Department of Otolaryngology – Head and Neck Surgery
Henry Ford Hospital
Detroit, MI
USA

ISBN 978-1-4939-5347-9 ISBN 978-1-4614-9011-1 (eBook)
DOI 10.1007/978-1-4614-9011-1
Springer New York Heidelberg Dordrecht London

Printed on acid-free paper

Springer is part of Springer Science+Business Media (www.springer.com)

I dedicate this book to my patients, my residents, and my fellows, from whom I have learned a tremendous amount and am humbly grateful. I also owe a debt of gratitude to my 3 children (Trevor, Garrett, and Kyle) – who have endured countless missed parties, late dinners, and shortened vacations in sacrifice for commitment to my career.

–David J. Terris

To my parents, David and Judy, who have always lovingly supported us as we pursued our interests.
To my mentor, Dave Terris, who is always open to challenging questions and new ideas.
To my wife, Ora, and sons, Jonas, Emmett, Leo, and Caleb, whose love is irreplaceable.

–Michael C. Singer

Foreword

It is a privilege to write the Foreword for the book *Minimally Invasive and Robotic Thyroid and Parathyroid Surgery*, edited by David J. Terris and Michael C. Singer.

We are living in an era of remarkable increase in the detection of both thyroid and parathyroid diseases, due to more precise laboratory and imaging methods. In addition, recent technological advances offer better surgical visualization through optical magnification and more precise dissection of the delicate anatomical structures within the central neck compartment.

This book brings a significant new contribution for all health professionals interested in the surgical treatment of thyroid and parathyroid diseases. In fact, it represents a formidable effort to minimize the operative invasiveness while keeping the solid scientific basis of the surgical treatment of these diseases established long ago by the landmark work of Kocher and his followers.

Drs. Terris and Singer, both world-class head and neck surgeons, were able to invite outstanding authors, who produced a comprehensive and very up-to-date collection of chapters, covering all aspects of minimally invasive thyroid and parathyroid surgery.

It is important to emphasize that some of the techniques described in this book are not universally applicable, due to several geographical and socioeconomic peculiarities of different countries around the world. Nevertheless, all surgeons must be aware of the newest available technical developments, in order to offer their patients the most effective, yet least aggressive, operative treatment for their thyroid and parathyroid diseases.

São Paulo, Brazil — Claudio R. Cernea, MD, PhD

Preface

In the last 15 years, thyroid and parathyroid surgery has undergone revolutionary changes. While the fundamental principles of these delicate surgeries have remained unchanged, tenets from the fields of laparoscopic, minimal invasive, and plastic surgery have led to dramatic innovations in technique and approaches. These minimally invasive approaches are designed to reduce the functional and cosmetic impact of surgery on patients undergoing thyroid and parathyroid surgery. In an effort to optimize the benefits for patients, surgeons have developed a wide array of minimally invasive techniques.

While minimally invasive thyroid and parathyroid techniques have been adopted on a widespread scale, no attempt has been made to compile these different techniques into one practical guide. This book serves as a resource for surgeons, fellows, residents, and students who are interested in learning about both the philosophy and technical details of the different robotic and endoscopic techniques available. Each chapter is authored by a surgeon writing about an area in which they hold a particular expertise. In many of the chapters, pioneers of surgical techniques describe their procedures in detail. Numerous figures and drawings serve to facilitate the understanding of the details of these procedures.

While the surgical approaches covered in this book vary greatly in technique and details, they all share one common element. All of these procedures were developed by thyroid and parathyroid surgeons trying to improve the surgical outcomes for their patients. Perhaps through a greater knowledge and understanding of these techniques, further innovation will be spurred.

Augusta, GA, USA — David J. Terris, MD, FACS
Detroit, MI, USA — Michael C. Singer, MD

Contents

Contributors

Peter Angelos, MD, PhD, FACS Department of Surgery, The University of Chicago Medicine, Chicago, IL, USA

Carrie Bush, MD Department of Otolaryngology, Georgia Regents University, Augusta, GA, USA

Michael J. Campbell, MD Department of Surgery, University of California, Davis, CA, USA

Herbert Chen, MD Division of General Surgery, Department of Surgery, University of Wisconsin, Madison, WI, USA

Eun Chang Choi Department of Otorhinolaryngology, Yonsei University College of Medicine, Severance Hospital, Yonsei University Health System, Seoul, Republic of Korea

June Young Choi Department of Surgery, Seoul National University Hospital, Seoul, Republic of Korea

Woong Youn Chung, MD Department of Surgery, Yonsei University College of Medicine, Seoul, Republic of Korea

E. Ashlie Darr, MD Division of Thyroid and Parathyroid Surgery, Department of Otolaryngology-Head and Neck Surgery, Massachusetts Eye and Ear Infirmary, Boston, MA, USA

Leigh Delbridge, MD Endocrine Surgical Unit, University of Sydney, Sydney, NSW, Australia

Quan-Yang Duh, MD Department of Surgery, University of California, San Francisco, San Francisco, CA, USA

VA Medical Center, San Francisco, CA, USA

William S. Duke, MD Department of Otolaryngology, Georgia Regents University, Augusta, GA, USA

Raymon Grogan, MD Endocrine Surgery Research Program, Department of Surgery, The University of Chicago Medicine, Chicago, IL, USA

Keith S. Heller, MD, FACS Department of Surgery, New York University Langone Medical Center, New York, NY, USA

F. Christopher Holsinger, MD, FACS Division of Head and Neck Surgery, Stanford University Medical Center, Stanford CA

Jeffrey J. Houlton, MD Department of Otolaryngology–Head and Neck Surgery, Medical University of South Carolina, Charleston, SC, USA

Yoshifumi Ikeda, MD, FACS Department of Surgery, Teikyo University School of Medicine, Tokyo, Japan

Lana Jackson, MD, PharmD Department of Otolaryngology, Georgia Regents University, Augusta, GA, USA

Yoon Woo Koh, MD, PhD Department of Otorhinolaryngology, Yonsei University College of Medicine, Severance Hospital, Yonsei University Health System, Seoul, Republic of Korea

Schelto Kruijff, MD Endocrine Surgical Unit, University of Sydney, Sydney, NSW, Australia

Kyu Eun Lee, PhD Department of Surgery, Seoul National University Hospital, Seoul, Republic of Korea

Sohee Lee, MD Division of Breast-Thyroid Surgery, Department of Surgery, Seoul St. Mary's Hospital, The Catholic University of Korea, Seoul, Republic of Korea

Celestino P. Lombardi, MD Division of Endocrine and Metabolic Surgery, Department of Surgery, Istituto di Semeiotica Chirurgica, Università Cattolica del Sacro Cuore, Rome, Italy

Valeria Matteucci, MD Department of Surgery, Endocrine Surgery Unit, Azienda Ospedaliero-Universitaria Pisana, Pisa, Italy

Paolo Miccoli, MD Department of Surgery, Azienda Ospedaliero-Universitaria Pisana, University of Pisa, Pisa, Italy

Michele N. Minuto, MD, PhD Department of Surgical Sciences and Applied Diagnostics (DISC), IRCCS, Azienda Ospedaliero-Universitaria San Martino-IST, University of Genoa, Genoa, Italy

Salem I. Noureldine, MD Division of Head and Neck Endocrine Surgery, Department of Otolaryngology – Head and Neck Surgery, Johns Hopkins University School of Medicine, Baltimore, MD, USA

Sarah C. Oltmann, MD Department of Surgery, University of Wisconsin, Madison, WI, USA

Lisa A. Orloff, MD Department of Otolaryngology/Head and Neck Surgery, University of California, San Francisco, San Francisco, CA, USA

Janice L. Pasieka, MD, FRCSC, FACS Department of Surgery, North Tower, Calgary, lberta, Canada

J. Drew Prosser Department of Otolaryngology, Georgia Regents University, Augusta, GA, USA

Marco Raffaelli, MD Division of Endocrine and Metabolic Surgery, Department of Surgery, Istituto di Semeiotica Chirurgica, Università Cattolica del Sacro Cuore, Rome, Italy

Gregory Randolph, MD, FACS, FACE Division of Thyroid and Parathyroid Surgery, Massachusetts Eye and Ear Infirmary, Harvard Medical School, Boston, MA, USA

Michael C. Singer, MD Division of Thyroid and Parathyroid Surgery, Department of Otolaryngology-Head and Neck Surgery, Henry Ford Hospital, Detroit, MI, USA

C. Arturo Solares, MD Department of Otolaryngology, Department of Neurosurgery, Georgia Skull Base Center, Georgia Health Sciences University, Augusta, GA, USA

David L. Steward, MD Department of Otolaryngology–Head and Neck Surgery, University Hospital, Cincinnati, OH, USA

David J. Terris, MD, FACS Department of Otolaryngology – Head and Neck Surgery, GRU Thyroid Center, Georgia Regents University, Augusta, GA, USA

Ralph P. Tufano, MD, MBA, FACS Division of Head and Neck Endocrine Surgery, Department of Otolaryngology – Head and Neck Surgery, Johns Hopkins University School of Medicine, Baltimore, MD, USA

Neelima Tummala, MD Department of Otolaryngology/Head and Neck Surgery, University of California, San Francisco, San Francisco, CA, USA

1 The Evolution of Thyroid Surgery

E. Ashlie Darr and Gregory Randolph

The early history of thyroid surgery is closely related to the manifestation of iodine deficiency as goitrous glandular enlargement. The first mention of goiter as a disease entity occurred in 2700 B BC in China. However, it was not until AD 500 that Abdul Kasan Kelibis Abis reportedly performed the first surgical excision of the thyroid gland in Baghdad. Despite significant postoperative hemorrhage, the patient survived.

Understanding of the nature of thyroid diseases was, of course, limited in ancient times, and attempts at surgery were rare. Early nonsurgical treatments for goiter included the application of toad's blood or placement of a cadaver's hand on the neck. In the twelfth and thirteenth centuries in Salerno, Italy, heated setons were placed at right angles into the substance of the gland and turned twice daily until they pierced the skin. In some cases, a large hook was placed into the goiter, the overlying skin dissected away, and a segment of tissue was extirpated. A boot lace was sometimes used to strangulate a portion of the gland prior to removal. Patients were strapped to tables and held down during these procedures, and many of them expired due to sepsis or massive bleeding. Indications for surgery during those times were primarily large goiters causing airway impingement or suppurating glands. The latter may have in fact been representative of tuberculous lymphadenitis.

Surgical advances occurred slowly and were limited by lack of anesthesia, antisepsis, and poor instrumentation. The first thyroidectomy using scalpels was performed by Wilhelm Fabricus in 1646 on a 10-year-old girl, who died, leading to his imprisonment. A successful partial thyroidectomy was achieved in Paris in 1791 by Pierre Joseph Desault, followed in 1808 by a total thyroidectomy by Guillaume Dupuytren. The latter led to the patient's demise due to postoperative "shock" despite low blood loss. A German surgeon named Johann Hedenus was the most prolific thyroid surgeon of that era, reporting on a series of six successful goiter excisions in 1821.

The first experimental use of iodine as a treatment for goiter was performed in 1820 by Johann Straub and Francois Coindet of Switzerland. Coindet suggested the preoperative use of iodine as a means to decrease the size and vascularity of goiters. Iodine was hailed as a miracle drug, and its widespread use often led to toxicity. With regard to surgical technique, a variety of incisional styles, including oblique, longitudinal, and Y-shaped, were used during that era. Incision was followed by blunt dissection, often leading to significant hemorrhage, and wounds were typically left open and packed. Bloodletting was a

E.A. Darr, MD (✉)
Division of Thyroid and Parathyroid Surgery,
Department of Otolaryngology-Head and Neck Surgery,
Massachusetts Eye and Ear Infirmary,
243 Charles Street, Boston, MA 02114, USA
e-mail: ashlie.darr@gmail.com

G. Randolph, MD, FACS, FACE
Division of Thyroid and Parathyroid Surgery,
Massachusetts Eye and Ear Infirmary,
Harvard Medical School, Boston, MA, USA

D.J. Terris, M.C. Singer (eds.), *Minimally Invasive and Robotic Thyroid and Parathyroid Surgery*,
DOI 10.1007/978-1-4614-9011-1_1, © Springer Science+Business Media New York 2014

treatment used for postoperative complications despite significant blood losses during surgery.

The surgical revolution began in the mid-1800s with the development of anesthesia. The first to use sulfuric ether during surgery was Crawford W. Long in Georgia in 1842. In 1847, the first thyroidectomy using anesthesia was performed in Russia by Nikolai Pirigov. Joseph Lister introduced the concept of antisepsis in 1867, which was further promoted by the initiation of cap and gown wearing in the operating room by Gustav Neuber in 1883. This, together with the advent of steam sterilization of surgical instruments in 1886 by Ernst von Bergmann in Germany, contributed to lower postoperative infection rates and laid the foundation for current antiseptic surgical practice. Further progress in thyroid surgery was achieved due to the introduction of improved hemostatic tools, such as the self-retaining arterial forceps designed by Spencer Wells in 1872. These improvements led to the reduction of mortality from thyroid surgery from 40 % in 1850 to 20 % in 1875.

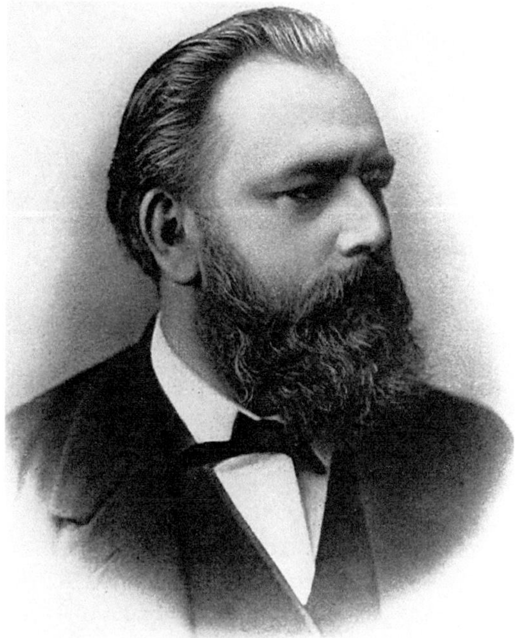

Fig. 1.1 Albert Theodor Billroth, 1867 (Reproduced with permission from Institut für Medizingeschichte, Universität Bern, Buehlstrasse 26, CH 3012 Bern)

Modern Thyroid Surgery

The age of modern thyroid surgery followed from the developments of the surgical revolution. As mortality rates declined, increased numbers of thyroid surgeries were performed, and greater understanding and teaching of thyroid physiology, anatomy, and surgical technique ensued. Among the most notable surgeons of the nineteenth century is Albert Theodor Billroth (1829–1894), who served as chair in both Zurich and Vienna, published the textbook *General Surgical Pathology and Therapeutics*, and created the *Archives of Clinical Surgery* (Fig. 1.1). He also disseminated his thyroidectomy techniques, such as division of the sternocleidomastoid muscle and incision and drainage of thyroid cysts, by founding a school of surgery. A variety of methods for hemostasis were also taught, including arterial ligation using aneurysmal needles and the use of penghawar djambi, an Indian vegetable hemostatic agent. Billroth initially abandoned thyroid surgery for over a decade due to high mortality rates. With advancement in hemostasis and antisepsis, however, patient mortality rates in Billroth's practice decreased from 40 to 8 % over his career.

In spite of Billroth's myriad achievements, Theodor Kocher (1841–1917) stands alone as the father of modern thyroid surgery (Fig. 1.2). He completed more than 5,000 thyroidectomies during his career as chair at the University of Bern. Mortality rates in his hands were 0.2 % by 1898 due to his adoption of antiseptic and hemostatic techniques. Kocher pioneered the standard collar incision, which now carries his name, and utilized local anesthesia with cocaine.

Kocher abandoned performing total thyroidectomy for benign disease when he discovered that patients developed the postoperative sequelae of hypothyroidism, namely myxedema, shedding light on thyroid physiology. He also established partial thyroidectomy as a treatment for Graves' disease. William Halsted, an American surgeon, visited the clinics of both Kocher and Billroth and noted that Kocher's patients often developed myxedema postoperatively but rarely tetany, whereas the opposite was true for Billroth. This speaks to the notoriety Kocher achieved for his bloodless field, attention to detail, and completeness of surgery. In 1908, he was awarded the Nobel Prize for his contributions to the understanding of thyroid physiology and thyroid surgery. He was the first surgeon to be awarded this honor.

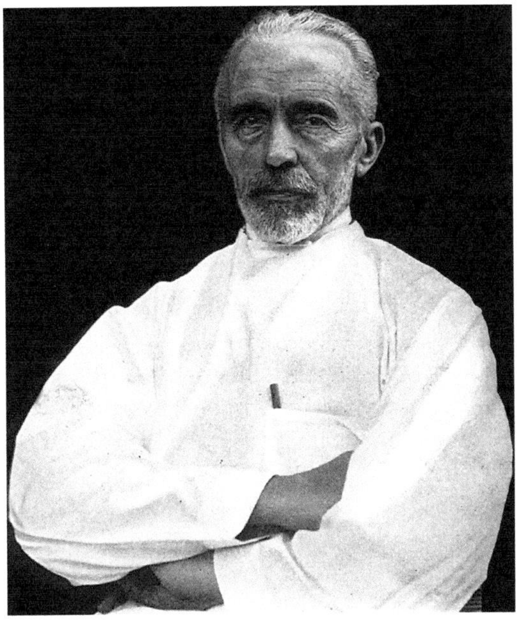

Fig. 1.2 Theodor Kocher, 1912 (Reproduced with permission from Institut für Medizingeschichte, Universität Bern, Buehlstrasse 26, CH 3012 Bern)

As a student of both Billroth and Kocher, Halsted brought his education home to the United States, where he wrote *The Operative Story of Goiter* in 1920. He helped to found Johns Hopkins Hospital, where he developed the first residency program and became the first professor of surgery. He trained many distinguished surgeons, including Cushing, Dandy, Reed, Lahey, and Crile. Among his various contributions to surgery, Crile devised an antishock garment for patient use during thyroid surgery (Fig. 1.3).

Postoperative tetany was first described by Wolfler in 1879, but it was Eugene Gley who first associated this symptom with disruption or removal of the parathyroid glands in 1891. An understanding of parathyroid physiology as it relates to calcium was discovered in 1900 by Mccallum and Carl Voegtlin. They discovered that postthyroidectomy tetany was associated with low levels of calcium in the tissues and that this could be reversed by injection of parathyroid extracts or calcium. Pfieffer and Mayer were the first to demonstrate success in the treatment of tetany with parathyroid autotransplantation. Frank Lahey further advanced the concept of autotransplantation in 1926 by advising its placement into the sternocleidomastoid muscle, while Sam Wells in 1976 showed the efficacy of subtotal parathyroidectomy with forearm autotransplantation for four-gland hyperplasia. A significant advancement in parathyroid surgery

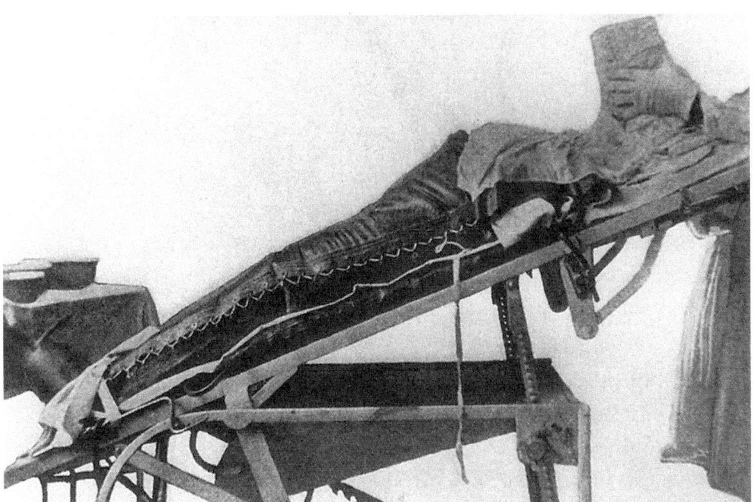

Fig. 1.3 Pneumatic antishock suit devised by Crile, used to prevent shock during thyroid surgery (From Park R. Principles and practice of modern surgery. Philadelphia: Lea and Brothers; 1907. Used with permission)

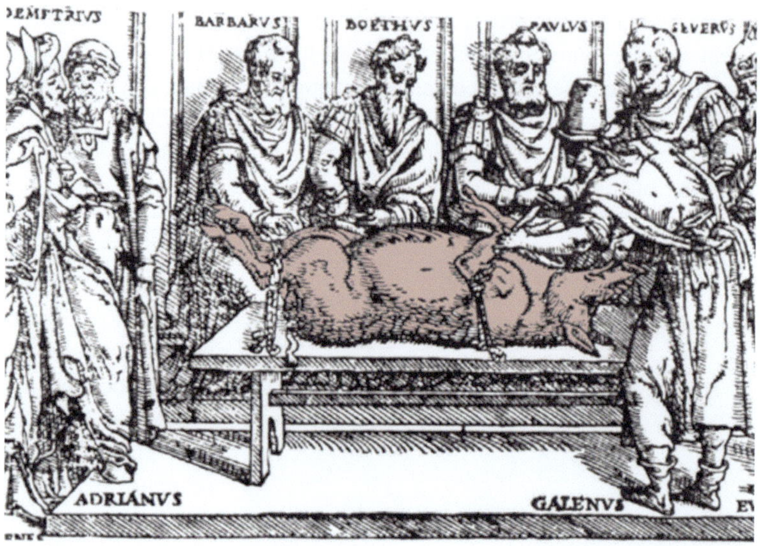

Fig. 1.4 Galen teaching Roman elders the anatomy of the recurrent laryngeal nerve in a living pig. Upon severing the nerve, the squealing pig became mute (From Galeni Liborum Quinta Classis EAM Medicinae Partem, edited by Fabius Paulinus. Published by Guinta Family of Venice, 1625. IM Rutkow. In: Surgery: an illustrated history, St. Louis: Mosby; 1993. p. 40)

occurred with the advent of the immunoassay measurement of parathyroid hormone (PTH) by Solomon Berson and Rosalyn Yalow in 1963, which earned them a Nobel Prize.

The anatomy of the recurrent laryngeal nerves was first detailed by Galen in the second century (Fig. 1.4). Due to his widespread influence, this knowledge was transmitted to generations of scholars and surgeons to come. A great deal was thus known by the 1700s about both the anatomy of the recurrent nerves and the sequelae of injury. The original approach of Kocher and Billroth to preserve the nerve was to ligate the inferior thyroid artery, away from the nerve–artery crossing point. Both Kocher and Miculicz advised leaving a small portion of thyroid tissue behind to cover and protect the nerve. Many other surgeons, including Prioleau, believed that the best strategy for avoiding nerve injury was to avoid visualizing it. It was Lahey in 1938 who demonstrated the importance and safety of nerve identification and dissection when he reported on a series of 3,000 thyroidectomies performed by he and his colleagues over a 3-year period. The significance of the superior laryngeal nerve was not recognized until much later in 1935 when goiter surgery brought an end to singer Amelita Galli-Curci's operatic career.

The turn of the twentieth century led to significant advancement in thyroid disease management with the advent of blood transfusions, frozen section pathology, improvement in patient follow-up and research, and thyroid cancer staging systems. Treatment of hypothyroidism began with the transplantation of thyroid tissue into the spleen of a patient's myxedematous daughter by E. Payr in 1906. Thereafter, surgeons began the practice of thyroid tissue transplantation to control symptoms of hypothyroidism after thyroidectomy. This was replaced by the development of animal thyroid extracts and later thyroxine, which was isolated by Edward C. Kendall in 1914. The treatment of hyperthyroidism was advanced with the development of antithyroid drugs and radioiodine therapy in the 1940s, providing alternatives to surgical excision, and propranolol was introduced for perioperative management in 1965. In the last quarter of the twentieth century, scintigraphy was developed and utilized as a diagnostic tool in thyroid disease workup but was largely supplanted by ultrasound in the 1980s. This allowed for discovery of small, subcentimeter nodules that were not clinically palpable. Further advancements in imaging, including with computed tomography and magnetic resonance imaging (MRI), allowed for assessment of substernal extension of goiters and for evaluation of metastatic lymphadenopathy in cases of thyroid cancer. N. Söderström was the first to develop fine-needle aspiration cytology for thyroid disease in 1952. This became widely available in the 1970s, allowing for the preoperative diagnosis of cancer to be made, resulting in improved surgical decision-making and prioritization. Improved anesthetic agents, lighting, and instrumentation, such as advanced energy devices for hemostasis, further modernized the field. Development of the intraoperative PTH assay led to additional real-time assessment of parathyroid status during surgery for hyperparathyroidism.

Riddell in 1970 first described the use of recurrent laryngeal nerve (RLN) stimulation as a method for intraoperative detection of neural functionality. This was performed by using a finger to feel for laryngeal twitch as well as visualizing cricothyroid contraction upon stimulation of the laryngeal nerves with a handheld stimulator. Riddell also described direct laryngoscopic evaluation of vocal fold motion with RLN stimulation intraoperatively after completion of surgery on the first side. At the same time, Flisburg and Lindholm introduced the technique of insertion of intramuscular electrodes through the cricothyroid membrane into the vocalis muscle for intraoperative EMG monitoring. In 1978, Rea and Davis instead used an endoscopically placed vocal fold electrode. Intramuscular electrode placement required separate endoscopic or other procedures to be performed, as well as expertise and precision of placement in order for them to function properly. Intramuscular electrodes were also easily dislodged and thus difficult to use. These shortcomings were improved upon with the advent of noninvasive surface electrodes. This technology was first described by Davis in 1979, who reported on a gold foil electrode wrapped around an endotracheal tube in dog studies. In 1990, Goldstone used an endotracheal tube with two paired wires connected to electrodes that were exposed at the level of the vocal folds. These, in turn, were connected to an electromyogram (EMG) monitor. This became the basis for the development of the modern RLN endotracheal tube-based monitoring system, which has enhanced the capability of the surgeon both to identify the nerve intraoperatively and to detect its function in real time.

Other recent additions to thyroid disease management include the use of molecular genetic analysis and testing. The discovery of the *ret* proto-oncogene has led to its use in the prophylactic management of the children of patients with multiple endocrine neoplasia 2 (MEN-2) syndrome. Continued discoveries and understanding of genetic mutations associated with aggressive phenotypes of differentiated thyroid cancer show promise in improving the diagnostic accuracy of fine-needle aspiration biopsy (FNAB) and in predicting prognosis.

Over the last decade, there has been an increasing interest in minimally invasive thyroid and parathyroid techniques. These all represent extensions of previous innovations in the field. This book focuses on these concepts and techniques.

Recommended Reading

Becker WF. Presidential address: pioneers in thyroid surgery. Ann Surg. 1977;5:493–504.

Berson SA, Yalow RS, Aurbach GD, et al. Immunoassay of bovine and human parathyroid hormone. Proc Natl Acad Sci U S A. 1963;49:613.

Davis WE, Rea JL, Templer J. Recurrent laryngeal nerve localization using a microlaryngeal electrode. Otolaryngol Head Neck Surg. 1979;87(3):330–3.

Flisburg K, Lindholm T. Electrical stimulation of the human recurrent laryngeal nerve during thyroid operation. Acta Otolaryngol. 1970;263:63.

Garrison FH. An introduction to the history of medicine. 4th ed. Philadelphia: WB Saunders; 1929.

Goldstone A, Schettino RL. The electrode endotracheal tube: a state of the art method for monitoring recurrent laryngeal nerve vocal cord muscle integrity in the intubated patient. Otolaryngol Head Neck Surg. 1990;103:249.

Halstead WS. The operative story of goitre. Johns Hopkins Hosp Rep. 1920;19:71.

Kendall E. The isolation in crystalline form of the compound which occurs in the thyroid: its chemical nature and physiologic activity. JAMA. 1915;64:2042.

Lahey F. Routine dissection and demonstration of the recurrent laryngeal nerve in subtotal thyroidectomy. Surg Gynecol Obstet. 1938;66:775.

MacCallum WJ, Voegtlin C. On the relations of tetany to the parathyroid glands and to calcium metabolism. J Exp Med. 1900;11:118.

McGreevy PS, Miller FA. Biography of Theodor Kocher. Surgery. 1969;65:990.

Merke F. History and iconography of endemic goitre and cretinism. Lancaster/Boston: MTP Press; 1984. xi, 339 p.

Nuland SB. Doctors: the biography of medicine. New York: Alfred A. Knopf; 1988.

Organ Jr CH. The history of parathyroid surgery, 1850–1996: The Excelsior Surgical Society 1998 Edward D. Churchill Lecture. J Am Coll Surg. 2000; 191:284.

Randolph G. Surgery of the thyroid and parathyroid glands. 2nd ed. Philadelphia: Saunders/Elsevier; 2013.

Riddell V. Thyroidectomy: prevention of bilateral recurrent nerve palsy. Results of identification of the nerve over 23 consecutive years (1946–69) with a description of an additional safety measure. Br J Surg. 1970;57(1):1–11.

Roses DF. Traditions in surgery, vol. 2. New York: The Exeter Group; 1996.

Schlich T. The origins of organ transplantation: surgery and laboratory science, 1880–1930. Rochester: University of Rochester Press; 2010. p. 355.

Shedd DP. Historical landmarks in head and neck cancer surgery. Pittsburgh: American Head and Neck Society; 1999.

Söderström N. Puncture of goiters for aspiration biopsy. Acta Med Scand. 1952;144(3):237–44.

Ureles AL, Freedman ZR. Thyroidology: reflections on twentieth century history. In: Falk S, editor. Thyroid disease: endocrinology, surgery, nuclear medicine, and radiotherapy. 2nd ed. Philadelphia: Lippincott-Raven; 1997.

Welbourn RB. The history of endocrine surgery. New York: Praeger; 1990 xvi, 385 p.

Wells S. The use of torsion in surgical operations. Br Med J. 1974;1:47.

Wells SA. Parathyroid autotransplantation in primary parathyroid hyperplasia. N Engl J Med. 1976;295:57.

2 Defining Minimally Invasive and Remote Access Surgery of the Thyroid and Parathyroid Glands

Michael J. Campbell and Quan-Yang Duh

Introduction

Minimally invasive and remote access surgery for the thyroid and parathyroid glands has evolved over the last two decades. The emphasis of minimally invasive surgery is limiting the amount of tissue dissection while achieving the same surgical results. Alternatively, the emphasis of remote access surgery is to achieve better cosmetic results by avoiding a cervical scar. Therefore, although minimally invasive surgery and remote access surgery may use similar tools, they ultimately provide different advantages and drawbacks.

The concept of minimally invasive parathyroidectomy (MIP) has been widely embraced, but includes a variety of operations, and the term may be confusing. The approaches and techniques of minimally invasive thyroidectomy (MIT) have been less universally adopted. MIP and MIT encompass an assortment of procedures ranging from simply shortening the cervical incision to using the endoscope and robot. In this chapter we review the evolution of the concepts, principles, and techniques of MIP, MIT, and remote access surgery for the thyroid and parathyroid surgery with the intent of giving surgeons a framework to understand these diverse and frequently misunderstood operations.

M.J. Campbell, MD
Department of Surgery,
University of California, Davis,
CA, USA

Q.-Y. Duh, MD (✉)
Department of Surgery,
University of California, San Francisco,
San Francisco, CA, USA

VA Medical Center,
4150 Clement Street, San Francisco,
CA 94121, USA
e-mail: quan-yang.duh@ucsfmedctr.org

Minimally Invasive and Remote Access Parathyroid Surgery

Background

Bilateral four-gland parathyroid exploration for patients with primary hyperparathyroidism (HPT) through a 5–6 centimeter (cm) lower neck incision has been the standard surgical approach for decades. With the widespread adoption of high-quality preoperative localization studies such as ultrasound (US) and sestamibi scanning (MIBI), as well as the introduction of intraoperative parathyroid hormone (ioPTH) monitoring to exclude hyperplasia or multiple adenomas, surgeons were able to modify their approach to use smaller incisions and focus on a single side of the neck or a single enlarged parathyroid adenoma. The term *minimally invasive parathyroidectomy* is used to convey the potential advantages of this approach over traditional bilateral exploration, with shorter hospital stays, less pain, and better cosmesis.

In the mid-1990s, concurrent with the development of laparoscopic abdominal surgery, some neck surgeons began to explore the possibility of

D.J. Terris, M.C. Singer (eds.), *Minimally Invasive and Robotic Thyroid and Parathyroid Surgery*,
DOI 10.1007/978-1-4614-9011-1_2, © Springer Science+Business Media New York 2014

using the endoscope for parathyroid operations. In contrast to the abdomen, the neck has no preformed space to accommodate the scope. Instead, this space is created bluntly and can be maintained with positive pressure, similar to laparoscopy, or by lifting up the superficial tissues with instruments or lifting devices. Endoscopic parathyroidectomy can thus be classified into two categories based on how the operative space in the neck is maintained. Totally endoscopic minimally invasive parathyroidectomy (EMIP) relies on gas insufflation, and minimally invasive video-assisted parathyroidectomy (MIVAP) uses instruments and lifting devices.

As the techniques of endoscopic parathyroidectomy matured, surgeons realized that the same operation could be accomplished by placing the port sites outside the neck, typically in the chest, breast, and axilla. This was the birth of remote access parathyroid surgery. Remote access surgery trades the potential advantage of not having any visible incision in the neck for the potential disadvantage of a larger dissection required for the instruments to reach the target. Figure 2.1 outlines the various approaches to minimally invasive and remote access parathyroidectomy.

Mini-open Parathyroidectomy

The open, focused parathyroidectomy has gained widespread acceptance as having statistically equivalent outcomes to traditional bilateral exploration. For a well-localized parathyroid adenoma, a focused approach can be performed through an incision of 2.5 cm with a success rate of 96 %.

One key to a successful focused parathyroidectomy is accurate preoperative localization. Patients with primary HPT and a concordant preoperative MIBI and US very likely have a single adenoma at that location (96 %). In contrast, those who have no parathyroid localized on MIBI and US have a 30 % chance of having multigland disease and usually require bilateral exploration.

An anterior mini-open parathyroidectomy is performed through a small skin crease incision in the central, inferior neck between the strap muscles and is well suited for exploring the lower parathyroid glands which tend to be more anterior. The lateral, or so-called back-door, approach is better for upper parathyroid adenomas which tend to be located posteriorly. In this approach the space between the strap muscles and sternocleidomastoid muscle is entered to expose the plane

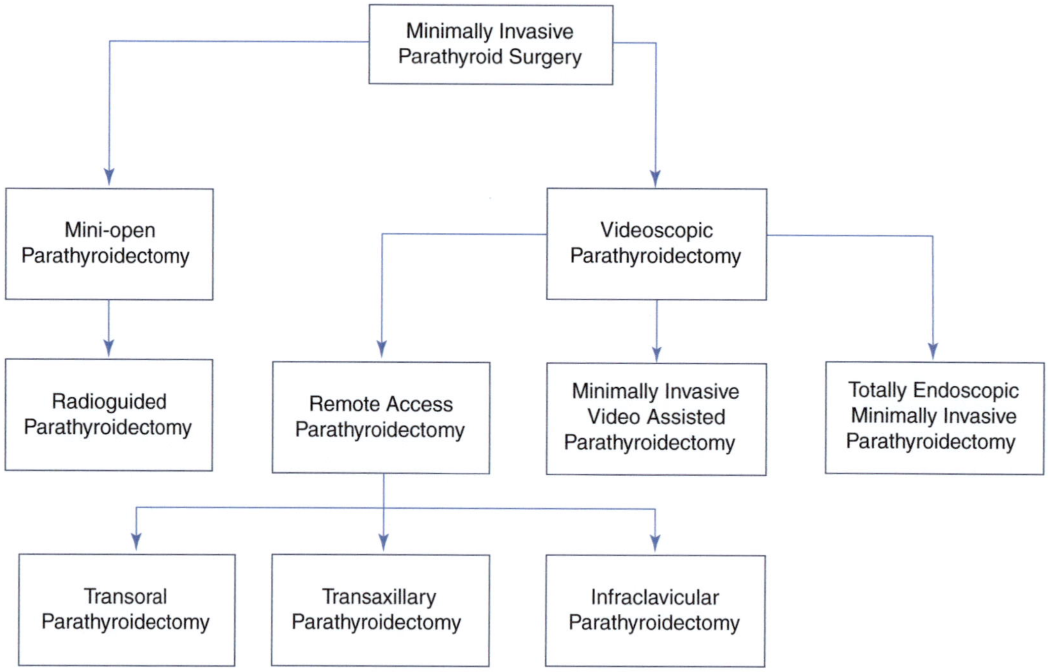

Fig. 2.1 Different approaches to minimally invasive and remote access parathyroid surgery

behind the thyroid. The disadvantage is the potential for a larger incision or bilateral incisions if the contralateral side needs to be explored.

Mini-open parathyroidectomy has an equivalent cure rate to the traditional bilateral exploration with shorter operative times and shorter hospital stays. Mini-open parathyroidectomy has also been shown to decrease the overall cost per procedure compared to traditional exploration. Its success depends on good preoperative imaging and ioPTH monitoring, which may not be universally available.

Radioguided Parathyroidectomy

Intraoperative radioguided localization, with sestamibi technetium-99m (TC-99m) can be used to aid the standard mini-open parathyroidectomy. In this technique, the patient is injected with a TC-99m radiotracer 1–2 h prior to surgery. The radiotracer collects preferentially in the mitochondria of enlarged parathyroid glands and can therefore be identified using a handheld gamma probe. The surgeon uses a gamma probe to explore the operative field, looking for counts greater than background.

Reports on the utility of radioguided parathyroidectomy have been mixed with localization rates between 40 and 100 %. Some of this variability may be due to the learning curve associated with this technology. Advocates suggest that using the gamma probe helps select the location of the skin incision and allows for identification of ectopic parathyroid tumors. Drawbacks may include the increased cost of the technology, its learning curve, and its lack of substantiated benefit.

Videoscopic Parathyroidectomy

Videoscopic parathyroidectomy has gained considerable attention over the last decade. The potential advantages of videoscopic techniques include the magnification provided by the optics, improved cosmesis, and reduced postoperative pain. Gagner et al. performed the first videoscopic parathyroidectomy in 1996. The procedure took almost 5 h to perform, and the patient developed hypercarbia and subcutaneous emphysema from his eyelids to his scrotum that took 3 days to resolve. Since Gagner's initial description, videoscopic parathyroidectomy has continued to evolve and currently can be divided into two subgroups, EMIP and MIVAP, depending on how the operating space in the neck is maintained.

Endoscopic Minimally Invasive Parathyroidectomy

Henry et al. described endoscopic minimally invasive parathyroidectomy (EMIP) using a lateral approach in 1999. One 12-mm and two 2.5-mm trocars are inserted at the anterior border of the sternocleidomastoid muscle. The plane between the strap muscles and the carotid is bluntly dissected and carbon dioxide (CO_2) insufflation is used to maintain the working space. The posterior surface of the thyroid is approached and the parathyroid adenoma is dissected free using 2-mm endoscopic instruments. A modified approach was report by Ikeda et al. in 2002.

Several large series comparing EMIP to open parathyroidectomy demonstrate equivalent cure rates with minimal morbidity. EMIP is generally reserved for single-gland disease with adequate preoperative localization. The major advantage of EMIP is the improved lighting and view provided by the endoscope and the limited size of incision regardless of the patient's body habitus. The major drawbacks are the cost of endoscopy, increased operative time, and possible gas insufflation complications such as hypercarbia, subcutaneous emphysema, and gas embolism.

Minimally Invasive Video-Assisted Parathyroidectomy

MIVAP differs from EMIP in that it does not require gas insufflation. MIVAP was first described by Miccoli et al. in 1998. In MIVAP, a small transverse skin incision is made 1 cm above the sternal notch. The strap muscles are separated. A 5-mm, 30° scope is inserted through the incision, and dissection is done using specially designed open instruments and external retractors, but under a videoscopic view. The operation is similar to mini-open parathyroidectomy, except special instruments and a videoscope are used, which allows the operation to be performed through a 1.5-cm instead of a 2.5-cm incision.

As with endoscopic MIP, MIVAP can be performed with high cure rates and minimal morbidity. The videoscope provides improved lighting and a magnified view. Because of the anterior central approach, it can be used to perform a bilateral exploration. One major drawback is the need for two experienced assistants, one to maintain external retraction and the other to handle the scope. Large parathyroid adenomas, large goiters, prior neck operations, lack of preoperative localization, and suspicion of hyperplasia are relative contraindications to MIVAP.

Remote Access Parathyroidectomy

Remote access parathyroidectomy developed as an extension of endoscopic parathyroidectomy by moving the trocar sites and incisions away from the anterior neck to achieve better cosmetic results. In 2000, Ikeda and Takami reported on six patients who underwent successful parathyroidectomy via an axillary approach and four patients that underwent exploration via an anterior chest approach. Although the operative time was long (180 min for a unilateral axillary approach), all the operations were successful with no significant morbidity. Small series by Landry et al. and Foley et al. also suggested successful outcomes can be achieved via the transaxillary approach but that it is associated with longer operative times and increased costs. In 2011, Karakas et al. described successful transoral parathyroidectomy in two patients.

Conclusion

In summary, MIP, especially mini-open parathyroidectomy, is available in most high-volume endocrine surgery centers and is associated with high success rates and minimal morbidity. It has become a costandard with traditional bilateral four-gland exploration for treating patients with primary HPT. The mini-open technique, with a 2.5-cm neck incision, is the most commonly performed parathyroid procedure. Endoscopic parathyroidectomy and MIVAP are performed at fewer centers, but also have excellent outcomes. Remote access parathyroidectomy appears safe and may have cosmetic advantages, but requires more extensive dissection and is more expensive. Successful MIP and remote access parathyroidectomy depends on accurate preoperative localization studies and intraoperative adjuncts such as ioPTH monitoring. Table 2.1 summarizes the advantages and drawbacks to the various approaches.

Table 2.1 Benefits and drawback to various approaches to parathyroidectomy and thyroidectomy

Approach	Incision length	Benefit	Drawback
Parathyroidectomy			
Traditional	4–5 cm	Excellent exposure to both sides of thyroid. Gold standard with cure rates in excess of 95 %	Relatively long incision. Bilateral exploration is often unnecessary
Mini-open "focused" parathyroidectomy	2–3 cm	Shorter incision. Able to explore both sides with aid of retraction. Reduced operative times and costs	Can be difficult in obese patients. Relies on adequate preoperative localization and ioPTH which may not be available
Radioguided parathyroidectomy	2–3 cm	Helps focus skin incision. May help localize ectopic adenomas	Difficult to learn. May increase patient costs
Totally endoscopic parathyroidectomy	(a) 5 mm ×3 (anterior approach) (b)1.2 cm, 2.5 mm x2 (lateral approach)	Improved magnification and lighting with the endoscope. Shortest incision	Gas insufflation can cause subcutaneous emphysema, air embolism, hypercapnea. Increased cost and operative time

Table 2.1 (continued)

Approach	Incision length	Benefit	Drawback
Minimally invasive video-assisted parathyroidectomy (MIVAP)	1.5 cm	Improved magnification and lighting with videoscope. No need for insufflation. Easy to convert to bilateral operation	Requires two experienced assistants to maintain exposure
Axillary approach to parathyroidectomy	4.5–6 cm	No neck scar	More extensive dissection. Increased operative times and cost. Difficult learning curve
Transoral approach to parathyroidectomy	1.5 cm	No neck scar	Concerns for infection. Minimal reported experience
Thyroidectomy			
Standard open thyroidectomy	4–6 cm	Excellent exposure. Able to perform neck bilateral exploration and lymph node dissection	Relatively long scar in the neck
Mini-open thyroidectomy	2.5 cm	Easy to learn. Easy to convert to bilateral thyroidectomy	Limited to thyroid lobes <7 cm. Lateral approach only for thyroid lobectomy
Completely endoscopic thyroidectomy			
Anterior approach	5 mm ×4	Short neck incisions and quicker return to normal activity. Magnified view	Limited to selected patients. Longer operative time. Insufflation may cause complications (hypercarbia, subcutaneous emphysema)
Lateral approach	10 mm ×1; 2.5 mm ×2	Short neck incisions and quicker return to normal activity. Magnified view	Limited to selected patients. Only hemithyroidectomy. Insufflation may cause complications
Minimally invasive video-assisted thyroidectomy (MIVAT)	1.5 cm	Use open instruments. Easy to learn. Less pain and better cosmetic outcomes	Requires two experienced assistants to maintain exposure
Remote access thyroidectomy – infraclavicular approach	3 cm; 5 mm ×2	No scar in the neck	More extensive dissection. Risk of subcutaneous hemorrhage
Remote access thyroidectomy – axillary approach	3–6 cm	No scar in the neck. Ipsilateral central neck dissection possible	More extensive dissection. Longer operative time. More expensive. Difficult to dissect contralateral thyroid lobe
Remote access thyroidectomy – breast approach	15 mm ×1; 12 mm ×1; 5 mm ×1	No scar in the neck	More extensive dissection. Scar in the breast
Remote access thyroidectomy – axillo-bilateral breast approach	2.5 cm areolar; 10 mm ×2 axillary	Improved angles of dissection between instruments and thyroid	More extensive dissection. Scar in the breast
Remote access thyroidectomy – bilateral axillo-breast approach	12 mm ×2 in each areolar; 5 mm × 2 in each axilla	Improved angles of dissection between instruments and thyroid. Bilateral dissection easy	More extensive dissection. Scar in the breast
Transoral thyroidectomy	2.5 cm in the floor of the mouth	No neck scar	Very limited data on the utility and complications of this procedure
Robotic facelift thyroidectomy	N/A	No neck scar. Supine position	Greater auricular nerve at risk

ioPTH intraoperative parathyroid hormone monitoring, *mm* millimeters, *cm* centimeters

Minimally Invasive and Remote Access Thyroid Surgery

Background

Traditional thyroid surgery was developed by Theodor Kocher at the beginning of twentieth century and was performed through an 8–10 cm collar incision. Currently open thyroidectomies are routinely performed through an incision that is 4–6 cm. Minimally invasive thyroidectomy (MIT) strives to minimize the length of incision in the neck, sometimes with the help of an endoscope. MIT encompasses a diverse set of procedures including (1) completely endoscopic thyroidectomy with CO_2 insufflation, (2) minimally invasive video-assisted thyroidectomy (MIVAT) without gas insufflation, and (3) mini-open thyroidectomy. All three approaches can be performed using an anterior (between the strap muscles) or lateral (between strap muscles and the sternocleidomastoid muscle) approach. Remote access thyroidectomy moves the incision from the neck to the chest, breast, axilla, upper back of the neck, or the mouth, but it is not truly minimally invasive surgery because of the additional surgical dissection required from the remote site. Figure 2.2 shows the various approaches of MIT and remote access thyroidectomy.

Mini-open Thyroidectomy

The typical incision for an open thyroidectomy is about 4–6 cm. Several institutions have reported performing thyroidectomies through mini-open incisions ranging from 2.5 to 3 cm. Ferzli et al. used a 2.5-cm incision in a skin crease above the isthmus. Subplatysmal flaps are raised, the upper pole is retracted inferiorly, and the superior pole vessels are ligated. This is followed by dividing the inferior pole vessels and the lateral attachments. Gosnell and colleagues described a similar technique through a small incision over a palpable thyroid nodule using the standard lateral approach to dissect the thyroid lobe.

The advantage of the mini-open thyroidectomy is that it is easily teachable because of its similarities to a traditional thyroidectomy with shorter operative times compared to endoscopic thyroidectomy. The size of gland, which should be less than 7 cm, is the major limiting factor to performing a mini-open thyroidectomy.

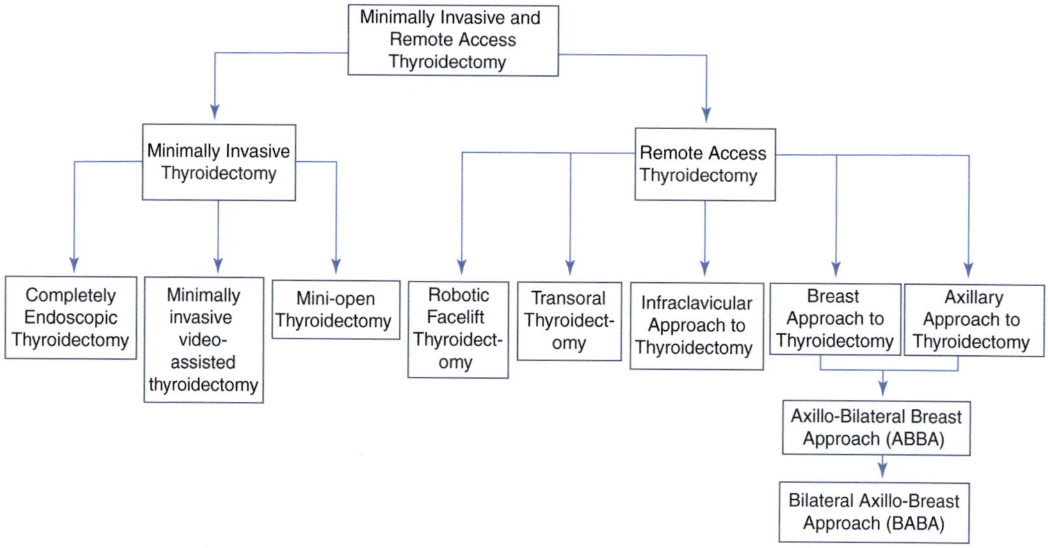

Fig. 2.2 Different approaches to minimally invasive and remote access thyroid surgery

Completely Endoscopic Thyroidectomy

The first completely endoscopic thyroidectomy was performed by Huscher et al. in 1997. In 2001, Gagner et al. presented a series of 18 patients who underwent endoscopic thyroidectomy via an anterior approach. Endoscopic thyroidectomy commonly uses a 5-mm scope at the sternal notch to bluntly create a subplatysmal space. The working space is maintained using CO_2 insufflation, and three additional working trocars are used. Using this approach, Gagner et al. reported no major complications, better cosmetic results, and an earlier return to activity when compared to conventional thyroidectomy. They recommended the technique for benign nodules smaller than 3 cm, and the technique may not be used in the reoperative setting, in obese patients or those patients with short, wide necks, and the elderly who could not tolerate CO_2 insufflation.

Henry described the lateral approach for endoscopic thyroidectomy in 2006. In this approach, the trocars are placed at the anterior border of the ipsilateral sternocleidomastoid muscle. Endoscopic thyroidectomy via the lateral approach is used for benign nodules smaller than 3 cm in size. Contraindications are previous neck surgery and neck irradiation.

Minimally Invasive Video-Assisted Thyroidectomy

The technique of MIVAT is similar to that of MIVAP. It uses traditional instruments that have been modified to fit through a smaller incision and does not require insufflation. MIVAT uses a 1.5-cm skin crease incision above the sternal notch. The working space is created by blunt dissection without gas insufflation and maintained with external retractors. The thyroid is mobilized and pulled through the incision and the remainder of the thyroidectomy is performed under direct vision without the endoscope. Because of the smaller neck incision and decreased dissection, MIVAT is associated with improved patient satisfaction, less postoperative pain, a shorter postoperative stay, decreased wound healing time, and improved "voice and swallowing" measures compared to traditional open thyroidectomy. A lateral MIVAT has been described by Yamashita et al. in Japan.

Remote Access Thyroid Surgery

Some surgeons, especially those in Asia where even a small scar in the neck is a significant cosmetic concern, adapted the tools of endoscopic thyroidectomy to move the trocar incisions to sites remote from the neck. Shimizu and colleagues reported the first remote access thyroidectomy in 1998 when they reported on five patients who underwent thyroidectomies via incisions below the ipsilateral clavicle. Subsequently remote access thyroidectomy has been described via incisions in the axilla, breast, mouth, and posterior upper neck. Because remote access surgery is technically more challenging, some surgeons began to use robotic assistance to improve the surgical view and instrument movement.

Infraclavicular Approach

Shimizu and colleagues described the infraclavicular approach for remote access thyroidectomy. Three infraclavicular incisions are used, and two Kirschner wires are used to lift up and expose the subplatysmal space and allow for gasless dissection of the thyroid. The strap muscles are divided and the thyroid lobe is dissected using open and endoscopic instruments.

Shimizu and colleagues reported excellent results in 193 patients. All underwent a unilateral thyroidectomy. The maximum tumor size was 7 cm. The mean operative time was 97 min. Four patients had temporary recurrent laryngeal nerve (RLN) palsies, and three had seromas that required aspiration. Shimizu et al. reported improved cosmetic results compared to open thyroidectomy as well as a shorter hospital stay and rehabilitation.

Axillary Approach

Ikeda and colleagues reported the first transaxillary remote access thyroidectomy in 2000. This approach can be performed with or without gas insufflation. When using gas insufflation, the subplatysmal space is insufflated to 4 mmHg, and a flexible endoscope is inserted. Three additional ports are inserted in the ipsilateral axilla. The thyroid gland is exposed by splitting the sternothyroid muscle. In the gasless approach, an external lift retractor is inserted through a 6-cm incision in the axilla to maintain the operative space.

Kang and colleagues reported their results using the transaxillary approach on 581 patients. In addition to improved cosmesis, they were also able to dissect the ipsilateral central lymph nodes when necessary. The disadvantages included a larger dissection for the remote access and difficulty seeing the contralateral thyroid lobe. There were no conversions to a traditional cervical incision and the mean operative time 129 min. Transient hypocalcemia occurred in 19 patients (3 %), temporary RLN palsy in 13 patients (2 %), and permanent RLN injury in 2 patients (0.3 %).

The assistance of the robot (da Vinci Surgical System, Intuitive Surgical, Sunnyvale, California) alleviated some of the limitations of remote access thyroidectomy. The benefits of using the robot include a three-dimensional view of the operating field, more flexible articulated instruments with greater degrees of freedom of movement and filtering of hand tremors. Robotic thyroidectomy is more expensive, requires training, and has not yet proven to be better than non-robotic remote access thyroidectomy in outcomes or cosmesis.

Breast Approach

Ohgami and colleagues were the first to describe using circumareolar incisions for trocar sites in remote access thyroidectomy. Two incisions are made on each breast at the upper areolar margin, and the subplatysmal space is bluntly created. The working space is maintained using gas insufflation. The inferior and superior pole vessels are ligated using ultrasonic shears, and the specimen is retrieved through one of the circumareolar port sites.

Park and colleagues reported their results of 100 patients using the breast approach for remote access thyroidectomy. They found no complications from gas insufflation and an overall excellent cosmetic result. Initially it was felt that patients with known malignancy or previous neck surgery or radiation were not good candidate for this operation, but subsequently several surgeons have reported excellent short-term oncological results with remote access thyroidectomy.

Hybrid Approaches

There are several hybrid approaches using both the breast and axilla for access to improve the angle between the endoscopic instruments and the thyroid gland. Shimazu and colleagues described the axillo-bilateral breast approach (ABBA) in 2003. In the ABBA, a trocar is placed in the ipsilateral axilla in addition to the breast port sites. Choe and colleagues described the bilateral axillo-breast approach (BABA) in 2007, in which a port is used in each axilla. With this approach, a central neck dissection is technically more feasible than with other remote access approaches. Some have criticized BABA for being overly invasive due to its extensive dissection.

Transoral Thyroidectomy

In 2010 Wilhelm and Metzig reported the first endoscopic transoral thyroidectomy. In this approach, a sublingual incision is made, and a trocar is placed into the subplatysmal layer, anterior to the thyroid cartilage, and insufflation is established. Two additional trocars are placed in the mouth. The surgeon then meticulously divides the isthmus and uses ultrasonic shears to ligate the upper and lower pole vessels. Once dissected free the thyroid is removed out of the sublingual incision.

In 2013, Nakajo and colleagues reported on a gasless transoral video-assisted neck surgery for thyroid resection. While similar to the approach reported by Wilhelm and Metzig, Nakajo et al. use an incision at the vestibulum and dissect anterior to the mandible and create the subplatysmal space. The working space is maintained using Kirschner wires to suspend the anterior cervical area. While both of these approaches by Wilhelm et al. and Nakajo et al. are promising, it is important to note that they are still in their infancy and have yet to be widely adopted by thyroid surgeons.

Robotic Facelift Thyroidectomy

In 2011, Terris et al. reported on a novel, remote access approach to performing a thyroidectomy using a postauricular facelift incision. The patient is positioned supine on the operating table, and an incision is made in the postauricular crease and continued within the occipital hairline. A musculocutaneous flap is raised, and a fixed retractor system is introduced to maintain the working space. The da Vinci surgical system is used to facilitate the dissection of the ipsilateral thyroid lobe.

The benefits of the robotic facelift thyroidectomy when compared to other remote access techniques such as the axillary approach include its easier positioning and shorter distance to the thyroid. The primary disadvantage includes dissection near the greater auricular nerve which may develop temporary or permanent hypesthesia. Only the ipsilateral thyroid lobe can be removed through a unilateral facelift incision, while a total thyroidectomy requires bilateral incisions.

Conclusions

Minimizing or completely avoiding a scar in the anterior neck is appealing to many patients who need thyroidectomy. Surgical invasiveness, however, is not just related to the length of or site of the incision, but includes the surgical trauma rendered to create the space for dissection. The standard open thyroidectomy has excellent results and minimal morbidity and complications. MIT and remote access thyroidectomy continue to evolve. Efforts to improve cosmesis, by shortening the incision or moving it from the neck must be balanced against the increased operative time and cost. For now, these techniques are limited to high-volume centers with specific interest and experience to achieve good results.

Recommended Reading

Assalia A, Inabnet WB. Endoscopic parathyroidectomy. Otolaryngol Clin North Am. 2004;37:871–86.

Beyer TD, et al. Parathyroidectomy outcomes according to operative approach. Am J Surg. 2007;193(3): 368–72.

Brunaud L, et al. Incision length for standard thyroidectomy and parathyroidectomy: when is it minimally invasive? Arch Surg. 2003;138:1140–3.

Choe JH, Kim SW, Chung KW. Endoscopic thyroidectomy using a new bilateral axillo-breast approach. World J Surg. 2007;31(3):601–6.

Cougard P, et al. Videoendoscopic approach for parathyroid adenomas: results of a prospective study of 100 patients. Ann Chir. 2001;126:314–9.

Ferzli GS, et al. Minimally invasive, nonendoscopic thyroid surgery. J Am Coll Surg. 2001;192(5):665–8.

Foley CS, et al. Robotic transaxillary endocrine surgery: a comparison with conventional open technique. Surg Endosc. 2012;26(8):2259–66.

Gagner M, Inabnet 3rd WB. Endoscopic thyroidectomy for solitary thyroid nodules. Thyroid. 2001;11(2): 161–3.

Gosnell JE, et al. Minimal access thyroid surgery: technique and report of the first 25 cases. ANZ J Surg. 2004;74(5):330–4.

Henry JF. Minimally Invasive thyroid and parathyroid surgery is not a question of length of the incision. Langenbecks Arch Surg. 2008;393:621–6.

Henry JF, Sebag F. Lateral endoscopic approach for thyroid and parathyroid surgery. Ann Chir. 2006;131(1): 51–6.

Henry JF, et al. Minimally invasive videoscopic parathyroidectomy by lateral approach. Langenbecks Arch Surg. 1999;384:298–301.

Henry JF, et al. Indications and results of video-assisted parathyroidectomy by a lateral approach in patients with primary hyperparathyroidism. Surgery. 2001; 130(6):999–1004.

Huscher CSG, et al. Endoscopic right thyroid lobectomy. Surg Endosc. 1997;11:877.

Ikeda Y, Takami H. Endoscopic parathyroidectomy. Biomed Pharmacother. 2000;54 Suppl 1:52–6.

Ikeda Y, et al. Endoscopic neck surgery by the axillary approach. J Am Coll Surg. 2000;191(3):336–40.

Ikeda Y, et al. Total endoscopic parathyroidectomy. Biomed Pharmacother. 2002;56:22s–5.

Inabnet 3rd WB. Robotic thyroidectomy: must we drive a luxury sedan to arrive at our destination safely? Thyroid. 2012;22(10):988–90.

Kang SW, et al. Gasless endoscopic thyroidectomy using trans-axillary approach; surgical outcome of 581 patients. Endocr J. 2009;56(3):361–9.

Karakas E, et al. Transoral thyroid and parathyroid surgery – development of a new transoral technique. Surgery. 2011;150(1):108–15.

Kebebew E, et al. Predictors of single-gland vs. multigland parathyroid disease in primary hyperparathyroidism: a simple and accurate scoring model. Arch Surg. 2006;141(8):777–82.

Kunstman JW, Udelsman R. Superiority of minimally invasive parathyroidectomy. Adv Surg. 2012;46:171–89.

Landry CS, et al. Robot assisted transaxillary surgery (RATS) for the removal of thyroid and parathyroid glands. Surgery. 2011;149(4):549–55.

Lang BH. Minimally invasive thyroid and parathyroid operations: surgical techniques and pearls. Adv Surg. 2010;44:185–98.

Linos D. Minimally invasive thyroidectomy: a comprehensive appraisal of existing techniques. Surgery. 2011;150:17–24.

Miccoli P, et al. Endoscopic parathyroidectomy by a gasless approach. J Laparoendosc Adv Surg Tech A. 1998;8(4):189–94.

Miccoli P, et al. Minimally invasive video-assisted thyroidectomy. Am J Surg. 2001;181(6):567–70.

Miccoli P, et al. Minimally invasive video assisted parathyroidectomy (MIVAP). Eur J Surg Oncol. 2003;29(2):188–90.

Naitoh T, et al. Endoscopic endocrine surgery in the neck. An initial report of endoscopic subtotal parathyroidectomy. Surg Endosc. 1998;12:202–5.

Nakajo A, Arima H, Hirata M, et al. Trans-Oral Video-Assisted Neck Surgery (TOVANS). A new transoral technique of endoscopic thyroidectomy with gasless premandible approach. Surg Endosc. 2013;27(4):1105–10.

Norman J, Chheda H, Farrell C. Minimally invasive parathyroidectomy for primary hyperparathyroidism: decreasing operative time and potential complications while improving cosmetic results. Am Surg. 1998;64(5):391–5.

Ohgami M, et al. Scarless endoscopic thyroidectomy: breast approach for better cosmesis. Surg Laparosc Endosc Percutan Tech. 2000;10(1):1–4.

Palazzo FF, Sebag F, Henry JF. Endocrine surgical technique: endoscopic thyroidectomy via the lateral approach. Surg Endosc. 2006;20:339–42.

Park YL, Han WK, Bae WG. 100 cases of endoscopic thyroidectomy: breast approach. Surg Laparosc Endosc Percutan Tech. 2003;13(1):20–5.

Satchie B, Chen H. Radioguided techniques for parathyroid surgery. Asian J Surg. 2005;28(2):77–81.

Shimazu K, et al. Endoscopic thyroid surgery through the axillo-bilateral-breast approach. Surg Laparosc Endosc Percutan Tech. 2003;13(3):196–201.

Shimizu K, Tanaka S. Asian perspective on endoscopic thyroidectomy – a review of 193 cases. Asian J Surg. 2003;26(2):92–100.

Shimizu K, Akira S, Tanaka S. Video-assisted neck surgery: endoscopic resection of benign thyroid tumor aiming at scarless surgery on the neck. J Surg Oncol. 1998;69:178–80.

Shimizu K, et al. Video-assisted neck surgery: endoscopic resection of thyroid tumors with a very minimal neck wound. J Am Coll Surg. 1999;188(6):697–703.

Sosa JA, Udelsman R. Minimally invasive parathyroidectomy. Surg Oncol. 2003;12:125–34.

Terris DJ, Singer MC, Seybt MW. Robotic facelift thyroidectomy: patient selection and technical considerations. Surg Laparosc Endosc Percutan Tech. 2011;21(4):237–42.

Wilhelm T, Metzig A. Video. Endoscopic minimally invasive thyroidectomy: first clinical experience. Surg Endosc. 2010;24(7):1757–8.

Wilhelm T, Metzig A. Endoscopic minimally invasive thyroidectomy (eMIT): some clarifications regarding the idea, development, preclinical studies, and application in humans. Surg Endosc. 2010 Aug 24.

Principles and Philosophy of Minimally Invasive and Remote Access Endocrine Surgery

3

David J. Terris

Minimally Invasive Thyroid and Parathyroid Surgery

Laparoscopically trained endocrine surgeons at the University of Pisa described in 1998 a technique of endoscopic-assisted thyroid surgery in which a very small incision in the cervical neck is made, and a gasless retractor-based video-assisted thyroidectomy is performed. Paolo Miccoli and his colleagues introduced a number of novel procedural concepts with their technique (Fig. 3.1). One of the first, and among the most important, is avoidance of the raising of subplatysmal flaps. This minimizes both the time required for surgery and the dissection-associated trauma to the tissues which predisposes to seroma formation and skin flap edema. Blunt dissection is used heavily and undertaken with elevators rather than sponges or peanuts. The technique eventually relied substantially on ultrasonic technology which affords the ability to ligate vessels reliably in a small space. Retraction on the thyroid gland itself is not intuitive but paramount to the successful performance of the procedure. Nerve dissection is accomplished by the use of the same blunt elevators, in a direction perpendicular to the course of the nerve. A final nonintuitive step is the placement of clamps on the superior pole in order to deliver the dissected gland through the incision. No drains are necessary, and in the Italian health system, the patients are kept in the hospital overnight.

Substantial modifications to the Miccoli technique were described by our group in an effort to facilitate its performance by lower-volume surgeons. The very first difference is that the location of the incision is identified with the patient sitting upright in the holding area in order to be certain the incision is in the proper location for when the patient is upright and in public. Some of the technical changes included the utilization of nerve monitoring as an additional safety measure, implementation of a slave monitor to improve the ergonomics especially for the camera assistant, and bundle ligation of the superior pedicle (Fig. 3.2) which reduces the time required to mobilize the superior pole. Patients are uniformly managed without a drain and on an outpatient basis. For those undergoing total thyroid surgery, routine calcium supplementation is provided to obviate the need for blood tests and to minimize the likelihood of symptomatic hypocalcemia.

An intermediate approach to minimally invasive surgery was also described in which a small incision is used but without the need for endoscopic assistance. The incision size for these

D.J. Terris, MD, FACS
Department of Otolaryngology – Head and Neck Surgery, GRU Thyroid Center,
Georgia Regents University,
120 Fifteenth Street, BP-4109, Augusta,
GA 30912-4060, USA
e-mail: dterris@georgiahealth.edu

D.J. Terris, M.C. Singer (eds.), *Minimally Invasive and Robotic Thyroid and Parathyroid Surgery*,
DOI 10.1007/978-1-4614-9011-1_3, © Springer Science+Business Media New York 2014

procedures is generally between 25 and 40 mm, and the patients benefit from all of the same procedural innovations, although with a slightly longer incision.

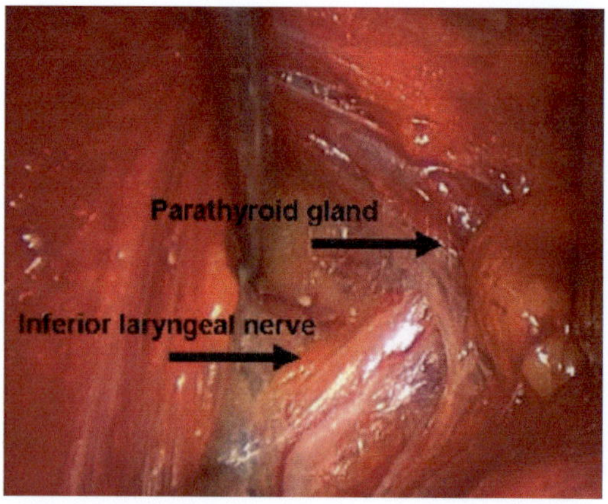

Fig. 3.1 Paolo Miccoli and his colleagues in Pisa developed a minimally invasive cervical approach that relies on endoscopic assistance to achieve and incision as small as ¾ in., with excellent visualization of the critical structures, such as the recurrent laryngeal nerve and parathyroid glands, as shown. Importantly, their innovations helped to demonstrate that the conventional approaches (and incision sizes) were no longer necessary for many patients (Reprinted with permission from Miccoli P, Berti P, Ambrosini CE. Perspectives and lessons learned after a decade of minimally invasive video-assisted thyroidectomy. ORL J Otorhinolaryngol Relat Spec. 2008;70(5):282–6)

Remote Access and Robotic Thyroid and Parathyroid Surgery

In the inexorable movement toward smaller and more easily hidden scars, and especially in cultures where a neck scar is particularly undesirable (including a number of Asian countries), Yoshifumi Ikeda from Japan made substantial contributions by innovating and refining a totally endoscopic insufflation-based axillary thyroidectomy. Although this technique is lengthy and challenging for even very skilled laparoscopic and endocrine surgeons, it paved the way for future creative surgeons who modified this approach in a number of different ways and with a number of different portals.

By 2013, the most popular technique that has emerged has been a gasless axillary approach which was refined by several different South Korean groups. Deserving of much credit in advancing this field, Woong Youn Chung merged robotic technology with remote access principles (Fig. 3.3) and was able to substantially shorten the duration of axillary thyroidectomy. This group has quickly accumulated a vast experience with this approach and proven its safety and completeness, at least in a South Korean population. A more extensive bilateral axillary and breast approach has

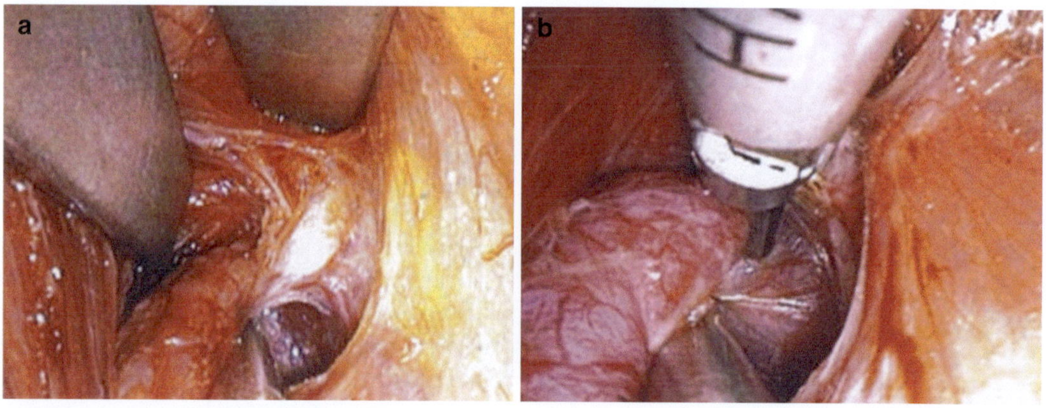

Fig. 3.2 An important modification of the Miccoli minimally invasive thyroidectomy was the application of bundle ligation of the superior vascular pedicle, which is faster and easier in the confined space of the upper pole of the thyroid gland. After the upper pole is fully mobilized (**a**), and advanced energy device is used to ligate the entire upper pedicle (**b**) in a single bundle (Reprinted with permission from Terris DJ, Seybt MW. Modifications of Miccoli minimally invasive thyroidectomy for the low-volume surgeon. Am J Otolaryngol. 2011;32(5):392–7)

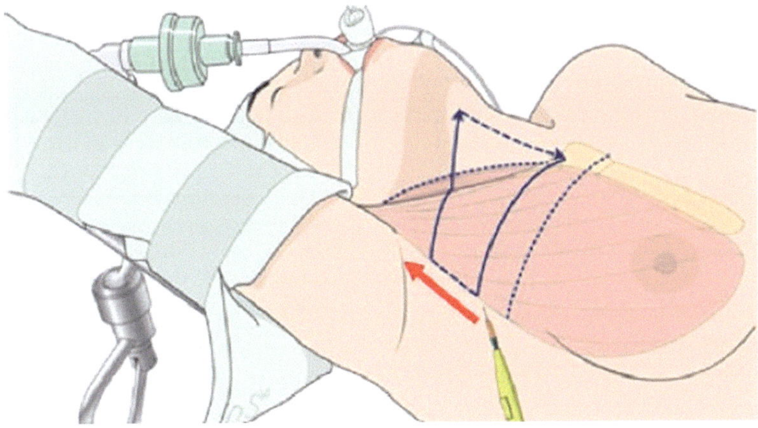

Fig. 3.3 Particularly in many Asian countries where the skin type predisposes to hypertrophic scarring and there is a cultural aversion to neck scars, remote access surgery has been extraordinarily popular. Woong Youn Chung made substantial contributions by innovating a gasless transaxillary approach that is retractor based and eventually incorporated the use of the robot (Reprinted with permission from Kang SW, Jeong JJ, Yun JS, Sung TY, Lee SC, Lee YS, Nam KH, Chang HS, Chung WY, Park CS. Robot-assisted endoscopic surgery for thyroid cancer: experience with the first 100 patients. Surg Endosc. 2009;23(11):2399–406)

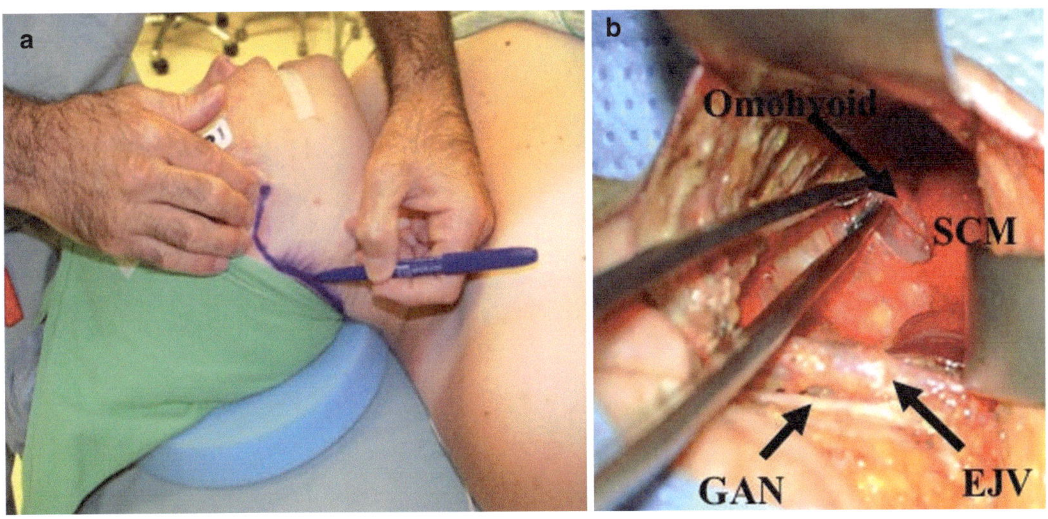

Fig. 3.4 Profound differences in patient populations hampered the extrapolation of the axillary thyroidectomy to North American patients. An alternative procedure using a facelift incision (**a**) was therefore described that is associated with easier positioning and a shorter distance to the thyroid gland. The exposure of the thyroid gland is achieved by reflecting the omohyoid muscle ventrally (**b**). *GAN* greater auricular nerve, *EJV* external jugular vein, *SCM* sternocleidomastoid muscle (Reprinted with permission from Terris DJ, Singer MC, Seybt MW. Robotic facelift thyroidectomy: II. Clinical feasibility and safety. Laryngoscope. 2011;121(8):1636–41)

also proven to be popular in the South Korean patient environment. Because of challenges in extrapolating these approaches to a North American population, an alternative approach that uses a facelift incision has recently been described (Fig. 3.4).

Future Considerations

Probably the only certain prediction that can be made with regard to the future of endocrine neck surgery is that it is bound to change. Technology continues to improve, surgical techniques continue to evolve, and the expectations of society continue to motivate innovation and enhancements. Perhaps the thyroid will be removed through small puncture holes. Perhaps a transcutaneous noninvasive technique that is safe and effective will be described. Perhaps the need for thyroid surgery will be eliminated altogether. Regardless of the directions, the future is certainly exciting.

Recommended Reading

Holsinger FC, Kuppersmith RB, Chung WY. Robotic and extracervical approaches to the thyroid and parathyroid glands: a modern classification scheme. In: Randolph GW, editor. Surgery of the thyroid and parathyroid glands. Philadelphia: Saunders; 2013.

Ikeda Y, Takami H, Sasaki Y, Kan S, Niimi M. Endoscopic neck surgery by the axillary approach. J Am Coll Surg. 2000;191(3):336–40.

Kang SW, Jeong JJ, Yun JS, Sung TY, Lee SC, Lee YS, Nam KH, Chang HS, Chung WY, Park CS. Robot-assisted endoscopic surgery for thyroid cancer: experience with the first 100 patients. Surg Endosc. 2009a;23(11):2399–406.

Kang SW, Lee SC, Lee SH, Lee KY, Jeong JJ, Lee YS, Nam KH, Chang HS, Chung WY, Park CS. Robotic thyroid surgery using a gasless, transaxillary approach and the da Vinci S system: the operative outcomes of 338 consecutive patients. Surgery. 2009b;146(6):1048–55.

Lee KE, Rao J, Youn YK. Endoscopic thyroidectomy with the da Vinci robot system using the bilateral axillary breast approach (BABA) technique: our initial experience. Surg Laparosc Endosc Percutan Tech. 2009; 19(3):e71–5.

Lee KE, Koo do H, Kim SJ, Lee J, Park KS, Oh SK, Youn YK. Outcomes of 109 patients with papillary thyroid carcinoma who underwent robotic total thyroidectomy with central node dissection via the bilateral axillo-breast approach. Surgery. 2010;148(6):1207–13.

Lee S, Ryu HR, Park JH, Kim KH, Kang SW, Jeong JJ, Nam KH, Chung WY, Park CS. Early surgical outcomes comparison between robotic and conventional open thyroid surgery for papillary thyroid microcarcinoma. Surgery. 2012;151(5):724–30.

Miccoli P, Berti P, Conte M, Bendinelli C, Marcocci C. Minimally invasive surgery for thyroid small nodules: preliminary report. J Endocrinol Invest. 1999;22(11): 849–51.

Miccoli P, Berti P, Ambrosini CE. Perspectives and lessons learned after a decade of minimally invasive video-assisted thyroidectomy. ORL J Otorhinolaryngol Relat Spec. 2008;70(5):282–6.

Pothier DD. The use of drains following thyroid and parathyroid surgery: a meta-analysis. J Laryngol Otol. 2005;119(9):669–71.

Seybt MW, Terris DJ. Outpatient thyroidectomy: experience in over 200 patients. Laryngoscope. 2010;120(5): 959–63.

Snyder SK, Hamid KS, Roberson CR, Rai SS, Bossen AC, Luh JH, Scherer EP, Song J. Outpatient thyroidectomy is safe and reasonable: experience with more than 1,000 planned outpatient procedures. J Am Coll Surg. 2010;210(5):575–82, 582–4.

Terris DJ, Seybt MW. Modifications of Miccoli minimally invasive thyroidectomy for the low-volume surgeon. Am J Otolaryngol. 2011;32(5):392–7.

Terris DJ, Bonnett A, Gourin CG, Chin E. Minimally invasive thyroidectomy using the Sofferman technique. Laryngoscope. 2005;115(6):1104–8.

Terris DJ, Singer MC, Seybt MW. Robotic facelift thyroidectomy: II. Clinical feasibility and safety. Laryngoscope. 2011;121(8):1636–41.

Ambulatory Endocrine Surgery

4

Jeffrey J. Houlton and David L. Steward

Over the past four decades, the healthcare system has seen a tremendous increase in the acceptance of ambulatory surgery. This trend toward outpatient procedures has affected nearly every surgical specialty (general surgery, orthopedics, urology, otolaryngology, etc.) and continues to include increasingly more complex procedures. In this chapter we will review the current standards and controversies specific to ambulatory endocrine surgery. This discussion will primarily involve outpatient thyroid surgery, as it continues to be a more significant source of discussion, but will also include issues unique to outpatient parathyroid surgery.

Ambulatory Surgery

In the United States, the first significant increases in ambulatory surgery began in the 1980s. In 1983, only 239 stand-alone ambulatory surgical centers existed in the United States. By 2003, this number had swelled to over 3,300 centers. Similarly, the number of outpatient procedures performed dramatically increased from 380,000 in 1983, to 31.5 million in 1996, to an estimated 53.3 million in 2006 (as reported by the National Survey of Ambulatory Surgery).

This dramatic increase in outpatient surgery is generally attributed to two influential factors: (1) a national focus on decreasing the burgeoning costs of healthcare and (2) innovations in surgical and anesthetic techniques which reduce patient recovery time.

In an effort to reduce healthcare costs, several government-mandated changes to Medicare were introduced in the 1980s which provided financial incentives to beneficiaries performing operations in ambulatory centers. This began with the Omnibus Budget Reconciliation Act of 1980 which increased reimbursement for facility fees at ambulatory centers, reduced Part B deductibles for patients undergoing ambulatory surgery, and increased surgeon reimbursement for ambulatory procedures. The Social Security Act Amendments of 1983 further created strong Medicare-based incentives toward shifting operative care to hospital outpatient centers, ambulatory centers, and surgeon's offices. Following these Medicare trends, private insurance companies and state-mandated healthcare plans began to provide similar financial incentives over the next several decades. Currently, a myriad of less explicit policies continue to provide financial incentives for ambulatory surgery to third-party payers, healthcare providers, and patients in the current system. Additionally, and importantly, these early

J.J. Houlton, MD
Department of Otolaryngology–Head and Neck Surgery, Medical University of South Carolina, Charleston, SC, USA
e-mail: houltojy@ucmail.us.edu

D.L. Steward, MD (✉)
Department of Otolaryngology–Head and Neck Surgery, University Hospital, Cincinnati, OH 45267-0528, USA
e-mail: david.steward@uc.edu; stewardd@ucmail.uc.edu

D.J. Terris, M.C. Singer (eds.), *Minimally Invasive and Robotic Thyroid and Parathyroid Surgery*, DOI 10.1007/978-1-4614-9011-1_4, financial incentives helped shift attitudes toward the acceptance of ambulatory surgery by both patients and providers.

Ambulatory Thyroid Surgery

In 1986, Steckler became the first author to advocate outpatient thyroidectomy. His rationale included cost savings, patient comfort, and a very acceptable safety profile in the selected group of patients operated. Initially met with mixed acceptance, outpatient thyroidectomy gained significant enthusiasm in the 1990s and 2000s. Initial reports advocated hemi-thyroidectomy, but more contemporary studies concluded that completion and total thyroidectomy were safe outpatient procedures in selected patients. This includes a 2007 report of over 1,000 outpatient thyroidectomies in which Snyder concluded that ambulatory surgery was safe and cost-effective.

In the context of this review, outpatient or ambulatory surgery is defined as any procedure that does not require postoperative overnight observation or admission. This includes both standard postanesthesia care unit (PACU) recovery and planned short-stay recovery (4–6-h observation period) at an ambulatory care center or hospital-based outpatient center. The primary goals of ambulatory thyroidectomy are to maximize patient comfort, to reduce resource allocation/healthcare cost, and to maintain patient safety.

Patient Comfort

Generally, hemi-thyroidectomy, completion thyroidectomy, and total thyroidectomy (with or without central node dissection) are relatively well-tolerated procedures. Pain is usually described as modest, especially if the strap musculature is preserved. Anecdotally, patients seem to tolerate pain with the use of combination hydrocodone/acetaminophen tablets and seem to use similar amounts of these analgesics whether at home or in hospital. The majority of patients, but not all, seem to value the comfort of home and prefer same-day discharge when given a preference. In a report by Sampson, 646 of 655 patients undergoing outpatient thyroidectomy reported being "very pleased" with their treatment and discharge strategy. In a study published by Houlton et al. in 2009, only 20 % of 137 patients undergoing total or completion thyroidectomy were admitted for overnight observation due to either patient preference or comorbidities.

In addition, the use of newer surgical techniques and technologies may be resulting in improved patient comfort. Over the past several decades, surgical trends away from the classic low-collar incision, with wide elevation of subplatysmal flaps, toward minimal invasive techniques have resulted in less postoperative pain according to several studies. Also, the use of the harmonic scalpel and other ultrasonic technologies, which are an important aspect of minimally invasive surgery according to Miccoli et al., has been reported to decrease postoperative pain when compared to a suture ligature technique.

On the other hand, though the majority of patients fair well with same-day discharge, there is a significant subset of patients that are more comfortable with overnight observation. This may be because they require intravenous medications for nausea or pain control, have little help at home, or may simply be personal preference. Ultimately, the decision about patient comfort should be discussed with, and left up to, the patient.

Cost Savings

There is little doubt that ambulatory thyroidectomy results in decreased healthcare expenditures. This includes reductions in nursing care, overnight variable expenses, and hospital bed allocation. While these reductions ultimately translate into to a decreased hospital charge and cost, the exact amount of savings is fairly difficult to calculate. In 2007, a $2,474 reduction in hospital charge (as opposed to reimbursed cost) per outpatient surgery was reported by Seybet et al. In 1995, Marohn et al. reported a $1,500 decrease in dollars spent by the US military hospital system per same-day discharge. Similarly, Mowschenson et al. reported a 30 % reduction in cost with outpatient surgery. Regardless of the exact dollars saved, outpatient surgery is more efficient for hospital system, third-party payers, and government agencies. In addition, a portion of these savings are passed onto the patient, depending on their healthcare plan and insurance deductible.

Patient Safety

Patient safety remains the principal concern when contemplating outpatient surgery. In fact, the ability to manage postoperative complications on an outpatient basis remains the central point of contention in the outpatient discussion. Safety concerns can generally be divided into two categories: (1) managing postoperative complications inherent to thyroid surgery and (2) managing complications inherent to ambulatory surgery and general anesthesia.

Significant surgical complications associated with thyroid surgery include hypocalcemia, postoperative bleeding/hematoma, recurrent laryngeal nerve injury, superior laryngeal nerve injury, tracheal injury, airway compromise, and wound infection.

Hypocalcemia

The management of post-thyroidectomy hypocalcemia has traditionally been a barrier to ambulatory surgery. Transient hypocalcemia is the most common complication of total, or completion, thyroidectomy, affecting approximately 25 % of patients (though rates of hypocalcemia vary widely across series). Permanent hypoparathyroidism is much less frequent, affecting less than 1 % of patients in experienced hands. Patients undergoing first time hemi-thyroidectomy are not at significant risk of hypoparathyroidism as long as contralateral parathyroid glands are left undisturbed. In addition, hemi-thyroidectomy results in virtually no risk of bilateral vocal cord paralysis and less risk of hematoma formation, ultimately making this a safer outpatient procedure than completion or total thyroidectomy. Alternatively, patients undergoing central node dissection are at increased risk of hypocalcemia compared to total thyroidectomy alone.

A variety of supplementation strategies have been developed for the prevention and treatment of post-thyroidectomy hypocalcemia. These strategies can generally be divided into three groups: (1) watchful waiting, (2) routine prophylactic supplementation, and (3) the more contemporary, PTH-based selective supplementation.

Watchful waiting refers to the traditional method of checking calcium levels every 6–8 h during a hospital stay and only supplementing patients after a trend toward hypocalcemia develops. This frequently requires a 48–72-h hospitalization to both recognize and adequately treat hypocalcemia. Alternatively, an early, routine supplementation strategy involves supplementing all patients prophylactically with calcium and/or vitamin D. Routine supplementation has been shown to reduce the rate of postoperative hypocalcemia compared with a watchful waiting approach and results in little, if any, negative effects. As such, the watchful waiting technique has largely been supplanted by most authors.

More recently, several groups have published on PTH-based selective supplementation strategies that use postoperative PTH levels (generally drawn 1 h after surgery in the PACU) to predict a patient's risk of developing hypocalcemia. Those patients that are hypoparathyroid (defined variably as PTH less than 8–20 pg/mL) are then supplemented selectively and fairly aggressively. This strategy has several advantages that lend itself toward outpatient surgery. Most importantly, by identifying those patients most at risk for hypocalcemia, patients can be treated more generously with calcium and calcitriol (PTH-activated vitamin D). Also, a PTH-based protocol may be able to predict which patients benefit from overnight observation instead of same-day discharge. In a study published by the authors of this manuscript in 2011, 180 patients underwent completion or total thyroidectomy and were subject to a discharge criterion that included a postoperative PTH >20 pg/mL. Sixty-six percent of patients met this criterion, and ultimately 95 patients underwent outpatient surgery. None of these outpatients suffered from symptomatic hypocalcemia. This is in contrast to several ambulatory thyroidectomy series which, somewhat consistently, report a 5 % incidence of symptomatic hypocalcemia when using routine supplementation.

Regardless of technique, properly educating patients is paramount to the successful management of hypocalcemia. The avoidance of symptomatic calcium-related complications relies on patients seeking medical care when symptoms occur. Fortunately, the symptoms of hypocalcemia, including perioral paresthesias and muscle spasm, occur consistently and significantly earlier than life-threatening tetany or cardiac arrhythmias. As such, reports of post-thyroidectomy tetany, arrhythmia, or hypocalcemia-related death are devoid in the ambulatory literature. It is critical that patients be educated about the symptoms of hypocalcemia verbally and with a written handout. Access to a physician or representative should be provided 24 h a day. A 48-h calcium check may be warranted in patients at high-risk for hypocalcemia, though the authors typically check calcium levels 5–7 days following surgery.

In summation, both routine calcium supplementation (1 g TID or QID with or without vitamin D) and PTH-based supplementation are fairly safe replacement strategies and may be adapted to outpatient completion or total thyroidectomy. Watchful waiting, however, is not an advisable strategy for managing ambulatory patients. Ultimately, patient education and access to a medical care are critical components to the successful management of outpatient hypocalcemia.

Hematoma

The risk of postoperative hematoma and potential airway compromise remains the largest apprehension to outpatient surgery. Hematoma is generally accepted to occur and become symptomatic less than 1 % of the time.

Traditionally, patients were admitted postoperatively with a suction drain in order to monitor and prevent hematoma. In addition, some surgeons have placed hemostatic neck wraps or pressure dressings at the time of surgery to mitigate hematoma formation. Unfortunately, neither drain placement nor pressure dressings have been shown to decrease the risk of hematoma formation when used routinely. In a 2008 study, 108 patients underwent thyroidectomy and were randomized to receive either pressure dressings or nonpressure dressings. The rate of hematoma formation was not different between the two groups and neck ultrasound did not show a difference in subcutaneous fluid collection.

In regard to drains, no less than 11 randomized controlled trials have evaluated the use of suction drains for the prevention of postoperative hematoma. No studies have consistently reported a reduction in hematoma formation, reoperation, or respiratory distress with the use of routine drains. In addition, several studies report an increase in postoperative pain and hospital stay with their use. As such, the authors do not routinely place suction drains, which contributes significantly to the feasibility of outpatient surgery. Instead drains are reserved for patients with coagulopathies, patients using anticoagulant/antiplatelet medications, large vascular Graves' glands, massive goiters, or those who had significant bleeding during surgery. Patients that have suction drains placed are observed overnight in the hospital and are not candidates for outpatient surgery. This allows nursing personnel to perform drain management and allows for the monitoring of those conditions that required drain placement.

Newer energy devices such as the harmonic scalpel (and other ultrasonic technologies) as well as energized vessel sealing devices have been reported to result in better hemostasis than classic suture ligature techniques. However, no studies have shown a reduction in hematoma formation with the use of these technologies. The same is true for the variety of hemostatic agents, whose use has become popular in endocrine surgery, including oxidized cellulose, thrombin, and fibrin glue.

At this point, the data would suggest that no intervention, other than meticulous intraoperative hemostasis, heralds a significant impact on hematoma formation. Observing patients in the hospital, however, likely leads to quicker recognition and treatment of postoperative hematomas. Monitoring is particularly pertinent given that a large majority of hematomas (but not all) occur within 24 h of surgery. While a significant portion of these hematomas could be recognized during recovery in the PACU (up to 4–6 h depending on protocol), it is clear that a certain percentage of hematomas will occur outside of this window. In a retrospective review by Burkey et al. in 2001, 43 % of hematomas occurred within 6 h of surgery, 38 % between 6 and 24 h, and 19 % greater than 24 h after surgery. However, patients with hematomas presenting greater than 6 h after surgery represented just 0.2 % of the entire 13,817 patient cohort. Similarly, in a review by Leyre et al. 53 % of hematomas presented within 6 h of surgery, 37 % occurred between 6 and 24 h, and 10 % occurred greater than 24 h after surgery.

In the end, the unpredictable nature of hematoma formation, though rare, remains the most important limiting factor to an outpatient approach. Though we are unaware of any devastating consequences resulting from post-ambulatory hematoma formation, this small but profound risk must be accepted by both surgeon and patient prior to undertaking outpatient surgery. Patient education, therefore, continues to be critical. As part of instruction, patients should have a contingency plan set forth if bleeding does occur. As such, same-day surgery is generally not recommended for those patients requiring distant travel or who lack family support at home.

Airway Compromise

The risk of airway compromise from bilateral cord paralysis or tracheal injury is very low following routine surgery. When these complications do occur, they are generally recognized intraoperatively or shortly after the emergence of anesthesia. If there is concern for bilateral cord paresis or paralysis (resection of a nerve, bilateral injury, etc.), patients should be observed overnight with central monitoring or cleared by flexible laryngoscopy. Intraoperative recurrent laryngeal nerve monitoring may also be useful in this regard. Though nerve monitoring has not been shown to reduce the incidence of cord paralysis or paresis (a large study of over 1,000 at risk nerves found no difference in rates of paralysis between monitored and unmonitored patients), it is frequently reliable in predicting nerve function at the end of the operation. If the recurrent laryngeal nerves were electrically stimulated at some point during the procedure, but failed to stimulate later in the thyroidectomy, it is the authors' experience that the vocal cord will likely not be functioning postoperatively. If both nerves fail to stimulate, a high level of concern for respiratory distress should be maintained, and extubation should be undertaken cautiously.

Comorbidities

Though several authors advocate the use of local and regional anesthesia for thyroidectomy, the majority of thyroidectomies are performed under general anesthesia. For many decades, same-day discharge following general anesthesia has been recognized as safe for the majority of patients, though significant complications do rarely transpire. In a 1993 report of 38,000 patients undergoing ambulatory surgery, 1 in 1,500 patients endured a serious medical complication within 30 days of ambulatory surgery. This includes myocardial infarction, stroke, and pulmonary embolism, most frequently. Several authors have attempted to provide guidelines for medical candidacy for outpatient thyroid surgery. Materazzi et al., in 2007, recommended that patients be of American Society of Anesthesiologists (ASA) class I or II, be easily intubatable, and have a BMI less than 32 kg/m^2. The American Thyroid Association is currently sponsoring in-press guidelines for patients undergoing outpatient thyroid surgery. They recommend that eligible patients be of ASA class I–III, without major comorbidities (free of seizure disorder,

Table 4.1 Relative contraindications to outpatient surgery

Distant travel
Significant comorbidities ASA IV or V Uncompensated cardiac/pulmonary disease Obstructive sleep apnea
Drain placement Graves' with large vascular goiters Antiplatelet/anticoagulant therapy Massive goiter Poor hemostasis
Airway concern
Poorly tolerating anesthetic
Secondary or tertiary hyperparathyroidism
PTH <15–20 pg/mL post thyroidectomy[a]

[a]Optional

obstructive sleep apnea, pregnancy, and uncompensated respiratory or cardiac disease), not use antiplatelet/anticoagulant therapy, and live within proximity of a skilled hospital facility. Correspondingly, a set of proposed relative contraindications to outpatient surgery are listed in Table 4.1.

In terms of complications, it is also mentionable that one benefit of an outpatient approach may be the reduction of certain in-hospital medical complications. Though this has not been studied adequately, it is conceivable that ambulatory endocrine surgery might reduce rare nosocomial infections (pneumonias, urinary tract infections, etc.) and overnight medical errors.

Ambulatory Parathyroid Surgery

Though the majority of controversy concerning ambulatory endocrine surgery involves thyroidectomy, there are several notable issues related to parathyroid surgery. Analogous to thyroidectomy, the classic approach to parathyroidectomy involved a low-collar incision, large subplatysmal flaps, and mandatory bilateral exploration, historically requiring suction drain placement and inpatient observation. With the advent of improved parathyroid adenoma localization (sestamibi localization and ultrasound imaging) and with the use of intraoperative PTH assays, limited unilateral dissections have become standard. With less dissection, surgery for well-localized adenomas is extremely well tolerated by the vast majority of patients. Virtually all healthy patients are candidates for outpatient surgery. Localized excisions are reported to be very safe even in morbidly obese and elderly patients.

Parathyroid operations that require four-gland exploration raise the risk of postoperative hypoparathyroidism and are slightly more uncomfortable than localized procedures, though they are still tolerated quite well. The majority of patients are eligible for outpatient surgery which is performed more liberally than for patients undergoing total thyroidectomy. This is because the risk of hypocalcemia (with solitary adenoma excision), hematoma, and vocal cord paralysis is significantly less following parathyroid surgery compared to total thyroidectomy.

There are several unique risks to parathyroid surgery, however. In addition to hemodilution, and parathyroid devascularization, postoperative hypocalcemia may uniquely result from hungry bone syndrome for patients with long-standing or severe hyperparathyroidism. The risk of post-parathyroidectomy hypocalcemia is directly proportional to preoperative hypercalcemia and is increased in patients with bone density scores ≤ -3 and when all four glands have been manipulated. Hypocalcemia can be quite significant, not infrequently reaching symptomatic levels, yet because calcium levels are high preoperatively, it may take 48–72 h for serum levels to reach a nadir. Therefore, overnight admission is not adequate to completely trend calcium levels. In general, we prefer outpatient management in patients with primary hyperparathyroidism, even in patients at increased risk of developing hypocalcemia. Calcium levels are drawn 48 h following surgery for patients at risk for hungry bone syndrome or when there is concern for significant devascularization. A PACU-drawn PTH level may also be helpful in this setting, though we have only found it to be predictive of hypocalcemia if PTH levels are very low or undetectable. This is because serum calcium levels typically remain high in the immediate postoperative period appropriately suppressing PTH levels.

Patients with renal failure and secondary or tertiary hyperparathyroidism also offer a unique challenge following surgery. These patients typically become hypocalcemic quickly and dramatically, following 3 ½ gland parathyroidectomy, typically requiring aggressive oral and intravenous calcium replacement. Therefore, patients with secondary and tertiary hyperparathyroidism should not undergo outpatient surgery and these conditions should generally be considered contraindications to an ambulatory approach.

Same-Day Discharge

Patients should meet the discharge criteria listed in Table 4.2 prior to same-day discharge. Patients must have received proper education and a discussion about risks of complications must be addressed. Education should be reinforced with written instructions provided by the surgeon or discharge nurse. Nurses must be trained to comfortably assess the neck and respiratory status of the patient if the surgeon is not present at the time of discharge. Adequate family support and adequate functional status should be assessed. The patient should receive either routine calcium therapy or supplementation based on a selective PTH protocol. Anesthesiology staff should clear the patient for discharge and assess for recalcitrant nausea and vomiting. Coordination of these steps should not be underestimated, and initially will take significant communication with anesthesiology and nursing staff. Ultimately, multidisciplinary care is paramount to successful outpatient endocrine surgery.

Table 4.2 Discharge criteria

Patient education completed
Neck exam reassuring
Calcium supplementation provided
Appropriate functional status
Ensure family member at home
Ensure access to a skilled hospital facility
Patient understands risks of complications

Conclusion

With the advent of less invasive surgical techniques, improved calcium supplementation strategies, and lower morbidity anesthetic techniques, outpatient endocrine surgery has become safer and better tolerated. Patient satisfaction with ambulatory surgery is high, and overall, the risks of symptomatic hypocalcemia, postoperative hematoma, and airway compromise are low in experienced hands. Patient education is paramount to the successful management of outpatient complications. Patients should be given both verbal and written instructions and must be given continuous access to a physician. Ultimately, despite meticulous precautions, complications are inevitable and both patient and surgeon alike must be willing to accept the low risk of potentially devastating consequences, including hematoma formation. Despite these inherent risks, ambulatory endocrine surgery should be considered safe, cost-effective, and efficient in selected patients.

Recommended Reading

Ancona-Berk VA, Chalmers TC. An analysis of the costs of ambulatory and inpatient care. Am J Public Health. 1986;76:1102–4.

Ayyash K, Khammash M, Tibblin S. Drain vs. no drain in primary thyroid and parathyroid surgery. Eur J Surg. 1991;157(2):113–4.

Burkey SH, van Heerden JA, Thompson GB, et al. Reexploration for symptomatic hematomas after cervical exploration. Surgery. 2001;130:914–20.

Casalino LP, Devers KJ, Brewster LR. Focused factories? Physician-owned specialty facilities. Health Aff. 2003; 22(6):56–67.

Chin CW, Loh KS, Tan KS. Ambulatory thyroid surgery: an audit of safety and outcomes. Singapore Med J. 2007;48(8):720–4.

Colak T, Akca T, Turkmenoglu O, et al. Drainage after total thyroidectomy or lobectomy for benign thyroidal disorders. J Zhejiang Univ Sci B. 2008;9: 319–23.

Cullen KA, Hall MJ, Golosinskiy A. Ambulatory surgery in the United States, 2006. Natl Health Stat Report. 2009;11:1–28.

Grodski S, Lundgren CI, Sidhu S, Sywak M, Delbridge L. Postoperative PTH measurement facilitates day 1 discharge after total thyroidectomy. Clin Endocrinol. 2009;70(2):322–5.

Hall MJ, Lawrence L. Ambulatory surgery in the United States, 1996. Adv Data. 1998;12(300):1–16.

Hallgrimsson P, Loven L, Westerdahl J, Bergenfelz A. Use of the harmonic scalpel versus conventional haemostatic techniques in patients with grave disease undergoing total thyroidectomy: a prospective randomised controlled trial. Langenbecks Arch Surg. 2008;393:675–80.

Harding J, Sebag F, Sierra M, et al. Thyroid surgery: postoperative hematoma – prevention and treatment. Langenbecks Arch Surg. 2006;391:169–73.

Henry JF, Gramatica L, Denizot A, Kvachenyuk A, Puccini M, Defechereux T. Morbidity of prophylactic lymph node dissection in the central neck area in patients with papillary thyroid carcinoma. Langenbecks Arch Surg. 1998;383(2):167–9.

Hopkins B, Steward DL. Outpatient thyroid surgery and the advances making it possible. Curr Opin Otolaryngol Head Neck Surg. 2009;17(2):95–9.

Houlton JJ, Pechter W, Steward DL. PACU PTH facilitates safe outpatient total thyroidectomy. Otolaryngol Head Neck Surg. 2011;144(1):43–7.

Hurtado-Lopez LM, Lopez-Romero S, Rizzo-Fuentes C, et al. Selective use of drains in thyroid surgery. Head Neck. 2001;23:189–93.

Koh YW, Park JH, Lee SW, Choi EC. The harmonic scalpel technique without supplementary ligation in total thyroidectomy with central neck dissection: a prospective randomized study. Ann Surg. 2008;247:945–9.

Kohn, LT, Corrigan JM, Donaldson MS. To err is human: building a safer health system. The National Academies Press, Washington, DC; 2001. p. 627.

Leader S, Moon M. Medicare trends in ambulatory surgery. Health Aff. 1989;8(1):158–70.

Lee SW, Choi EC, Lee YM, Lee JY, Kim SC, Koh YW. Is lack of placement of drains after thyroidectomy with central neck dissection safe? A prospective, randomized study. Laryngoscope. 2006;116(9):1632–5.

Leyre P, Desurmont T, Lacoste L, et al. Does the risk of compressive hematoma after thyroidectomy authorize 1-day surgery? Langenbecks Arch Surg. 2008;393(5):733–7.

Lo Gerfo P, Gates R, Gazetas P. Outpatient and short-stay thyroid surgery. Head Neck. 1991;13:97–101.

Marohn MR, LaCivita KA. Evaluation of total/near-total thyroidectomy in a short-stay hospitalization: safe and cost-effective. Surgery. 1995;118(6):943–8.

Materazzi G, Dionigi G, Berti P, et al. One-day thyroid surgery: retrospective analysis of safety and patient satisfaction on a consecutive series of 1,571 cases over a three-year period. Eur Surg Res. 2007;39:182–8.

Mezei G, Chung F. Return hospital visits and hospital readmissions after ambulatory surgery. Ann Surg. 1999;230(5):721.

Miccoli P, Bendinelli C, Berti P, et al. Video-assisted versus conventional parathyroidectomy in primary hyperparathyroidism: a prospective randomized study. Surgery. 1999;126(6):1117–22.

Miccoli P, Berti P, Dionigi G, et al. Randomized controlled trial of harmonic scalpel use during thyroidectomy. Arch Otolaryngol Head Neck Surg. 2006;132:1069–73.

Miccoli P, Minuto MN, Ugolini C, et al. Minimally invasive video-assisted thyroidectomy for benign thyroid disease: an evidence-based review. World J Surg. 2008;32:1333–40.

Mowschenson PM, Hodin RA. Outpatient thyroid and parathyroid surgery: a prospective study of feasibility, safety, and costs. Surgery. 1995;118:1051–3.

Norman J, Aronson K. Outpatient parathyroid surgery and the differences seen in the morbidly obese. Otolaryngol Head Neck Surg. 2007;236(2):282–6.

Piromchai P, Vatanasapt P, Reechaipichitkul W, Phuttharak W, Thanaviratananich S. Is the routine pressure dressing after thyroidectomy necessary? A prospective randomized controlled study. BMC Ear Nose Throat Disord. 2008;8(1):1.

Reeve TS, Babidge WJ, Parkyn RF, et al. Minimally invasive surgery for primary hyperparathyroidism: a systematic review. Aust N Z J Surg. 2000;70(4):244–50.

Sabour S, Manders E, Steward DL. The role of rapid PACU parathyroid hormone in reducing post-thyroidectomy hypocalcemia. Otolaryngol Head Neck Surg. 2009;141(6):727–9.

Samson PS, Reyes FR, Saludares WN, Angeles RP, Francisco RA, Tagorda Jr ER. Outpatient thyroidectomy. Am J Surg. 1997;173(6):499–503.

Sanabria A, Carvalho AL, Silver CE, et al. Routine drainage after thyroid surgery – a meta-analysis. J Surg Oncol. 2007;96:273–80.

Seybt MW, Terris DJ. Outpatient thyroidectomy: experience in over 200 patients. Laryngoscope. 2010;120:959–63.

Shin SH, Holmes H, Bao R, et al. Outpatient minimally invasive parathyroidectomy is safe for elderly patients. J Am Coll Surg. 2009;208(6):1071–6.

Shindo M, Chheda NN. Incidence of vocal cord paralysis with and without recurrent laryngeal nerve monitoring during thyroidectomy. Arch Otolaryngol Head Neck Surg. 2007;133:481–5.

Snyder SK, Hamid KS, Roberson C, et al. Outpatient thyroidectomy is safe and reasonable: experience with more than 1,000 planned outpatient procedures. J Am Coll Surg. 2010;210:575–84.

Steckler RM. Outpatient thyroidectomy: a feasibility study. Am J Surg. 1986;152:417–9.

Terris DJ, Moister B, Seybt MW, et al. Outpatient thyroid surgery is safe and desirable. Otolaryngol Head Neck Surg. 2007;136:556–9.

Terris DJ, Snyder S, Carneiro-Pla D, et al. American Thyroid Association Statement on Outpatient Thyroidectomy. Thyroid. 2013;23(10):1193–1202.

Trottier DC, Barron P, Moonje V, et al. Outpatient thyroid surgery: should patients be discharged on the day of their procedures? Can J Surg. 2009;52:182–6.

Vaiman M, Nagibin A, Olevson J. Complications in primary and completed thyroidectomy. Surg Today. 2010;40(2):114–8.

Vasher M, Goodman A, Politz D, Norman J. Postoperative calcium requirements in 6,000 patients undergoing outpatient parathyroidectomy: easily avoiding symptomatic hypocalcemia. J Am Coll Surg. 2010;211(1):49–54.

Warner MA, Shields SE, Chute CG. Major morbidity and mortality within 1 month of ambulatory surgery and anesthesia. JAMA. 1993;270(11):1437–41.

Winter A. Comparing the mix of patients in various outpatient surgery settings. Health Aff. 2003;22(6):68–75.

Wu G, Pai SI, Agrawal N, et al. Profile of patients with completion thyroidectomy and assessment of their suitability for outpatient surgery. Otolaryngol Head Neck Surg. 2011;145(5):727–31.

Zedenius J, Wadstrom C, Delbridge L. Routine autotransplantation of at least one parathyroid gland during total thyroidectomy may reduce permanent hypoparathyroidism to zero. Aust N Z J Surg. 1999;69(11):794–7.

Non-endoscopic Minimally Invasive Thyroid Surgery

5

Schelto Kruijff and Leigh Delbridge

Background

In the past decade, the drive towards minimally invasive surgery has caused an evolution in various surgical specialties. The emergence of minimally invasive endocrine surgical techniques has made procedures such as minimally invasive thyroid surgery and minimally invasive parathyroidectomy a part of daily surgical practice.

This chapter will discuss the emergence and evolution of non-endoscopic minimally invasive thyroid surgery (MITS), indications for the procedure and a step-by-step description of the surgical technique of MITS. A variety of the so-called "minimally invasive" approaches to the thyroid have been developed. These can generally be categorised as those that take a cervical approach, both endoscopic and non-endoscopic, or those that utilise an extra-cervical approach, either chest wall, trans-mammary or axillary. However, it should be noted that the extra-cervical endoscopic approaches, while they have the advantage of avoiding a cervical incision, require major dissection that exceeds that of conventional surgery, and so the term "minimally invasive" should be applied with caution. The various cervical approaches, which may or may not utilise endoscopic or video assistance, have been described by many different centres and have now been demonstrated to be both safe and feasible. The two most commonly utilised cervical techniques are minimally invasive video-assisted thyroidectomy (MIVAT) and minimal invasive thyroid surgery through a direct lateral mini-incision approach (MITS). Both of these techniques have proven to be feasible with comparable morbidity rates as conventional surgery. MITS, using the lateral mini-incision approach, was first described by the University of Sydney Endocrine Surgical Unit in 2002.

The major application of this surgical approach is for the diagnostic excision of small thyroid nodules with atypical follicular cytology or excision of toxic nodules (particularly given that the majority of these are benign follicular adenomas or hyperplastic thyroid nodules). Depending upon the location of the nodule within the thyroid gland, this can be achieved with either a complete lobectomy or a partial lobectomy, especially for nodules located either in the upper part of the superior pole or inferiorly within the lower pole. These patients are ideal candidates for a minimal access approach given the potential advantages of a small incision, less tissue trauma, less postoperative pain, shorter hospital stay and lower health-care cost combined with improved comfort and cosmetic results. MITS in diagnostic excision situations should be seen as procedure positioned between fine-needle aspiration biopsy (FNAB) and conventional standard thyroidectomy achieved through a 5–6-cm incision. MITS follows exactly the same principles as a

S. Kruijff, MD • L. Delbridge, MD (✉)
Endocrine Surgical Unit,
University of Sydney, Reserve Road, St Leonards,
Sydney, NSW 2065, Australia
e-mail: leigh.delbridge@sydney.edu.au

D.J. Terris, M.C. Singer (eds.), *Minimally Invasive and Robotic Thyroid and Parathyroid Surgery*,
DOI 10.1007/978-1-4614-9011-1_5, © Springer Science+Business Media New York 2014

conventional thyroid surgical procedure but is performed with less trauma.

Development of the MITS Technique

In the mid-1990s, the emergence of reliable preoperative parathyroid localisation facilitated the development of minimal access or minimally invasive parathyroidectomy (MIP). While the initial techniques employed endoscopic assistance, it soon became clear in our institution that a parathyroid adenoma could more easily be approached directly via a 2-cm open lateral mini-incision. This incision allowed dissection between the medial border of the sternocleidomastoid muscle and lateral border of the strap muscles without the use the endoscope.

As a consequence, focused lateral approach parathyroidectomy was adopted widely in our institution and provided a familiarity with a laterally based minimal access approach. When coexisting thyroid nodules required surgery during a minimal invasive parathyroidectomy, a resection or nodulectomy of the thyroid gland was a logic next step. Thus lobectomy and partial thyroidectomy as a MITS procedure slowly became incorporated as standard practice in our unit. The main advantage of the MITS procedure is that the approach maintains the conventional principles of open surgical technique. It uses a capsular dissection, requires identification of the laryngeal nerves and parathyroid glands and can be readily learned by experienced thyroid surgeons without requiring complex instrumentation and additional surgical assistance (such as is needed in endoscopic techniques). The simple MITS operative setup combined with its low costs has made it an attractive alternative treatment option to conventional thyroidectomy.

Indications and Patient Selection for MITS

Careful patient selection is essential for both benign and possibly malignant thyroid disease. The principal indications for MITS are (1) diagnostic excision of thyroid nodules when the fine-needle biopsy has demonstrated atypical or indeterminate features and formal excision is required and (2) excision of toxic or autonomous thyroid nodules. The principal exclusion criteria for MITS are (1) nodule diameter greater than 3 cm, (2) confirmed malignancy requiring a bilateral procedure and (3) bilateral multinodular goitre. The presence of Hashimoto's thyroiditis is considered a contraindication to MIVAT due to difficulties of safely dissecting the inflammatory capsule. However, there is no such problem with MITS during which the dissection is no different to that undertaken during formal open thyroid surgery.

MITS and Atypical Thyroid Nodules

In relation to the diagnostic excision of atypical solitary nodules, MITS can be seen as an ideal investigative procedure. Placing the incision in the lateral aspect of the neck is preferred because it seems to result in scars that are less visible and less likely to form a keloid that an incision placed in the midline of the neck. Laterally placed incisions are often barely visible after 6 months. However, the rate of malignancy for a biopsy or hemithyroidectomy in diagnostic circumstances is estimated to be 15 %. Therefore, a potential criticism of the MITS lateral approach could be that if the resected nodule should turn out to be a thyroid cancer, the incision would not be well positioned for the completion thyroidectomy. However, in our experience, depending upon patient preference and habitus, a completion thyroidectomy can be readily performed either by a matching contralateral mini-incision or by converting the initial lateral mini-incision into a standard cervicotomy (Fig. 5.1). We have previously demonstrated that in patients requiring a completion thyroidectomy, the mean final incision length, scar appearance and patient satisfaction with scar do not differ from those having an initial open procedure through a standard cervicotomy.

MITS and Toxic Nodules

Solitary autonomous or toxic nodules are ideally suited to a MITS procedure. The principle aim of

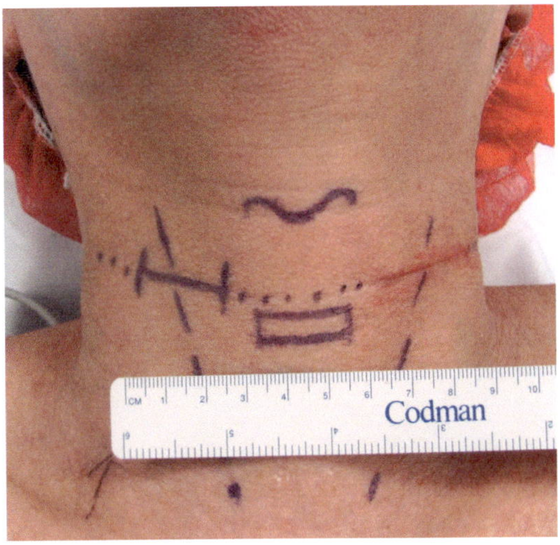

Fig. 5.1 Preoperative photograph demonstrating both a healed mini-incision at 3 weeks on the left and matching skin crease 2.5-cm mini-incision placement on the right in a patient undergoing completion thyroidectomy for follicular cancer (From Palazzo FF, et al. Safety and feasibility of thyroid lobectomy via a lateral 2.5-cm incision with a cohort comparison of the first 50 cases: evolution of a surgical approach. Langenbecks Arch Surg. 2005;390:230–5; with permission)

surgery (as distinct from the use of radioiodine ablation for toxic nodules) is to maximise preservation of normal thyroid tissue and avoid long-term hypothyroidism. Radioiodine has a significant risk of inducing long-term hypothyroidism, while thyroid lobectomy has reported rates of postoperative hypothyroidism between 15 and 35 %. This risk is even lower with MITS because only part of the thyroid lobe containing the toxic nodule is excised.

Surgical Technique of MITS

The Central Mini-incision Approach for Thyroid Lobectomy

Minimal invasive thyroidectomy with a central mini-incision is a technique that is performed through a small central incision, usually 3 cm or less. This is placed higher in the neck compared to the classic Kocher collar incision, usually directly over the cricoid. The surgeon needs to have a headlamp, as good illumination is critical, and usually magnified glasses. Because of the higher incision location, it is not necessary to develop large subcutaneous flaps, making this approach well suited for the use of local regional anaesthesia. A direct ligation of the superior pole vessels can be performed as a first step, as the incision is situated in the skin crease close to the cricoid cartilage. This procedure is best undertaken as a sutureless technique, using either electrothermal or ultrasonic energy devices for vessel ligation. Finally, the target lobe can be removed through the minimal incision by pulling it in a superior-medial direction, as the superior pole of the thyroid is usually more rigid and fixed than the mobile inferior pole. At this stage the opportunity arises to identify the recurrent laryngeal nerve (RLN). To improve exposure and allow identification of the key anatomical structures, the incision must be moved around the operative field and maintained in precise position with retractors.

The Lateral Mini-incision Approach

The major concern with the central mini-incision approach is the limited view of the lateral structures, in particular the RLN, especially if it is in an anatomically challenging relationship with the inferior thyroid artery or passes medial to an enlarged tubercle of Zuckerkandl. For this reason we prefer the lateral mini-incision approach for MITS procedures, providing, as it does, direct visualisation of the entire lateral anatomy related to the thyroid gland, including the RLN and the parathyroid glands. Concurrently it provides the cosmetic advantages of a laterally placed, high skin crease incision.

For the lateral approach general anaesthesia is used and the patient is placed in the supine position with the neck held in mild extension. A headlight is used to provide appropriate illumination of the operative field within the mini-incision. The procedure starts with a 2.5-cm lateral transverse incision made in a skin crease near the level of the thyroid nodule, directly over the medial border of the sternocleidomastoid (SCM) muscle. The sub-platysmal plane can be developed digitally to be able to fully use the mobility of the skin incision and move it

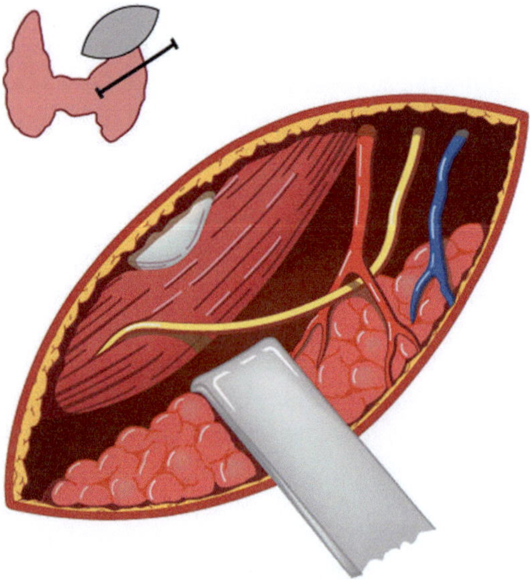

Fig. 5.2 Exposure and dissection of the superior pole achieved by retraction of the wound superiorly (From Palazzo FF, et al. Safety and feasibility of thyroid lobectomy via a lateral 2.5-cm incision with a cohort comparison of the first 50 cases: evolution of a surgical approach. Langenbecks Arch Surg. 2005;390:230–5; with permission)

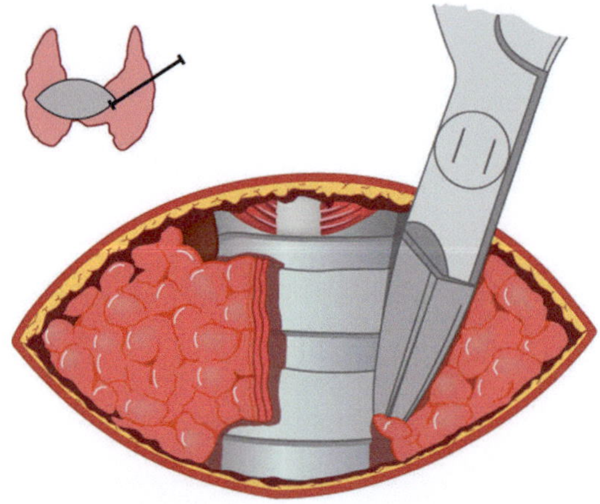

Fig. 5.3 Exposure and dissection of the isthmus achieved by retraction of the wound medially (From Palazzo FF, et al. Safety and feasibility of thyroid lobectomy via a lateral 2.5-cm incision with a cohort comparison of the first 50 cases: evolution of a surgical approach. Langenbecks Arch Surg. 2005;390:230–5; with permission)

over the relevant anatomy during the procedure. After the medial margin of the SCM is exposed together with the lateral border of the strap muscles, the SCM is retracted laterally and the space posterolateral to the strap muscles is developed to reveal the lateral border of the thyroid gland. This is then retracted medially to enable division of the middle thyroid vein. The space medial to the common carotid artery is then dissected down to the prevertebral fascial plane.

Superior Pole Dissection

The upper aspect of the dissection is achieved by moving the surgical field in the cranial direction and gently pulling the upper thyroid pole laterally to open up the avascular plane between the medial border of the upper pole and the cricothyroid muscle. In this way the external branch of the superior laryngeal nerve can be visualised and preserved. The superior thyroid artery is then divided (Fig. 5.2).

Trachea and Isthmus

The skin incision is now repositioned to the midline to expose the trachea and to allow division of the isthmus. This results in increased mobility of the thyroid gland and permits the lateral dissection to be completed. It must be emphasised that routine division of the isthmus at this stage is a vital manoeuvre, in order to provide sufficient mobility of the thyroid lobe to enable it to be subsequently delivered through the mini-incision for the final stage of dissection (Fig. 5.3).

Lower Pole Dissection

The skin incision is now moved caudally to facilitate mobilisation of the lower pole of the thyroid gland and to undertake a capsular dissection. At this stage it is important to identify and preserve the inferior parathyroid gland. If the parathyroid gland cannot be preserved on a vascularised pedicle, it is autotransplanted by injection into the adjacent SCM muscle (Fig. 5.4).

Lateral Dissection

The last step is to return the skin incision to its initial lateral position to enable delivery of the thyroid lobe, thereby improving the exposure of lateral gland (Figs. 5.5 and 5.6). This is performed, as with any open thyroid procedure, with capsular dissection encountering the recurrent laryngeal nerve as it passes medial to the tubercle of Zuckerkandl. At this stage the superior parathyroid is preserved if possible on a vascularised pedicle, or else autotransplanted. Finally, from the medial side, the ligament of Berry is progressively divided allowing the entire thyroid lobe to be delivered through the mini-incision. The entire lobe can then be removed at this stage if the location of the nodule requires a lobectomy. Once haemostasis has been confirmed, the skin incision is closed with subcutaneous absorbable sutures.

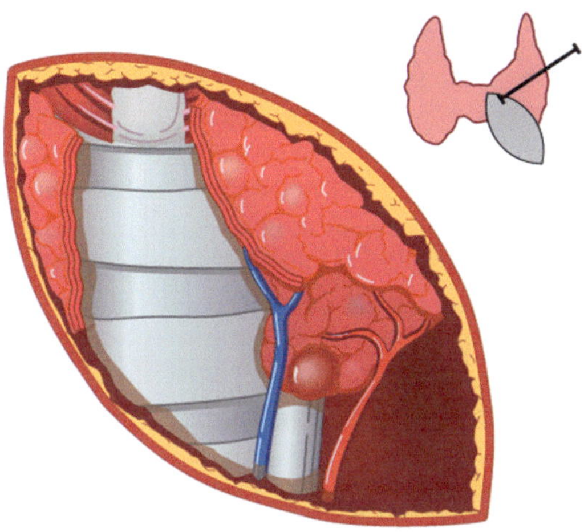

Fig. 5.4 Capsular dissection of the inferior pole of the thyroid achieved by retraction of the wound inferiorly (From Palazzo FF, et al. Safety and feasibility of thyroid lobectomy via a lateral 2.5-cm incision with a cohort comparison of the first 50 cases: evolution of a surgical approach. Langenbecks Arch Surg. 2005;390:230–5; with permission)

The Lateral Mini-incision Approach for Partial Thyroidectomy

Since most atypical nodules requiring diagnostic excision, and almost all toxic nodules, will turn out to be benign, an approach which allows preservation of the maximum residual normal thyroid tissue is preferred to avoid postoperative hypothyroidism (provided the anatomic location of the nodule is appropriate). For nodules at the cephalad part of the superior pole, it may be possible to resect just the upper pole. Likewise for those nodules located in an inferior position, resection of just the lower pole may be feasible. The technique of partial thyroidectomy is made possible by the advent of thermal sealing devices, which allow thyroid tissue to be divided in a bloodless manner. For both approaches, all the above steps are followed, with the exception that the superior pole vessels are not divided for inferior nodules and the inferior vessels also not divided for upper pole nodules. Otherwise division of the isthmus and formal identification of the recurrent laryngeal nerve and parathyroid glands is undertaken, and with those structures clearly visible, the upper or lower pole is resected. Once haemostasis has been confirmed, the skin incision is closed with subcutaneous absorbable sutures.

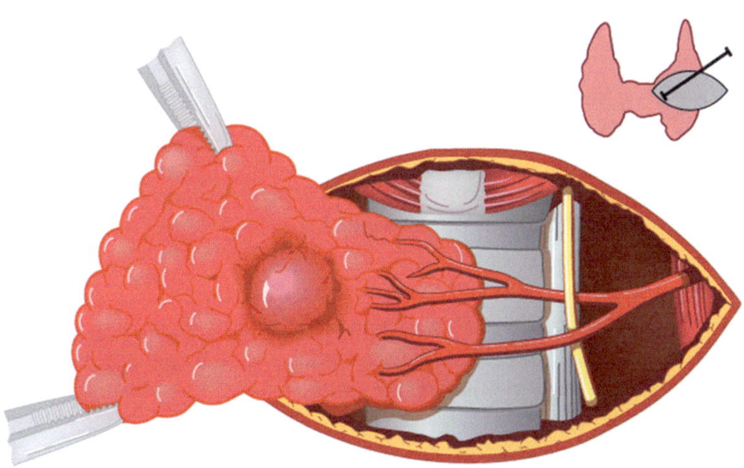

Fig. 5.5 The lateral aspect of the thyroid can be dissected after delivering the lobe through the mini-incision (From Palazzo, FF et al. Safety and feasibility of thyroid lobectomy via a lateral 2.5-cm incision with a cohort comparison of the first 50 cases: evolution of a surgical approach. Langenbecks Arch Surg. 2005;390:230–5; with permission)

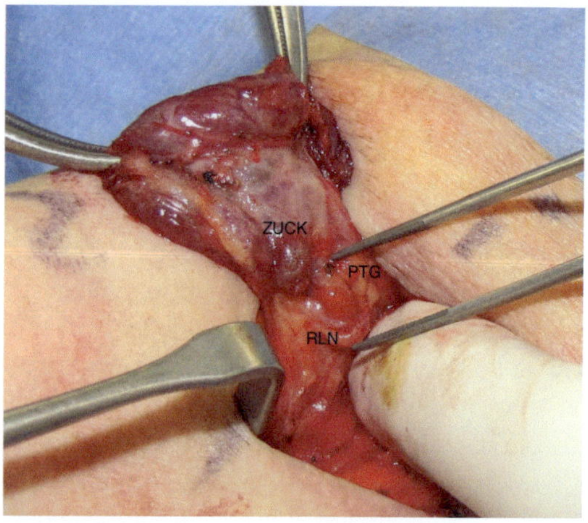

Fig. 5.6 Operative view – with the right lobe having been delivered through the mini-incision, the recurrent laryngeal nerve (*RLN*) and superior parathyroid gland (*PTG*) in relation to the tubercle of Zuckerkandl (*ZUCK*) are clearly in full view of the operating surgeon (From Palazzo FF, et al. Safety and feasibility of thyroid lobectomy via a lateral 2.5-cm incision with a cohort comparison of the first 50 cases: evolution of a surgical approach. Langenbecks Arch Surg. 2005;390:230–5; with permission)

Outcomes of MITS

The first paper describing MITS using the lateral mini-incision approach was published over 10 years ago with the title "Minimal access thyroid surgery: is it feasible, is it appropriate?" The study described 26 patients having undergone minimally invasive parathyroidectomy via a lateral mini-incision approach. However, these patients also underwent unplanned thyroid surgery because of the incidental discovery of an unsuspected thyroid nodule at the time of parathyroidectomy. In all cases the thyroid resection was completed without difficulty or complication, leading us to propose it as a primary surgical approach to small thyroid nodules requiring excision. The encouraging results of the earlier feasibility study led to a number of subsequent cohort studies evaluating the MITS procedures and comparing it with the conventional technique. A prospective, single-blinded, randomised controlled trial was then undertaken which compared MITS using the lateral direct approach versus conventional hemithyroidectomy. Patients with atypical nodules less than 3 cm diameters were included and randomised to either MITS through a lateral 2.5-cm incision or a conventional hemithyroidectomy through a traditional cervicotomy. When the cosmetic results were evaluated after 3 months, MITS seemed cosmetically superior to the conventional approach. Also, as shown in other studies, the direct lateral approach resulted in less postoperative pain. These benefits are provided with the same complication profile as conventional surgery.

Conclusion

As a true minimally invasive procedure, MITS provides a number of significant benefits to patients. It is an ideal procedure for evaluation of the atypical or indeterminate thyroid nodule or for the removal of a toxic nodule. Its adoption broadens the surgical options thyroid surgeons can offer their patients.

Recommended Reading

Agarwal G, et al. Minimally invasive parathyroidectomy using the 'focused' lateral approach. Surgical technique. ANZ J Surg. 2002;72:147–51.

Alvarado R, et al. Minimally invasive thyroid surgery for single nodules: an evidence based review of the lateral mini-incision technique. World J Surg. 2008;32:1341–8. Review.

Bellantone R, et al. Video assisted vs. conventional thyroid lobectomy. Arch Surg. 2002;137:301–4.

Chao TC, et al. Video-assisted open thyroid lobectomy through a small incision. Surg Laparosc Endosc Percutan Tech. 2004;14:15–9.

Del Rio P, et al. Pain after minimally invasive video-assisted and after minimally invasive open thyroidectomy: results of a prospective outcome study. Langenbecks Arch Surg. 2008;393:271–3.

Delbridge LW. Minimally invasive parathyroidectomy: the Australian experience. Asian J Surg. 2003;26:76–81.

Gagner M. Endoscopic subtotal parathyroidectomy in patients with primary hyperparathyroidism. Br J Surg. 1996;83:875.

Gagner M, Inabnet WB. Endoscopic thyroidectomy for solitary thyroid nodules. Thyroid. 2001;11:161–3.

Gauger PG, et al. Endoscopically assisted, minimally invasive parathyroidectomy. Br J Surg. 1999;86:1563–6.

Gossnell JE, et al. Minimal access thyroid surgery: technique and report of the first 25 cases. ANZ J Surg. 2004;74:330–4.

Hegazy MA, et al. Minimally invasive video-assisted thyroidectomy for small follicular thyroid nodules. World J Surg. 2007;31:1743–50.

Henry JF. Minimally invasive surgery of the thyroid and parathyroid glands. Br J Surg. 2006;93:1–2.

Ikeda Y, et al. Are there significant benefits of minimally invasive endoscopic thyroidectomy? World J Surg. 2004;28:1075–8.

Inabnet WB, et al. Safety of same day discharge in patients undergoing suture less thyroidectomy: a comparison of local and general anaesthesia. Thyroid. 2007;18: 57–61.

Lombardi CP, et al. Safety of video-assisted thyroidectomy versus conventional surgery. Head Neck. 2005; 27:58–64.

Lundgren CI, et al. Minimally invasive thyroid surgery for diagnostic excision of solitary thyroid nodules. Asian J Surg. 2007;30:250–4.

Miccoli P, et al. Comparison between minimally invasive video-assisted thyroidectomy and conventional thyroidectomy: a prospective randomized study. Surgery. 2001;130:1039–43.

Miccoli P, et al. Minimally invasive video-assisted thyroidectomy for papillary carcinoma: a prospective study of its completeness. Surgery. 2002;132:1070–3.

Palazzo FF, Delbridge LW. Minimal-access/minimally invasive parathyroidectomy for primary hyperparathyroidism. Surg Clin North Am. 2004;84:717–34.

Palazzo FF, et al. Safety and feasibility of thyroid lobectomy via a lateral 2.5-cm incision with a cohort comparison of the first 50 cases: evolution of a surgical approach. Langenbecks Arch Surg. 2005;390: 230–5.

Patel D, Kebebew E. Pros and cons of robotic transaxillary thyroidectomy. Thyroid. 2012;22:984–5.

Perigli G, et al. Clinical benefits of minimally invasive techniques in thyroid surgery. World J Surg. 2008;32: 45–50.

Ruggieri M, et al. The minimally invasive surgical approach in thyroid diseases. Minerva Chir. 2007;62:309–14.

Sackett WR, et al. Minimal access thyroid surgery: is it feasible, is it appropriate? ANZ J Surg. 2002;72:777–8.

Stalberg P, et al. Minimally invasive parathyroidectomy and thyroidectomy – current concepts. Surgeon. 2007;5:301–8.

Sywak MS, et al. A randomized controlled trial of minimal invasive thyroidectomy using the lateral approach versus conventional hemithyroidectomy. Surgery. 2008;144:1016–21; discussion 1021–2.

Terris D, et al. Minimally invasive thyroidectomy: basic and advanced techniques. Laryngoscope. 2006;116: 350–6.

Yeh MW, et al. Completion of thyroidectomy for malignancy after minimal access thyroid surgery. ANZ J Surg. 2006;76:332–4.

Minimally Invasive Video-Assisted Thyroidectomy

6

Paolo Miccoli, Michele N. Minuto, and Valeria Matteucci

Introduction

The mid-1990s was a "golden" era for the development of endoscopic surgical techniques that followed the introduction of laparoscopic surgery. After first being used in minimally invasive parathyroid surgery, endoscopes were introduced into thyroid surgery. At first, endoscopes were used in the thyroid region to assess if their magnification might provide an advantage in a region where the identification of small structures was of paramount importance. Subsequently, a number of different, purely endoscopic operations were described. These procedures used gas insufflation and were completed in an entirely endoscopic manner. In 1998 the first minimally invasive video-assisted thyroidectomy (MIVAT) was performed in Pisa, Italy (Table 6.1). In this procedure the endoscope is held in position by an assistant, forgoing the need for gas insufflation. A year later the first series of MIVAT procedures was published. MIVAT was the only endoscopic technique that allowed performance of a total thyroidectomy through a single, minimal midline incision in the neck. This was perhaps the first example of a "single-port operation," well before this term was introduced.

While other complicated and often non-reproducible endoscopic techniques were abandoned, this operation has now become the most widespread technique for minimally invasive thyroidectomy. As a true minimally invasive approach, its popularity is partially attributable to the myriad advantages that it offers to patients over traditional thyroidectomy techniques. This procedure has been shown to result in less post-operative pain, faster recovery times, and greater patient satisfaction with their results while having a similar or better complication profile compared to conventional thyroidectomy. Further contributing to its attractiveness is MIVAT's standardization and thus reproducibility. As will be described, MIVAT largely recreates the steps of conventional thyroidectomy, making it relatively easy to learn and master.

P. Miccoli, MD
Department of Surgery, Azienda Ospedaliero-Universitaria Pisana, University of Pisa, Pisa, Italy

M.N. Minuto, MD, PhD (✉)
Department of Surgical Sciences and Applied Diagnostics (DISC), IRCCS, Azienda Ospedaliero-Universitaria San Martino-IST, University of Genoa, L.Go Rosanna Benzi 2, Genoa 16122, Italy
e-mail: micheleminuto@hotmail.com

V. Matteucci, MD
Department of Surgery, Endocrine Surgery Unit, Azienda Ospedaliero-Universitaria Pisana, Pisa, Italy

D.J. Terris, M.C. Singer (eds.), *Minimally Invasive and Robotic Thyroid and Parathyroid Surgery*, DOI 10.1007/978-1-4614-9011-1_6, © Springer Science+Business Media New York 2014

Table 6.1 Milestones in the development of the MIVAT technique

	Year	Ref.
First MIVAT performed in Pisa	1998	
First series reported in literature	1999	Miccoli et al.[1]
MIVAT and CT demonstrate similar surgical results	2001	Miccoli et al.[2]
MIVAT and CT demonstrate similar oncological results	2002	Miccoli et al.[3]
MIVAT and CT demonstrate a similar "manipulation" of the thyroid gland	2005	Lombardi et al.[4]
Central neck dissection is feasible with the MIVAT technique in selected cases	2007	Miccoli et al.[5]
MIVAT is demonstrated to be a safe and reproducible technique	2002, 2008	Miccoli et al.[6]; Terris et al.[7]
MIVAT and CT demonstrate similar oncological results after a 5-year follow-up	2009	Miccoli et al.[8]

[1]Miccoli P, Berti P, Conte M, Bendinelli C, Marcocci C. Minimally invasive surgery for thyroid small nodules: preliminary report. J Endocrinol Invest. 1999;22(11):849–51
[2]Miccoli P, Berti P, Raffaelli M, Materazzi G, Baldacci S, Rossi G. Comparison between minimally invasive video-assisted thyroidectomy and conventional thyroidectomy: a prospective randomized study. Surgery. 2001;130(6):1039–4
[3]Miccoli P, Elisei R, Materazzi G, Capezzone M, Galleri D, Pacini F, Berti P, Pinchera A. Minimally invasive video-assisted thyroidectomy for papillary carcinoma: a prospective study of its completeness. Surgery. 2002a;132(6):1070–3
[4]Lombardi CP, Raffaelli M, Princi P, Lulli P, Rossi ED, Fadda G, Bellantone R. Safety of video-assisted thyroidectomy versus conventional surgery. Head Neck. 2005;27(1):58–64
[5]Miccoli P, Elisei R, Donatini G, Materazzi G, Berti P. Video-assisted central compartment lymphadenectomy in a patient with a positive RET oncogene: initial experience. Surg Endosc. 2007;21(1):120–3
[6]Miccoli P, Bellantone R, Mourad M, Walz M, Raffaelli M, Berti P. Minimally invasive video-assisted thyroidectomy: multiinstitutional experience. World J Surg. 2002b;26:972–5
[7]Terris DJ, Angelos P, Steward DL, Simental AA. Minimally invasive video-assisted thyroidectomy. A multi-institutional North American experience. Arch Otolaryngol Head Neck Surg. 2008;134(1):81–4
[8]Miccoli P, Pinchera A, Materazzi G, Biagini A, Berti P, Faviana P, Molinaro E, Viola D, Elisei R. Surgical treatment of low- and intermediate-risk papillary thyroid cancer with minimally invasive video-assisted thyroidectomy. J Clin Endocrinol Metab. 2009;94(5):1618–22

Selection Criteria

The extent of the operation does not represent a limit of the technique as the surgeon can strictly adhere to the basic rules of a conventional thyroidectomy. As a result, when necessary, a near-total or an extracapsular total thyroidectomy can be achieved, according to the oncologic principles of thyroid surgery. A level VI (central neck) lymph node dissection can also be performed with the MIVAT technique. However, this should be limited to cases of prophylactic neck dissections.

The possibility of performing a thorough total thyroidectomy with the MIVAT technique was demonstrated during the years that followed its introduction. Its safety and efficacy documented, the indications for MIVAT expanded from benign disease to the treatment of low- and intermediate-risk papillary and follicular carcinomas. Subsequently, it has been shown to be appropriate for the treatment of medullary carcinoma in patients with a RET mutation, requiring not only a total thyroidectomy, but also a prophylactic central neck dissection.

In order to have successful outcomes, the following are broad inclusion and exclusion criteria:

- Benign thyroid nodules under 35 mm in their largest diameter or cytologically malignant (or suspicious) nodules under 20 mm, *together with*
- A thyroid volume (ultrasonographically estimated) under 25 ml
- No suspicion of metastatic lymph nodes in the central neck
- No evidence of metastatic or suspicious lymph nodes in the lateral neck
- No evidence of severe thyroiditis

As a suggestion, we always recommend to strictly adhere to the indications proposed, since every extension can cause unnecessary and undesired complications or conversions.

The Technique

The general principle behind the MIVAT technique is to perform a thorough thyroidectomy following the basic principles of the traditional thyroid surgery while gaining the advantages of endoscopic magnification. Critically, the endoscope is used only when it can improve the outcome of the procedure (thus the term "video-assisted" and not "endoscopic").

Instruments

The instruments specifically dedicated to MIVAT are a 30°, 7 or 5 mm, 29 cm long endoscope, a 21 cm long suction dissector (used to avoid the fogging of the endoscope resulting from the steam produced by the energy instrument), two 2 mm elevators of approximately the same length as the suction dissector, small grasping forceps (15 cm long), scissors (8 mm blades, 8 cm long), and two small retractors (16 cm long). Other instruments often utilized are an energy device of choice, titanium clips, and conventional forceps used for thyroid surgery. An insulated Bovie tip should be used to avoid skin burns and inadvertent injury to surrounding structures (given the limited working space).

Positioning

The operation can be conducted under general (either with orotracheal intubation or laryngeal mask airway) or locoregional anesthesia, following the surgeon's, anesthesiologist's, and patient's preferences.

The patient is placed in the supine position, with the neck only slightly hyperextended. Avoiding significant neck extension is one of the factors that explains the decreased pain associated with this procedure.

The primary surgeon will stand on the right side of the patient. Two assistants are employed. The camera assistant is positioned on the left side, across from the primary surgeon. The second assistant, who holds the retractors, stands at the head of the bed, facing the feet. The monitors are placed at both sides of the patient's head. The main monitor is in front of the primary surgeon. The second monitor is helpful but optional.

The camera assistant will always hold the endoscope looking toward the patient's head, positioned slightly away from the axis of the patient's midline, depending on the working side. The angled endoscope should always be used in one of two main positions: looking upside-down (30° lens looking inferiorly) and downside-up (30° angle looking upward), with no intermediate positions. This standardization allows the surgeon to always obtain the same visualization of the anatomy and orientation toward the neck. This is particularly crucial for non-experienced surgeons during all steps of the procedure.

Procedure Details

For teaching purposes we divide a MIVAT lobectomy into five steps:

Step 1: Incision and access to the thyroid region (performed under direct vision)

Step 2: Section of the upper pedicle (performed endoscopically)

Step 3: Identification of the critical structures: the recurrent nerve and the parathyroids (performed endoscopically)

Step 4: Extraction of the thyroid lobe outside the neck and completion of the near-total or total lobectomy (performed under direct vision)

Step 5: Suture of the access point

Step 1. Incision and Access to the Thyroid Region

The operation starts with a 2 cm, midline incision in a skin crease on the same line of the conventional Kocher's incision. This helps to maintain a satisfactory result in the case the operation needs a conversion to open surgery, when a short extension of the wound edges would convert the access to that of a conventional thyroidectomy.

Once the incision is made, the two smallest retractors should be positioned laterally. The "linea alba" should be carefully identified as in an open approach. The main challenge is

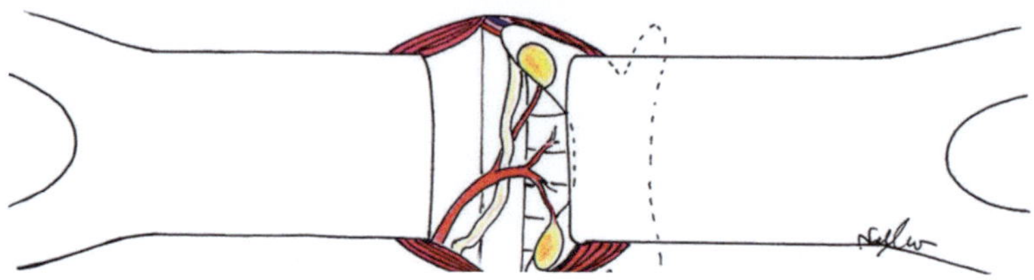

Fig. 6.1 The medial retractor is used to "hook" the thyroid lobe toward the trachea while also rotating it out of the trachea-esophageal groove

correctly identifying it in this limited space. We recommend palpating the tip of the thyroid cartilage to help find the midline.

Once identified, the midline should be opened by means of conventional electrocautery for a limited extent. The short aperture of the strap muscles will help avoid excessive retraction on the skin edges, focusing the majority of the tension on the muscles themselves. This allows the skin edges to remain vital and results in a good cosmetic outcome.

After visualization of the thyroid gland, the operative space of one side should be entered with blunt dissection utilizing the spatulas. As in open surgery, the virtual space between the strap muscles and the thyroid lobe should be entered with the small retractors at first and then with the conventional army-navy after the posterior aspect of the thyroid lobe and the carotid sheath are visualized.

The correct positioning of the retractors is one of the key points of this operation. The lateral retractor should be retracting the carotid sheath and all its contents laterally (preventing an undesired thermal injury to those structures when the energy devices are used in the small operative space). The medial retractor should "hook" the thyroid lobe medially, while at the same time trying to slightly rotate it on the tracheal axis. The retractor should almost hide the lobe from the view of the endoscope (Fig. 6.1). The medial retractor mimics the role of the hand of the assistant during a conventional thyroidectomy. Be aware that, in this phase, the two retractors should always be placed in a symmetrical position, at the two edges of the incision.

Step 2. Section of the Upper Pedicle

This is the most challenging part of the endoscopic operation, and the only one step that is significantly different from the way it is performed in traditional surgery.

The largest retractors are still positioned on both sides of the incision. This positioning will be maintained throughout this entire step.

The endoscopic portion of the operation starts by introducing the tip of the endoscope through the incision to allow visualization of the operative field. The endoscope is a 30°, 7 mm in caliber scope that will initially be oriented caudally to allow division of the middle thyroid vein when present (Fig. 6.2a). Ligation can be achieved using either the energy instrument or a double clip (Fig. 6.2b).

Once this step is done, the endoscope can be rotated downside-up and, looking upward, the upper pedicle will be visualized at the top of the screen (Fig. 6.3).

The upper pedicle is then sectioned in one step. Alternatively, based on the surgeon's preference, the superior pedicle vessels can be divided individually. It is important to remember that for MIVAT, thyroid glands are of limited size, and consequently these vessels can be very small. Before sectioning the vessels of the upper pedicle, it is highly advised to carefully check for the presence of the branches of the superior laryngeal (or Galli-Curci's) nerve. The superior nerve creates a loop at various heights of the upper pedicle or higher, heading medially to enter the lateral side of the cricothyroid muscle (Fig. 6.4a–c). The magnification provided by the endoscope, together with the view it allows of the cephalic aspect of the surgical field, permits this nerve to be seen when it is in its lowest positions (which is often not recognized during conventional thyroidectomy). Once the branches of the nerve have been visualized, their safety should be guaranteed by avoiding excessive heat exposure from using an energy device too close to them.

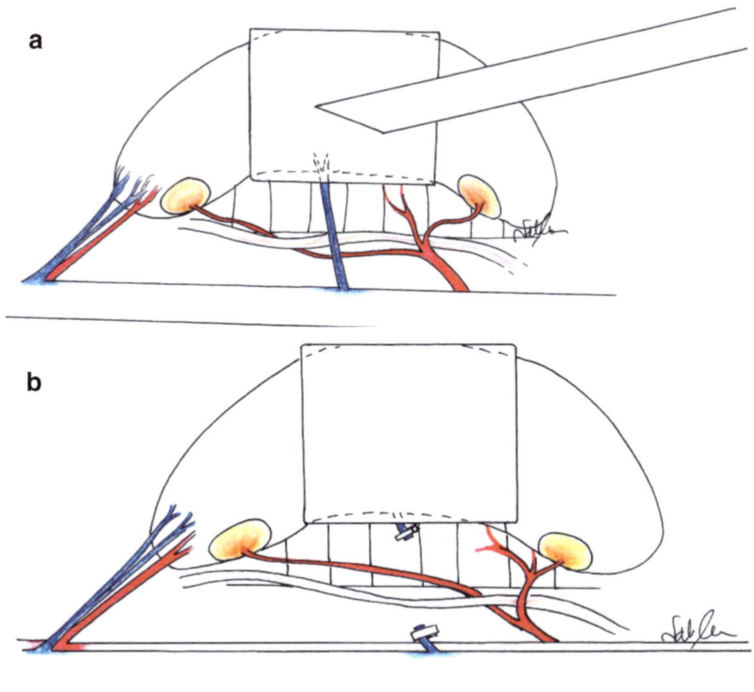

Fig. 6.2 The endoscope, oriented caudally, allows direct vision of the middle thyroid vein (**a**). This vein is then divided (**b**)

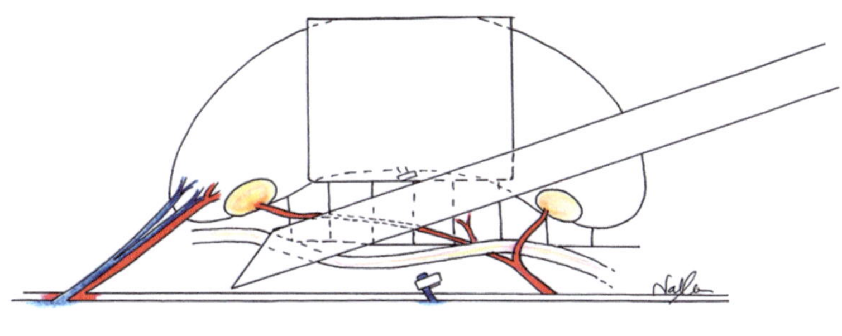

Fig. 6.3 In order to visualize the superior pedicle vessels, after division of the middle thyroid vein, the endoscope is faced cranially

Once the pedicle has been divided, hemostasis should be carefully verified. Any area of uncertain ligation should be immediately addressed for two reasons. Any acute bleeding can be very hard to manage endoscopically and can lead to undesired conversions. On the other hand, delayed bleeding can result in highly dangerous situations. As no drain will be left in the neck and the incision will be sealed, a spontaneous evacuation of the hematoma cannot be readily achieved.

Step 3. Identification of the Recurrent Nerve and the Parathyroid Glands

The great benefit of endoscopic magnification is the reason why this step is the easiest of the whole procedure. From conventional thyroid surgery, an experienced thyroid surgeon knows exactly where to search for the recurrent laryngeal nerve and the parathyroid glands. During MIVAT, having 20x magnification of these areas facilitates quick identification of these structures.

Proper positioning of all of the instruments is a key point during this step of the procedure. The retractors, in their lateral positions, should expose the space where the recurrent nerve and the parathyroid glands are located. The medial retractor is essential to "load" the thyroid lobe, also lifting it in order to visualize the area between the trachea and the esophagus

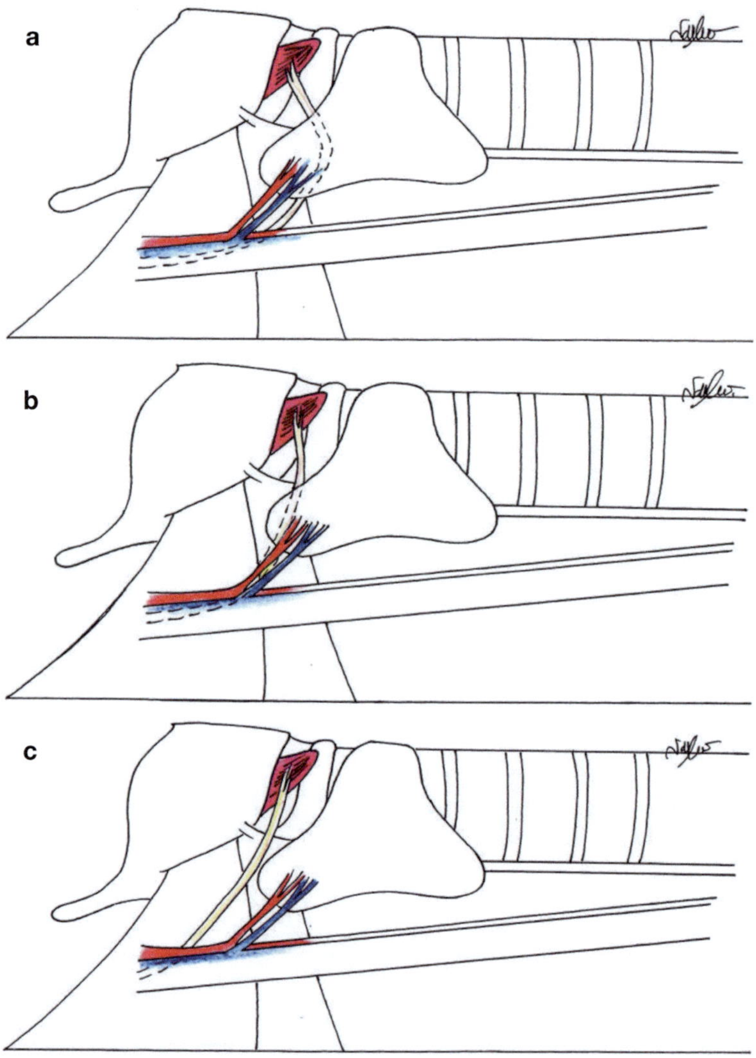

Fig. 6.4 The external branch of the superior laryngeal nerve can be visualized. This nerve can loop inferiorly to varying degrees (**a–c**)

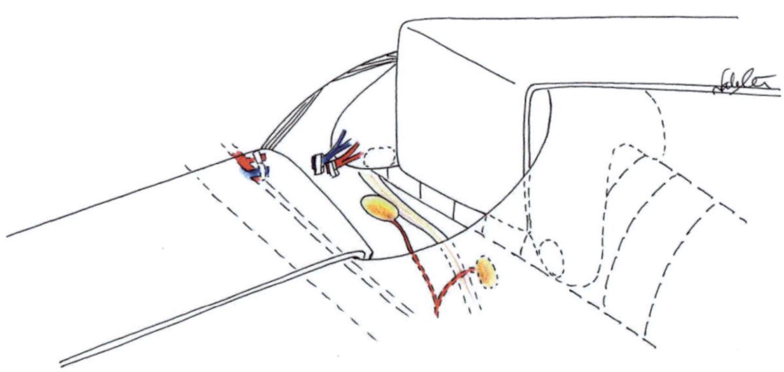

Fig. 6.5 The region where the recurrent laryngeal nerve and the superior parathyroid gland are located is exposed with medial retraction of the thyroid lobe

(Fig. 6.5). The endoscope should always be facing downward, with only a slight medial orientation.

During this step there is generally no need to divide anything, and the entire phase is performed with blunt dissection achieved with the two spatulas. First, the recurrent laryngeal nerve is identified and then dissected until its point of entry in the laryngeal muscles. There is no need, in our opinion, to dissect the nerve too extensively in the caudal direction (farther from its entry point), since the purpose of this dissection is to avoid any traction on the nerve during the step of the mobilization of the lobe. Adequately releasing the nerve allows it to lie on the posterior fascia of the neck when extracting the lobe. The same principle is applied to the parathyroid glands: once identified, they should be only minimally dissected to avoid injury to their vascular pedicles, which might limit their viability and function.

The main branch of the recurrent nerve lies on the anterior surface of the vertebral muscles covered by the deep cervical fascia on the right side and on the esophagus on the left side. On both sides the nerve can be easily visualized at the point it crosses the inferior thyroid artery. This exposure can be achieved with the two spatulas using blunt dissection. An additional anatomical clue to the location of the nerve is the many small lymph nodes that are almost always present in the area surrounding the recurrent nerve. These can be easily dissected, uncovering the nerve itself.

The most frequent position of the superior parathyroid gland is at the upper pole of the thyroid lobe, laterally to the lobe itself, or adherent to it. Familiarity with the typical shape and color of parathyroid glands is essential for their recognition. These characteristics are greatly enhanced by the endoscopic vision. Once identified the parathyroid gland can be gently dissected, always taking care to preserve its small pedicle, and delicately moved away from the thyroid gland. It is important to release the parathyroid glands adequately from the thyroid lobe to avoid any damage to their vascular supply during the mobilization and extraction of the lobe.

In regard to the inferior parathyroid gland, it can often be in a position where it can be hidden behind the blade of the retractor. In the case when an inferior parathyroid gland cannot be identified during the endoscopic exploration, the surgeon can move to the next step of the surgery and search for the inferior parathyroid gland once the lobe has been rotated outside the wound.

Step 4. Mobilization and Extraction of the Thyroid Lobe and Completion of the Lobectomy

This portion of the operation is performed under direct vision, basically following the rules of conventional open surgery.

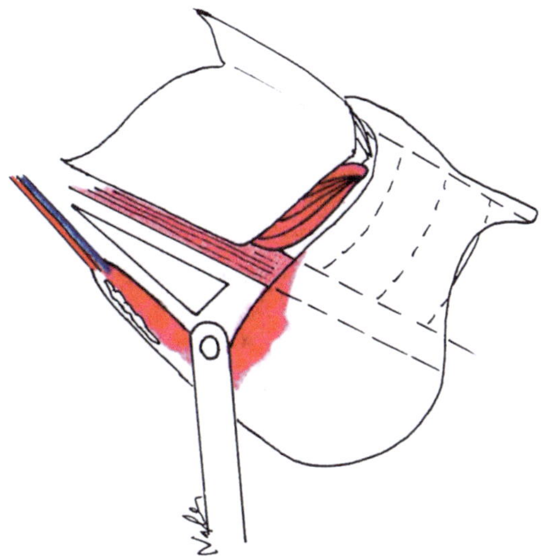

Fig. 6.6 The "triangle of Miccoli-Berti" is demonstrated. The *triangle* is bordered by the upper pedicle laterally, the pyramidal lobe or isthmus medially, and the prethyroidal muscles

This step starts by grasping the superior pole of the thyroid lobe (which has already been dissected) with a conventional forceps. It is then gently extracted through the incision by rotating the entire lobe on his longest axis, paying attention to avoid any damage to the vessels of the inferior pole, from where the vascular feeding of the inferior parathyroid gland may arise. If the upper pedicle has been properly and completely dissected, the surgeon will encounter no resistance in delivering the superior pole of the lobe. Once the upper pole is through the incision, it is necessary to increase the mobility of the lobe itself. This can be achieved by a step-by-step dissection, starting from the areas that are safer (with a minimal risk of creating any morbidity).

With this basic principle in mind, better mobility can be obtained by starting to dissect the lobe from the upper pole and descending toward the isthmus, ultimately dividing it. The critical point of this maneuver, in our experience, is to open the space between the posterior aspect of the upper pedicle (the origin of the ligament of Berry) and the isthmus itself. This area is known among those who perform the MIVAT procedure as the "triangle of Miccoli-Berti," after the surgeons who identified this point as an essential step for the correct extraction of the thyroid lobe (Fig. 6.6). The "triangle" is oriented downward, composed of the posterior aspect of the upper pedicle laterally, the pyramidal lobe medially, and the prethyroidal muscles forming the base. This area can be safely dissected prior to exposing the recurrent nerve and the parathyroid glands once again. It is necessary, once all the elements are identified, to cut the isthmus in a downward direction, completely dividing it and exposing the tracheal surface. The lobe is now free from its superior and medial attachments. The next step is to cut the vessels of the inferior pole, taking care to not damage the vessels supporting the inferior parathyroid gland. Once this step is complete, the lobe can be completely and delicately delivered through the incision. The surgeon can now expose the lateral side of the lobe, following, once again, the previously identified recurrent nerve and both the parathyroid glands in the traditional way.

If a problem is encountered while delivering the lobe (generally because of an underestimation of its size), the surgeon can use these two "tricks" to allow a tension-free extraction avoiding any rupture of the capsule. If there is an evident cystic component, aspirating the liquid with a syringe can significantly decrease the size of the lobe. If there is excessive tension on the strap muscles, these can act "like a curtain," hampering delivery of the lobe. This can often be solved by asking the anesthesiologist to provide a paralyzing agent. This will allow the strap muscles to relax and the entire trachea-larynx-thyroid lobe block to be more easily mobilized.

A total thyroidectomy can be performed by repeating the same steps on the opposite side. If the surgeon has started on the side with the largest lobe, as we always suggest, the opposite lobectomy will typically take less time to complete.

Step 5. Suture of the Access

Once the lobectomy/total thyroidectomy is finished and the hemostasis is carefully obtained, the surgeon should inspect the critical structures on both sides for the last time. The integrity of the recurrent nerve(s) should be verified as well as the viability of the parathyroid glands. When their vitality is uncertain, they should be autotransplanted. No drain is placed in MIVAT cases.

The strap muscles can then be reapproximated with one or two single stitch(es). Three single subcutaneous stitches are used to approach the skin edges. In our institution surgical glue is used to seal the skin.

Outcomes

Since its development, MIVAT has consistently been shown to result in extensive advantages for patients. These results have been exhibited in studies both from the group that developed MIVAT and subsequent groups who have adopted the technique.

The most commonly demonstrated advantages of MIVAT compared with other thyroidectomy techniques are decreased postoperative pain and improved cosmetic outcome. Other significant benefits of the technique include less frequent and less severe dysphonia and dysphagia, shorter recovery periods, and greater overall patient satisfaction with their surgical experience. The rates of complications, including laryngeal nerve injury and hypoparathyroidism, have been demonstrated to be as low as with conventional thyroidectomy.

Conclusion

MIVAT currently represents the most widespread minimally invasive technique for thyroidectomy, for reasons including its reproducibility, excellent clinical and oncological results, and the clear advantages it provides to patients.

Recommended Reading

Bärlehner E, Benhidjeb T. Cervical scarless endoscopic thyroidectomy: axillo-bilateral-breast approach (ABBA). Surg Endosc. 2008;22(1):154–7.

Berti P, Materazzi G, Conte M, Galleri D, Miccoli P. Visualization of the external branch of the superior laryngeal nerve during video-assisted thyroidectomy. J Am Coll Surg. 2002;195(4):573–4.

Cernea CR, Ferraz AR, Nishio S, Dutra Jr A, Hojaij FC, dos Santos LR. Surgical anatomy of the external branch of the superior laryngeal nerve. Head Neck. 1992;14(5):380–3.

Choe JH, Kim SW, Chung KW, Park KS, Han W, Noh DY, Oh SK, Youn YK. Endoscopic thyroidectomy using a new bilateral axillo-breast approach. World J Surg. 2007;31(3):601–6.

Del Rio P, Bezer L, Palladino S, Arcuri MF, Iotti E, Sianesi M. Operative time and postoperative pain following minimally invasive video-assisted parathyroidectomy. G Chir. 2010;31(4):155–8.

Foley CS, Agcaoglu O, Siperstein AE, Berber E. Robotic transaxillary endocrine surgery: a comparison with conventional open technique. Surg Endosc. 2012; 26(8):2259–66.

Gagner M. Endoscopic subtotal parathyroidectomy in patients with primary hyperparathyroidism. Br J Surg. 1996;83(6):875.

Gagner M, Inabnet 3rd WB. Endoscopic thyroidectomy for solitary thyroid nodules. Thyroid. 2001;11(2): 161–3.

Hartl DM, Ferlito A, Silver CE, Takes RP, Stoeckli SJ, Suárez C, Rodrigo JP, Sesterhenn AM, Snyderman CH, Terris DJ, Genden EM, Rinaldo A. Minimally invasive techniques for head and neck malignancies: current indications, outcomes and future directions. Eur Arch Otorhinolaryngol. 2011;268(9):1249–57.

Henry JF. Minimally invasive thyroid and parathyroid surgery is not a question of length of the incision. Langenbecks Arch Surg. 2008;393(5):621–6.

Hüscher CS, Chiodini S, Napolitano C, Recher A. Endoscopic right thyroid lobectomy. Surg Endosc. 1997;11(8):877.

Ikeda Y, Takami H, Sasaki Y, Kan S, Niimi M. Endoscopic neck surgery by the axillary approach. J Am Coll Surg. 2000;191(3):336–40.

Kandil EH, Noureldine SI, Yao L, Slakey DP. Robotic transaxillary thyroidectomy: an examination of the first one hundred cases. J Am Coll Surg. 2012;214(4): 558–64.

Kang SW, Lee SC, Lee SH, Lee KY, Jeong JJ, Lee YS, Nam KH, Chang HS, Chung WY, Park CS. Robotic thyroid surgery using a gasless, transaxillary approach and the da Vinci S system: the operative outcomes of 338 consecutive patients. Surgery. 2009;146(6): 1048–55.

Kim AJ, Liu JC, Ganly I, Kraus DH. Minimally invasive video-assisted thyroidectomy 2.0: expanded indications in a tertiary care cancer center. Head Neck. 2011;33(11):1557–60.

Landry CS, Grubbs EG, Warneke CL, Ormond M, Chua C, Lee JE, Perrier ND. Robot-assisted transaxillary thyroid surgery in the United States: is it comparable to open thyroid lobectomy? Ann Surg Oncol. 2012;19(4):1269–74.

Lee KE, Kim HY, Park WS, Choe JH, Kwon MR, Oh SK, Youn YK. Postauricular and axillary approach endoscopic neck surgery: a new technique. World J Surg. 2009;33(4):767–72.

Lombardi CP, Raffaelli M, Princi P, Lulli P, Rossi ED, Fadda G, Bellantone R. Safety of video-assisted thyroidectomy versus conventional surgery. Head Neck. 2005;27(1):58–64.

Lombardi CP, Raffaelli M, D'Alatri L, Marchese MR, Rigante M, Paludetti G, Bellantone R. Voice and swallowing changes after thyroidectomy in patients without inferior laryngeal nerve injuries. Surgery. 2006a;140(6):1026–32.

Lombardi CP, Raffaelli M, Princi P, De Crea C, Bellantone R. Video-assisted thyroidectomy: report on the experience of a single center in more than four hundred cases. World J Surg. 2006b;30(5):794–800.

Lombardi CP, Raffaelli M, D'alatri L, De Crea C, Marchese MR, Maccora D, Paludetti G, Bellantone R. Video-assisted thyroidectomy significantly reduces the risk of early postthyroidectomy voice and swallowing symptoms. World J Surg. 2008;32(5):693–700.

Lombardi CP, Raffaelli M, De Crea C, D'Alatri L, Maccora D, Marchese MR, Paludetti G, Bellantone R. Long-term outcome of functional post-thyroidectomy voice and swallowing symptoms. Surgery. 2009; 146(6):1174–81.

Lombardi CP, Raffaelli M, De Crea C, Sessa L, Rampulla V, Bellantone R. Video-assisted versus conventional total thyroidectomy and central compartment neck dissection for papillary thyroid carcinoma. World J Surg. 2012;36(6):1225–30.

Mattioli FP, Cagnazzo A, Varaldo E, Bianchi C, Spigno L, Gasparini C. An application of mini-invasive surface surgery: the thyroid. Ann Ital Chir. 1996;67(4):535–6.

Miccoli P, Minuto MN. Minimally invasive thyroidectomy: state of the art. Minerva Chir. 2009;64(6): 545–50.

Miccoli P, Berti P, Conte M, Bendinelli C, Marcocci C. Minimally invasive surgery for thyroid small nodules: preliminary report. J Endocrinol Invest. 1999;22(11): 849–51.

Miccoli P, Berti P, Raffaelli M, Materazzi G, Baldacci S, Rossi G. Comparison between minimally invasive video-assisted thyroidectomy and conventional thyroidectomy: a prospective randomized study. Surgery. 2001;130(6):1039–43.

Miccoli P, Elisei R, Materazzi G, Capezzone M, Galleri D, Pacini F, Berti P, Pinchera A. Minimally invasive video-assisted thyroidectomy for papillary carcinoma: a prospective study of its completeness. Surgery. 2002a;132(6):1070–3.

Miccoli P, Bellantone R, Mourad M, Walz M, Raffaelli M, Berti P. Minimally invasive video-assisted thyroidectomy: multiinstitutional experience. World J Surg. 2002b;26:972–5.

Miccoli P, Berti P, Materazzi G, Minuto M, Barellini L. Minimally invasive video-assisted thyroidectomy: five years of experience. J Am Coll Surg. 2004;199(2): 243–8.

Miccoli P, Barellini L, Monchik JM, Rago R, Berti PF. Randomized clinical trial comparing regional and general anaesthesia in minimally invasive video-assisted parathyroidectomy. Br J Surg. 2005;92(7):814–8.

Miccoli P, Minuto MN, Orlandini C, Galleri D, Massi M, Berti P. Ultrasonography estimated thyroid volume: a prospective study about its reliability. Thyroid. 2006a;16(1):37–9.

Miccoli P, Berti P, Frustaci GL, Ambrosini CE, Materazzi G. Video-assisted thyroidectomy: indications and results. Langenbecks Arch Surg. 2006b;391(2):68–71.

Miccoli P, Elisei R, Donatini G, Materazzi G, Berti P. Video-assisted central compartment lymphadenectomy in a patient with a positive RET oncogene: initial experience. Surg Endosc. 2007;21(1):120–3.

Miccoli P, Pinchera A, Materazzi G, Biagini A, Berti P, Faviana P, Molinaro E, Viola D, Elisei R. Surgical treatment of low- and intermediate-risk papillary thyroid cancer with minimally invasive video-assisted thyroidectomy. J Clin Endocrinol Metab. 2009;94(5):1618–22.

Miccoli P, Rago R, Massi M, Panicucci E, Metelli MR, Berti P, Minuto MN. Standard versus video-assisted thyroidectomy: objective postoperative pain evaluation. Surg Endosc. 2010;24(10):2415–7.

Miccoli P, Minuto MN, Miccoli M. Chapter 1: Incidence of morbidity following thyroid surgery: acceptable morbidity rates. In: Miccoli P, Terris D, Minuto MN, Seybt M, editors. Thyroid surgery: preventing and managing complications. Oxford: Wiley-Blackwell Ed; 2013.

Minuto MN, Berti P, Miccoli M, Ugolini C, Matteucci V, Moretti M, Basolo F, Miccoli P. Minimally invasive video-assisted thyroidectomy: an analysis of results and a revision of indications. Surg Endosc. 2012;26(3):818–22.

Ohgami M, Ishii S, Arisawa Y, Ohmori T, Noga K, Furukawa T, Kitajima M. Scarless endoscopic thyroidectomy: breast approach for better cosmesis. Surg Laparosc Endosc Percutan Tech. 2000;10(1):1–4.

Perigli G, Cortesini C, Qirici E, Boni D, Cianchi F. Clinical benefits of minimally invasive techniques in thyroid surgery. World J Surg. 2008;32(1):45–50.

Perrier ND, Randolph GW, Inabnet WB, Marple BF, VanHeerden J, Kuppersmith RB. Robotic thyroidectomy: a framework for new technology assessment and safe implementation. Thyroid. 2010;20(12):1327–32.

Terris DJ, Chin E. Clinical implementation of endoscopic thyroidectomy in selected patients. Laryngoscope. 2006;116:1745–8.

Terris DJ, Singer MC. Robotic facelift thyroidectomy: facilitating remote access surgery. Head Neck. 2012;34(5):746–7.

Terris DJ, Angelos P, Steward DL, Simental AA. Minimally invasive video-assisted thyroidectomy. A multi-institutional North American experience. Arch Otolaryngol Head Neck Surg. 2008;134(1):81–4.

Total Endoscopic Thyroidectomy: Axillary Approach

7

Yoshifumi Ikeda

Background

Endoscopic surgery reduces the level of surgical invasiveness and results in improved cosmetic outcomes. Consequently, endoscopic surgical techniques are rapidly being applied to thyroid and parathyroid surgery. Endoscopic procedures in the neck region can be classified as either "pure" endoscopic procedures, characterized by a steady gas insufflation with the use of trocars, or video-assisted techniques, which use external retraction instead of gas insufflation to maintain the operative space. Each approach has its own advantages and disadvantages. With the "pure" endoscopic techniques, the cosmetic results are often superior to those of video-assisted gasless techniques because the incision can be small in diameter and be placed remotely from the neck region. Remote access procedures, such as total endoscopic thyroidectomy by the axillary approach, allow for incisions to be placed in less-conspicuous, non-cervical locations.

First performed in 1999, there are several theoretical advantages of endoscopic thyroidectomy by the axillary approach. The thyroid gland is viewed from the lateral aspect in this method. Consequently the superior and inferior poles of thyroid gland can be easily dissected and the perithyroidal fascia can be carefully divided under direct vision. This is critical in avoiding injury to the recurrent laryngeal nerve or the parathyroid glands. In total endoscopic thyroidectomy by the axillary approach, since only the platysmal muscle needs to be displaced, CO_2 insufflation at the pressure of less than 4 mmHg is sufficient. Therefore, the potential complications of gas insufflation, including hypercapnia, respiratory acidosis, air embolus, and subcutaneous emphysema, are avoided.

It should be noted that thyroid lobectomies or subtotal thyroidectomies are possible with this operation. However, due to challenges related to anatomy and current technologies, a true total thyroidectomy cannot be safely performed because visualization of the contralateral recurrent laryngeal nerve is not easily achieved.

Selection Criteria

The indications for total endoscopic thyroidectomy by the axillary approach include the presence of a follicular nodule or adenomatous goiter with a maximum diameter of less than 6 cm. Patients with Graves' disease, with thyroid glands that have a volume less than 100 ml on preoperative evaluation, are also candidates for this approach. In regions in which lobectomy is an accepted practice for low-risk papillary thyroid carcinomas, total endoscopic thyroidectomy by the axillary approach can be performed. For these patients, with well-differentiated thyroid

Y. Ikeda, MD, FACS
Department of Surgery, Teikyo University
School of Medicine, 2-11-1 Kaga, Itabashi-ku,
Tokyo, 173-8605, Japan
e-mail: yikeda@med.teikyo-u.ac.jp

D.J. Terris, M.C. Singer (eds.), *Minimally Invasive and Robotic Thyroid and Parathyroid Surgery*,
DOI 10.1007/978-1-4614-9011-1_7, © Springer Science+Business Media New York 2014

carcinomas, this approach is an option when tumor size does not exceed 15 mm, there is no evidence of lateral lymph node metastasis, and there are no findings suggestive of possible local invasion.

Procedural Details

The patient is placed in the supine position on the operating table. After intubation, the neck is slightly extended. The arm on the side of the surgery is raised and the axilla is completely exposed. A 30-mm skin incision is made in the axilla. The incision is placed such that the scar in the axilla should be completely covered by the patient's arm when held in a neutral position. The deep layer of the platysma muscle is then exposed through the upper portion of the pectoralis major muscle. This dissection under the skin is performed using Kelly forceps and PDB™ Balloons (Tyco Healthcare, Mansfield, CT, USA). After the pocket is created, two 5-mm trocars are inserted through the skin incision, and a purse-string suture is placed to prevent the insufflation gas from leaking and the trocars from slipping out of the wound. Carbon dioxide is then insufflated up to 4 mmHg, and a flexible laparoscope (Olympus Corporation, Tokyo, Japan) is inserted through the trocar. After adequate space is created, one more 5-mm trocar is placed several centimeters caudal to the 30-mm skin incision in the axilla (Fig. 7.1). Additional blunt and sharp dissection, achieved with endoscopic scissors, is performed to enlarge the subplatysmal space. The anterior border of the sternocleidomastoid muscle is then separated from the sternohyoid muscle and a space is created between the sternothyroid muscle and the sternohyoid muscle (Fig. 7.2). By dividing the sternothyroid muscle with a Harmonic scalpel, the thyroid gland is exposed (Johnson-Johnson Medical, Cincinnati, OH, USA).

The upper pole of the thyroid gland can then be bluntly dissected and grasped. The superior thyroid artery and vein can then be identified. The superior pole vessels are then dissected away from the larynx medially to avoid injuring the external branch of the superior laryngeal nerve (Fig. 7.3). These vessels are then ligated with the Harmonic device. If the external branch of the nerve is identified close to the superior thyroid artery, the artery should be ligated with clips and then divided to avoid injuring the nerve. The lower pole of the gland is then grasped and retracted in a cephalad direction. This exposes the adipose tissue and cervical thymic tissue inferior to the thyroid gland, which can then be dissected and divided. Care should be taken to avoid injuring the inferior parathyroid gland, which often rests in this area. Allowing it to fall inferiorly with the surrounding adipose and thymic tissue can preserve the parathyroid gland.

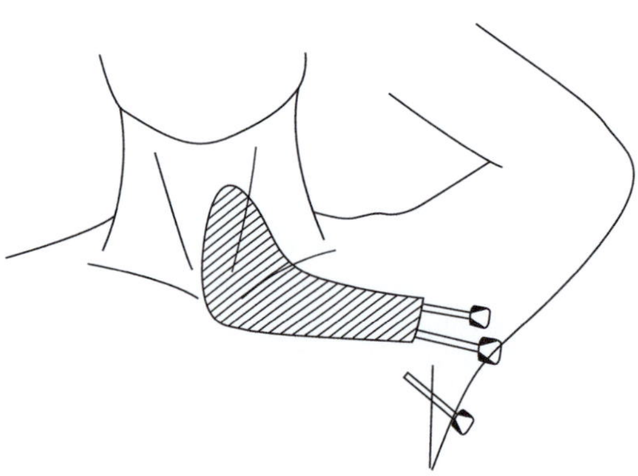

Fig. 7.1 Two trocars, one 12 mm and one 5 mm, are inserted through the 30-mm skin incision in the axilla. A second 5-mm trocar is then inserted just inferior to the incision

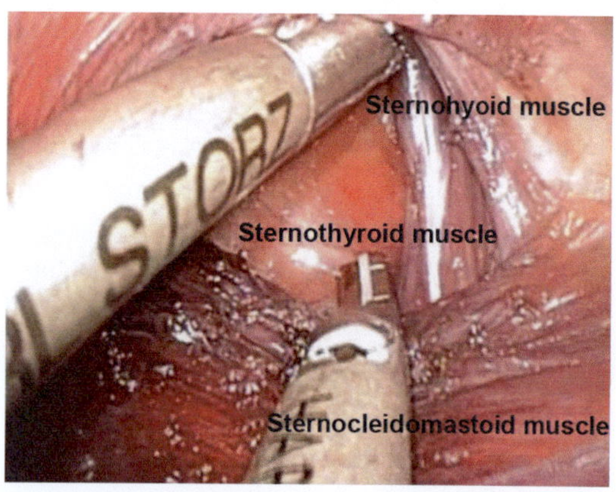

Fig. 7.2 The anterior border of the sternocleidomastoid muscle is separated from the sternohyoid muscle, and a space is created between the sternothyroid muscle and the sternohyoid muscle

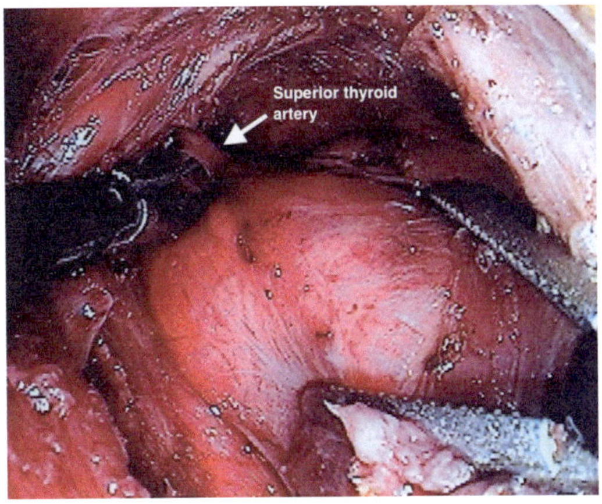

Fig. 7.3 The superior thyroid artery and vein are dissected to avoid injuring the external branch of the superior laryngeal nerve

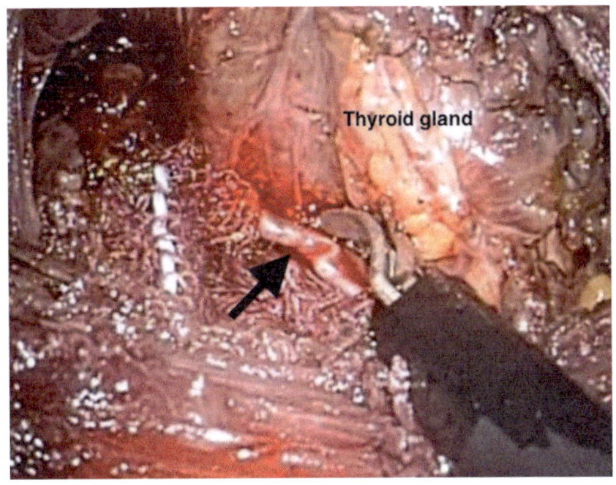

Fig. 7.5 The lateral view of the thyroid gland from the axillary port helped to ensure complete preservation and exposure of the nerve. The thyroid lobe is retracted medially. The *arrow* indicates the recurrent laryngeal nerve

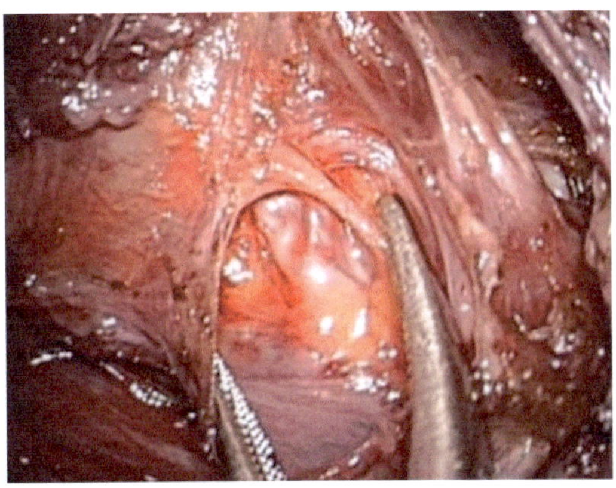

Fig. 7.4 The recurrent laryngeal nerve can usually be located between the trachea and the carotid artery. A right-sided nerve is shown

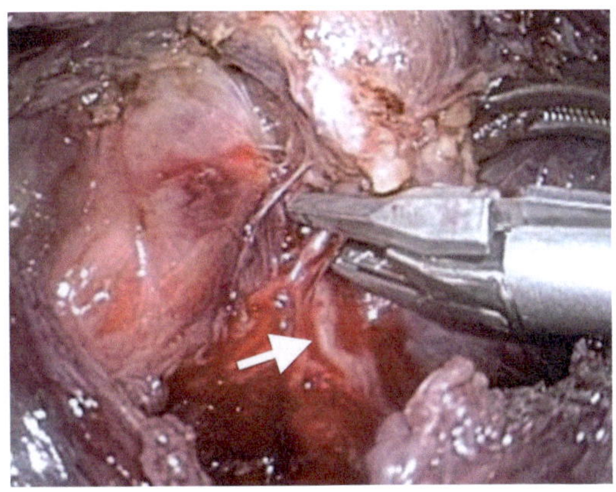

Fig. 7.6 When there is not adequate space to use the Harmonic scalpel to divide Berry's ligament because of concern about thermal injury, the ligament can be cut using endoscopic clips. A right thyroid lobe is retracted medially. The recurrent laryngeal nerve, marked by the *arrow*, is seen coursing distally

After releasing the inferior aspect of the gland, it is then retracted medially, and the perithyroidal fascia is incised using endoscopic scissors. In doing so, care must be taken to avoid injuring the recurrent nerve. The recurrent laryngeal nerve can usually be identified between the trachea and the carotid artery (Fig. 7.4), often in close proximity to the inferior thyroid artery. In this procedure, the lateral view from the axillary port helps to ensure complete visualization of the nerve (Fig. 7.5). After the nerve is clearly exposed, the inferior thyroid artery can be divided. The remaining attachments of the gland to Berry's ligament can then be dissected and divided with careful manipulation of the endoscopic scissors and the dissector. Berry's ligament then needs to be transected in order to complete the release of the thyroid gland from the trachea. To prevent thermal injury when using the dissector, great care is taken to maintain a distance of at least 5 mm from the major neurovascular structures and the trachea. When there is not adequate space to use the Harmonic device to manage Berry's ligament, endoscopic clips are placed across the ligament before it is divided (Fig. 7.6). Some patients are anxious about having clips left in the neck. In these patients, the clips are removed after tightening with a ligating loop just under the clip. During the course of this dissection, the superior

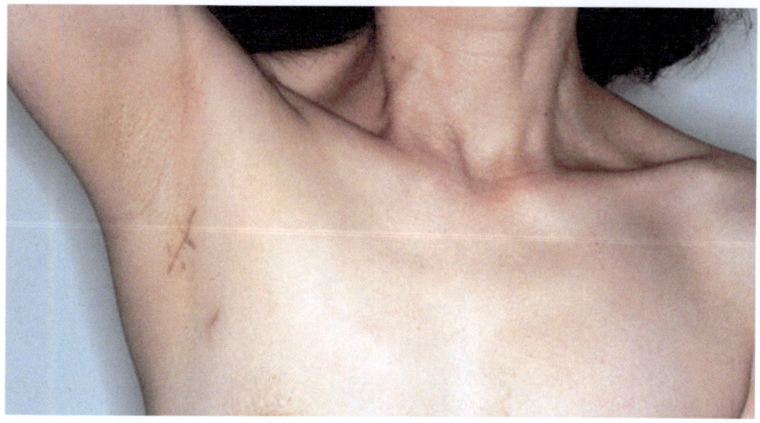

Fig. 7.7 The resulting scar typical of this approach is shown

parathyroid gland is typically identified and preserved. After the thyroid gland is freed from the trachea, the isthmus is divided using the Harmonic device. Complete hemostasis is then assured.

In patients who require a subtotal thyroidectomy, such as those with Graves' disease, the approach is slightly altered. When developing the working space prior to dissection of the thyroid gland, dissection of the operative pocket is extended to the level of the thyroid cartilage superiorly and to the medial border of the contralateral sternocleidomastoid muscle. After this is accomplished, the strap muscles are transversely divided along the width of the gland. While the contralateral recurrent laryngeal nerve can be identified from this approach, it cannot be fully dissected along its course.

Before completing the operation, a 3-mm closed suction drain is placed under the platysma muscle and brought out through the site of the most inferior 5-mm trocar in the axilla. The wound is then closed with 3-0 absorbable sutures. A 4-0 absorbable monofilament suture is then used to tightly suture the subcutaneous skin. Steri-Strips are then placed over the wound. The drain is removed 2 days after surgery.

Outcomes

Between August 1999 and July 2012, 244 patients underwent endoscopic thyroidectomy by the axillary approach. Of these patients, 194 underwent hemithyroidectomy for a thyroid nodule, 22 underwent subtotal thyroidectomy for Graves' disease, and 28 underwent hemithyroidectomy with ipsilateral central nodes dissection for thyroid papillary carcinoma. Average operative times were between 2 and 3 h and the need to convert to an open procedure occurred rarely. Rates of postoperative bleeding and laryngeal nerve dysfunction were similar to those of conventional thyroidectomy techniques. Of note, no complications related to gas insufflation occurred.

The cosmetic results have been excellent (Fig. 7.7), and patients report experiencing only minimal pain, hypesthesia, or paresthesia in the neck or chest.

Conclusion

As with many of the other remote access techniques, the indications for pure endoscopic thyroidectomy by the axillary approach are still limited. Nonetheless, in selected patients, it seems a valid option for thyroidectomy.

Recommended Reading

Amaral JF. The experimental development of an ultrasonically activated scalpel for laparoscopic use. Surg Laparosc Endosc. 1994;4:92–9.

Gagner M. Endoscopic subtotal parathyroidectomy in patients with primary hyperparathyroidism. Br J Surg. 1996;83:875.

Hüscher CS, Chiodini S, Napolitano C, Recher A. Endoscopic right thyroid lobectomy. Surg Endosc. 1997;11:877.

Ikeda Y, Takami H, Sasaki Y, Kan S, Niimi M. Endoscopic neck surgery by the axillary approach. J Am Coll Surg. 2000;191:336–40.

Ikeda Y, Takami H, Niimi M, Kan S, Sasaki Y, Takayama J. Endoscopic thyroidectomy by the axillary approach. Surg Endosc. 2001;15:1362–4.

Ikeda Y, Takami H, Sasaki Y, Takayama J, Niimi M, Kan S. Clinical benefits in endoscopic thyroidectomy by the axillary approach. J Am Coll Surg. 2003;196(2): 189–95.

Ikeda Y, Takami H, Sasaki Y, Takayama J, Kurihara H. Are there significant benefits of minimally invasive endoscopic thyroidectomy? World J Surg. 2004; 28(11):1075–8.

Maeda S, Uga T, Hayashida N, Ishigaki K, Furui J, Kanematsu T. Video-assisted subtotal or near-total thyroidectomy for Graves' disease. Br J Surg. 2006; 93(1):61–6.

Miccoli P, Berti P, Conte M, Raffaelli M, Materazzi G. Minimally invasive video-assisted parathyroidectomy: lesson learned from 137 cases. J Am Coll Surg. 2000;191:613–8.

Miccoli P, Berti P, Raffaelli M, Conte M, Materazzi G, Galleri D. Minimally invasive video-assisted thyroidectomy. Am J Surg. 2001;181:567–70.

Ohgami M, Ishii S, Arisawa Y, Ohmori T, Noga K, Furukawa T, Kitajima M. Scarless endoscopic thyroidectomy: breast approach for better cosmesis. Surg Laparosc Endosc Percutan Tech. 2000;10:1–4.

Sasaki A, Nakajima J, Ikeda K, Otsuka K, Koeda K, Wakabayashi G. Endoscopic thyroidectomy by the breast approach: a single institution's 9-year experience. World J Surg. 2008;32(3):381–5.

Shimizu K, Akira S, Jasmi AY, Kitamura Y, Kitagawa W, Akasu H, Tanaka S. Video-Assisted neck surgery: endoscopic resection of thyroid tumors with a very minimal neck wound. J Am Coll Surg. 1999;188: 697–703.

Yamamoto M, Sasaki A, Asahi H, Shimada Y, Sato N, Nakajima J, Mashima R, Saito K. Endoscopic subtotal thyroidectomy for patients with Graves' disease. Surg Today. 2001;31(1):1–4.

Yeung GH. Endoscopic surgery of the neck: a new frontier. Surg Laparosc Endosc. 1998;8:227–32.

8 Bilateral Axillo-breast Approach (BABA) Endoscopic and Robotic Thyroid Surgery

Kyu Eun Lee and June Young Choi

Introduction

Since the introduction of endoscopic thyroid surgery in the late 1990s, numerous remote access thyroidectomy techniques have been reported, including those using cervical, axillary, breast, and anterior chest approaches. One of the most widely adopted is the bilateral axillo-breast approach (BABA), performed either endoscopically or with robotic assistance.

Background

BABA endoscopic thyroid surgery was developed at Seoul National University Hospital in 2004. The introduction of BABA robotic thyroidectomy in 2008 expanded the indications for this procedure.

The advantages of endoscopic or BABA robotic thyroidectomy include the following: (1) after exposure is obtained, the view and orientation to the thyroid and surrounding structures are similar to that of conventional thyroidectomy; (2) this exposure provides a symmetrical view of the thyroid gland and the major critical structures during the operation; (3) there is no interference between instruments during the procedure; and (4) excellent cosmetic results are obtained with no visible cervical scar.

Selection Criteria

Since its introduction in 2004, BABA endoscopic thyroidectomy has been consistently performed on patients with benign thyroid nodules less than 5 cm, fine-needle aspiration biopsies results suspicious for follicular neoplasm or Hurthle cell neoplasm, and patients in whom diagnostic lobectomy revealed a well-differentiated thyroid carcinoma and now require completion thyroidectomy.

Absolute contraindications for BABA include patients with previous open neck surgery, aggressive thyroid malignancies (medullary thyroid cancer, advanced papillary or follicular thyroid cancer, and poorly differentiated thyroid cancer), patients with a history of breast malignancy, and patients with substernal goiters. Other patients who should be approached hesitantly are men, those with Graves' disease, and those with well-differentiated thyroid carcinoma over 1 cm in diameter.

Procedural Details

The patient is placed in the supine position on the operating table with a pillow under the shoulders. The patient's neck is then extended to expose the surgical area properly. In order to expose both

K.E. Lee, PhD • J.Y. Choi (✉)
Department of Surgery, Seoul National University Hospital, Seoul 110-799, Republic of Korea
e-mail: aznagran@gmail.com

D.J. Terris, M.C. Singer (eds.), *Minimally Invasive and Robotic Thyroid and Parathyroid Surgery*, DOI 10.1007/978-1-4614-9011-1_8, © Springer Science+Business Media New York 2014

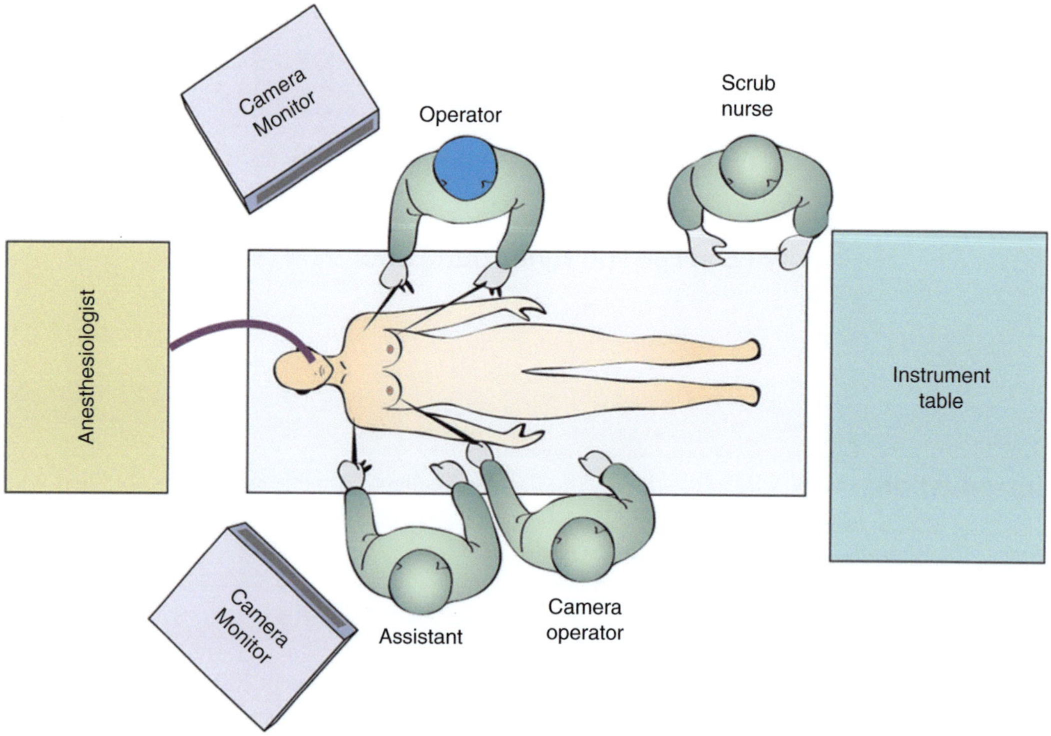

Fig. 8.1 Schematic depiction of the operating room setup for a BABA endoscopic right hemithyroidectomy

axillae, the arms should be abducted. Routine skin preparation is done with a standard antiseptic solution.

For room setup, the primary surgeon stands on the side contralateral to the side of the thyroid requiring surgery. The first assistant and camera operator stand across from the primary surgeon (Fig. 8.1).

After skin preparation, the surgeon marks the midline, the major anatomical landmarks (including the thyroid and cricoid cartilage, sternocleidomastoid muscles, clavicles, and suprasternal notch), and finally the different proposed incisions (Fig. 8.2). A 12-mm incision is marked in the axilla ipsilateral to the side of the thyroid pathology and a 5-mm incision is placed in the contralateral axilla. Symmetrical, 5-mm incisions are placed in the superomedial margins of the areolas.

A 1:200,000 epinephrine solution is then injected in the working area deep to the platysma muscle in the neck and the subcutaneous tissues on the anterior chest (Fig. 8.3a). In the neck area, a "pinch and raise" maneuver of the skin helps the injection of saline distribute into the subplatysmal space (Fig. 8.3b). This "hydrodissection" technique results in the formation of a saline pocket in the subplatysmal space, which can decrease bleeding in the flaps and makes the dissection easier.

After incisions are made in both axillae, blunt dissection is performed with a straight mosquito clamp and a vascular tunneler to elevate the flaps. The 12-mm incision is used to extract the specimen later in the case. After blunt dissection, the ports are inserted through the incisions. The working space is maintained with CO_2 gas insufflation at the pressure of 5–6 mmHg. Visualization is achieved with a 30° endoscope.

The next phase of the surgery requires sharp dissection which is achieved using a Harmonic device. The dissection should start in the infraclavicular area (Fig. 8.4). When this dissection is completed, the two 5-mm incisions in the superomedial margins of the areola of the breasts are made. The myocutaneous flap is then extended more cephalad, up to the thyroid cartilage.

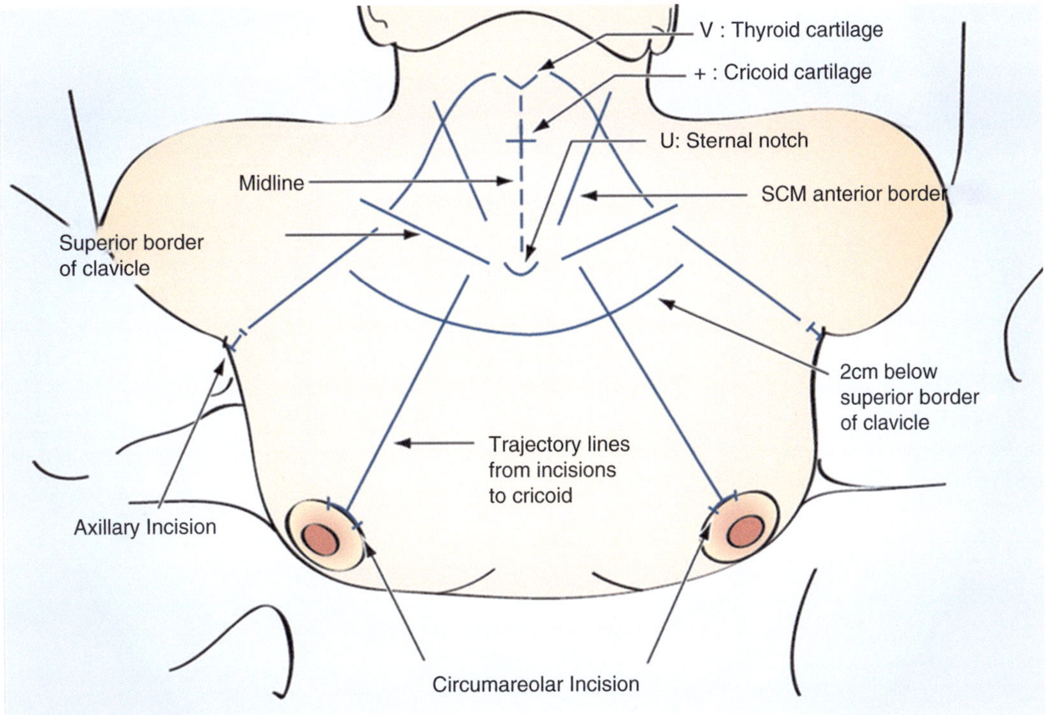

Fig. 8.2 Shown are the marks that should be made to prior to making the incisions

With the endoscope, the strap muscles and midline raphe can be well visualized. The midline is then divided with electrocautery from the thyroid cartilage to the suprasternal notch, exposing the isthmus of the thyroid gland (Fig. 8.5a, b). The thyroid isthmus is then divided in the midline using the Harmonic device. Prior to isthmectomy, the absence of isthmus lesions should be verified.

While the thyroid gland is retracted medially with an endo-clinch, the strap muscles should be retracted laterally with the forceps. Dissection is carried down to the deep aspect of the gland to expose its lateral surface. With a snake retractor drawing the strap muscles farther laterally (Fig. 8.6), additional lateral dissection can be accomplished. In order to expose the lateral part of the thyroid gland for dissection, the gland can be medially retracted with a "switching motion" of the instruments (Fig. 8.7). The middle thyroid vein is identified and divided during this stage of the procedure.

Before the inferior thyroid artery enters the thyroid glands, it passes directly under or over the recurrent laryngeal nerve. The inferior thyroid artery can thus be used as a guide to finding the recurrent laryngeal nerve. If the nerve cannot be exposed immediately, further dissection is needed of the loose fibrous tissue at the point of the artery near the tracheal esophageal groove. After the nerve is identified, it is traced from the area of the tubercle of Zuckerkandl to the ligament of Berry.

The inferior parathyroid gland can often be identified in this area. It is generally located near the branching point of the inferior thyroid artery. The gland is preserved by dissecting the gland in an inferior direction, maintaining the vascular pedicle. If the parathyroid gland cannot be preserved, reimplantation should be performed. The pectoralis major muscle serves as excellent option for reimplantation in BABA thyroidectomy.

Attention is then turned to the superior pole of the thyroid gland. Using Maryland forceps to retract the strap muscles laterally, the upper pole of the gland is dissected with the harmonic device. It is important to preserve the fascia of

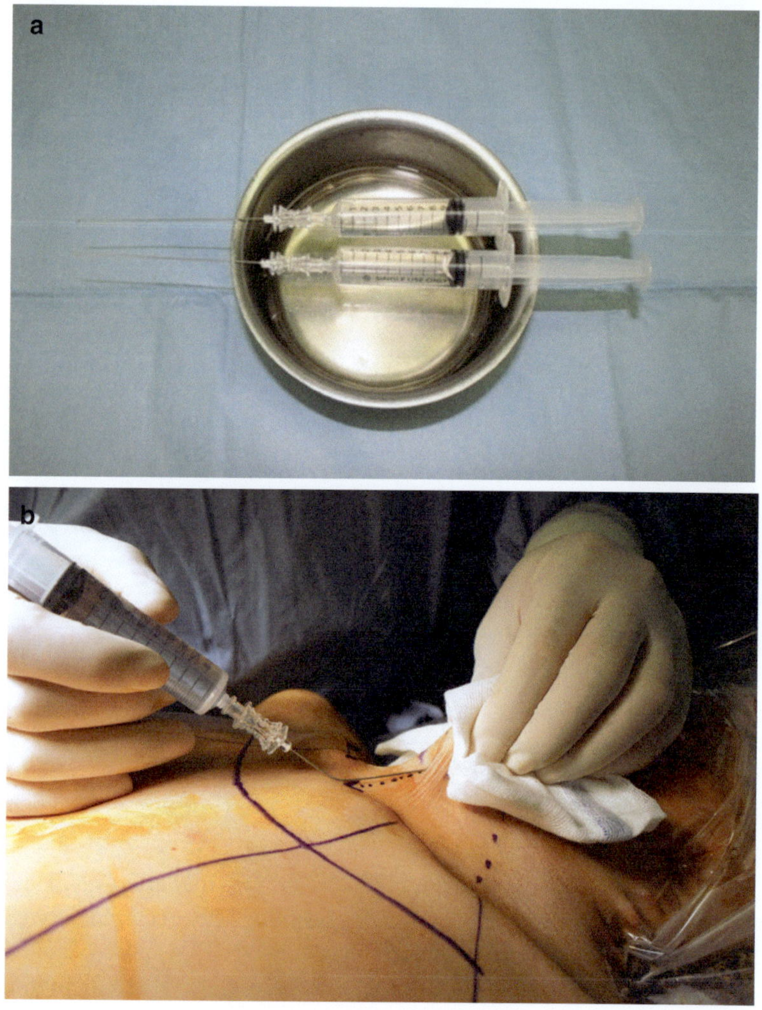

Fig. 8.3 (**a**) Saline injection preparation. (**b**) The "pinch and raise" maneuver facilitates injection into the subplatysmal plane

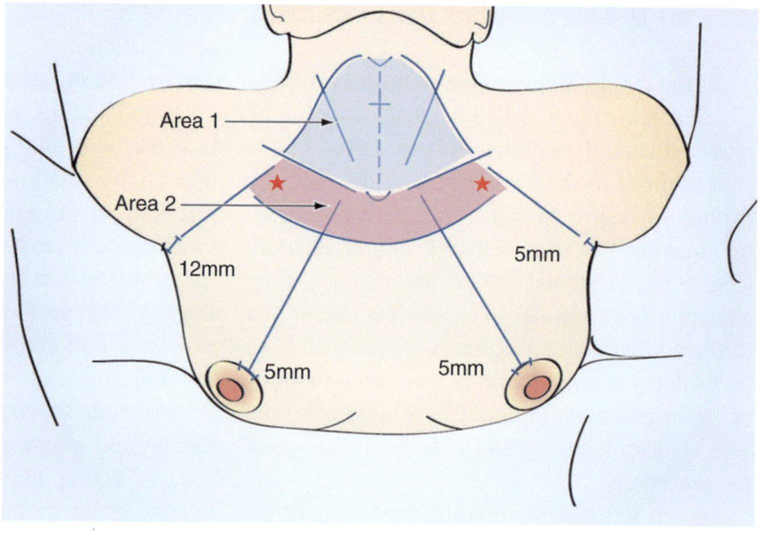

Fig. 8.4 Sharp dissection is used to elevate the flap through area 2 (marked by ★). The areolar incisions are then made and the flap is extended through area 1

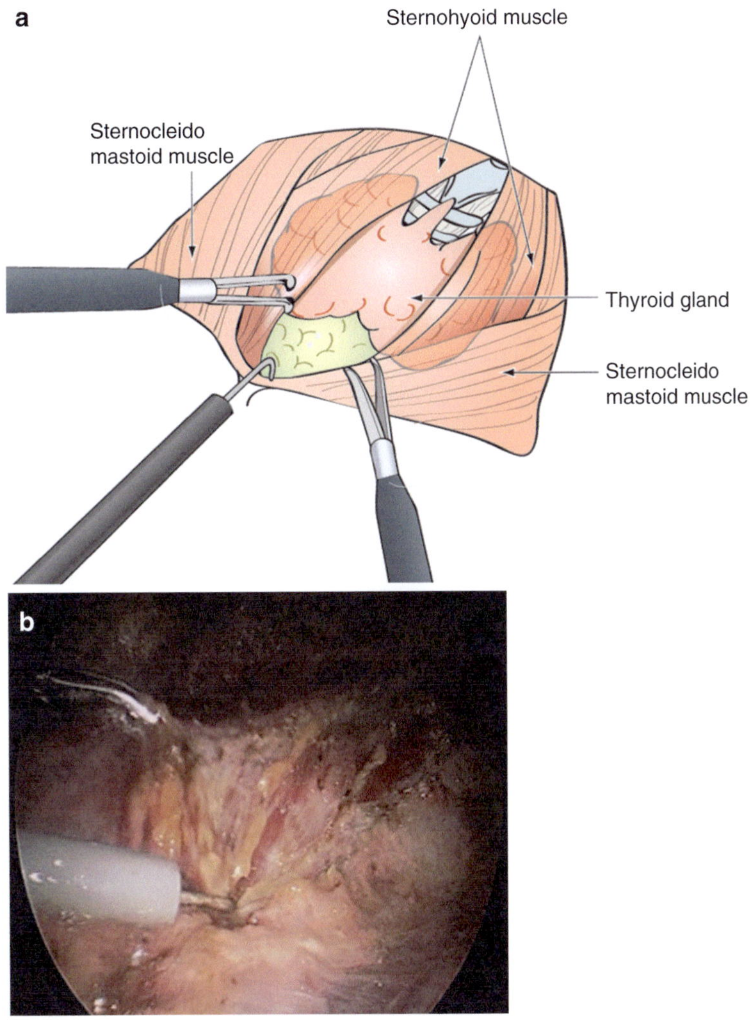

Fig. 8.5 (**a**) After flap development the midline raphe of the strap muscles is divided from the thyroid cartilage to the sternal notch. This exposes the thyroid isthmus. (**b**) The operative view

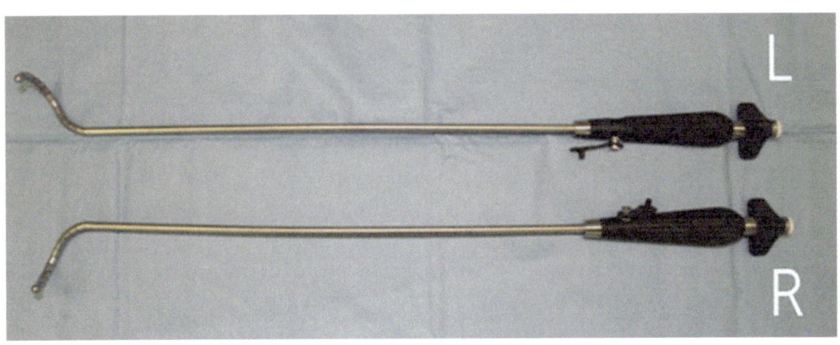

Fig. 8.6 Snake retractors used to retract the strap muscles laterally

the cricothyroid muscles, because the external branch of the superior laryngeal nerve is closely associated with it. The terminal branches of the superior thyroidal artery and vein are identified and carefully ligated with the harmonic shears. The branch that serves as the vascular supply to the superior parathyroid gland should be preserved (Fig. 8.8).

After dissecting the thyroid gland away from the trachea, the specimen is wrapped with a

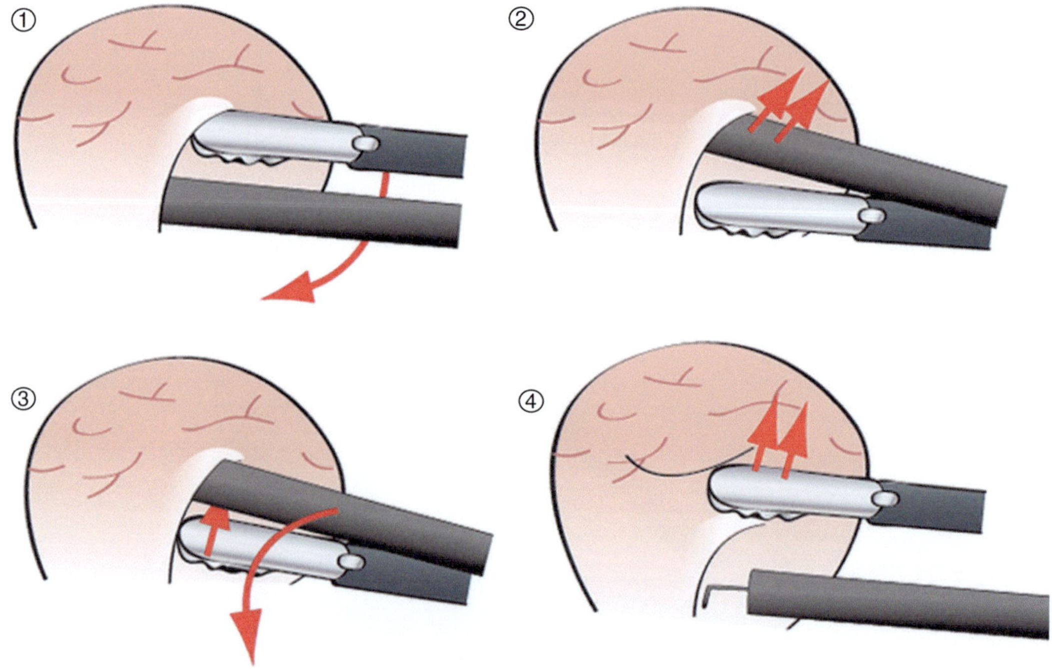

Fig. 8.7 A switching movement with the instruments can be used to draw the thyroid gland medially in order to expose its lateral aspect. *1–4* steps of the procedures (timeline)

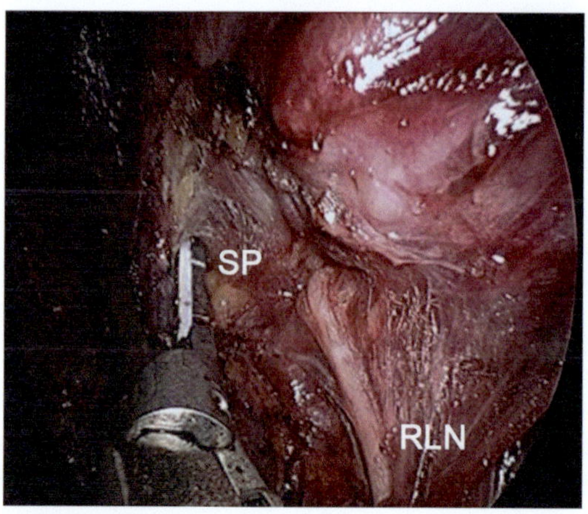

Fig. 8.8 With the right lobe of the thyroid gland retracted medially, the recurrent laryngeal nerve (*RLN*) is seen after its dissection. The superior parathyroid gland (*SP*) is deep to the nerve

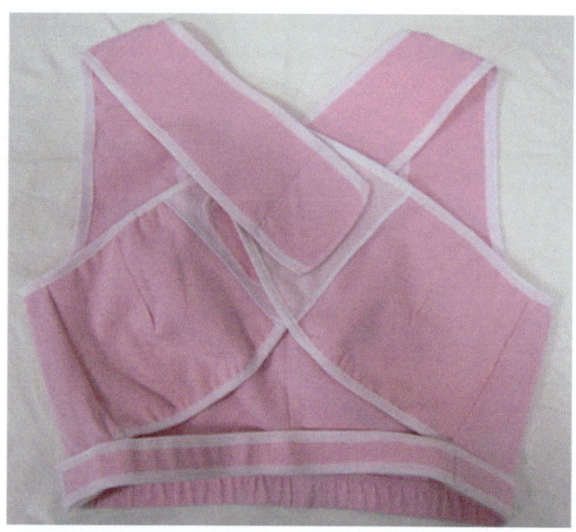

Fig. 8.9 The robo-bra helps with healing postoperatively

plastic bag and removed via the 12-mm axillary port. The specimen is inspected with care to identify any excised parathyroid gland. After meticulous hemostasis is achieved with electrocautery, the right and left strap muscles are reapproximated in the midline. One Jackson-Pratt (JP) drain is placed into the thyroid pocket via an axillary port. The skin of the breasts and axillae are sutured with buried stitches with absorbable sutures.

Finally the anterior chest is compressed with a robo-bra, which applies gentle pressure over the anterior chest flap, aiding healing and providing improved patient comfort (Fig. 8.9).

The patient is admitted for 3 days after the operation. In our institution, this is the same as patients undergoing open thyroid surgery.

The drain is removed on the day of discharge. Patients are asked to wear the robo-bra for 2 weeks after the operation.

Outcomes

Results with endoscopic BABA have been excellent. Patients undergoing endoscopic BABA thyroidectomy may experience higher rates of temporary hypocalcemia and transient vocal cord palsy, compared with patients undergoing open thyroidectomy. However, permanent complication rates are the same.

In regard to cosmetic results, patients have a very high level of satisfaction. Both the axillary and areolar incisions heal well and are typically well hidden.

BABA Robotic Thyroidectomy

Background

The surgical robot provides a number of powerful qualities that makes it an excellent tool for remote access surgeries, such as BABA, which require precise movements in deep and narrow operative fields. These assets include its flexible movements, 3-dimensional visualization, and tremor reduction ability. Starting in 2008 the robot was incorporated into BABA surgery.

The robot can make thyroid surgery more efficient, effective, and comfortable, especially dissecting the central neck compartment. In our institution, central neck dissection is performed in almost all patients with papillary thyroid carcinoma. BABA robotic thyroidectomy is thus particularly well suited for patients with papillary carcinoma.

Selection Criteria

With incorporation of the robot into the procedure, the indications for BABA have widened. In addition to the indications described earlier for endoscopic BABA, BABA robotic can be performed on patients with well-differentiated thyroid carcinomas less than 2 cm, patients with Graves' disease, male patients, and patients with benign nodules up to 8 cm in diameter. Prior to the introduction of the robot, men were not typically good BABA candidates due to the prominence of the clavicle and the absence of significant breast tissue (which limits the range and flexibility of the instruments).

Absolute contraindications for BABA robotic thyroidectomy are the same as for endoscopic BABA. Thyroid nodules over 8 cm can be challenging to remove with this technique. With BABA robotic thyroidectomy, lateral neck dissection can be effectively performed, so patients with suspicious lateral neck nodal disease remain eligible for this approach. Also, previous breast surgery for breast cancer or breast augmentation is not considered a contraindication.

Procedural Details

Many details of BABA robotic thyroidectomy are the same as with the endoscopic approach. The initial positioning, preparation of the patient, markings, and injections are identical in both techniques.

One element that is different from BABA endoscopic thyroidectomy is the length of incisions. For the robotic technique, the incision on the right areola is 12 mm, in order to accommodate the robotic camera. The two axillary incisions in BABA robotic are only 8 mm, through which are placed 8-mm ports (Fig. 8.10).

After flap elevation is completed in the same manner as in endoscopic BABA, the robot is docked from left shoulder of the patient. The anesthesiologist and the ventilator are placed on the right side of the patient. The head of the patient is positioned towards the robotic system and its center column is aligned with the camera port (12-mm port) of the right breast. After docking, the robotic arms are deployed through the axillary ports (Fig. 8.11).

The midline is divided and the isthmus transected in the same manner as endoscopic BABA. The thyroid gland is then retracted medially with ProGrasp forceps, and the strap muscles are retracted laterally with a Maryland forceps.

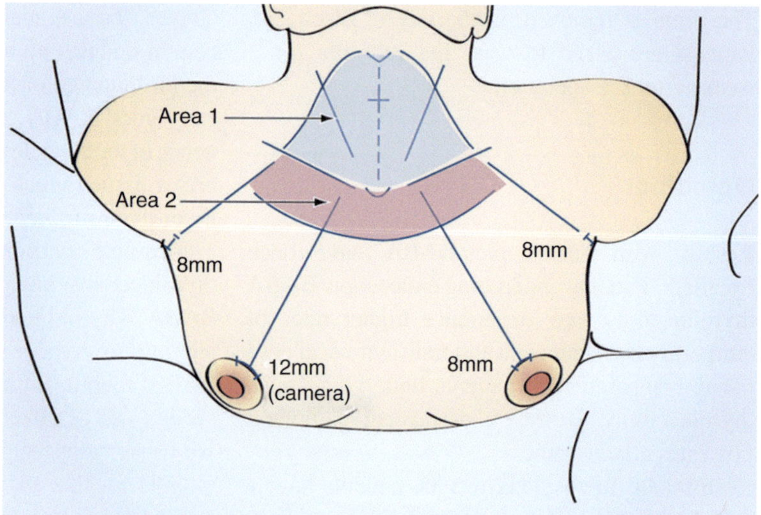

Fig. 8.10 The marks and incisions for BABA robotic thyroidectomy

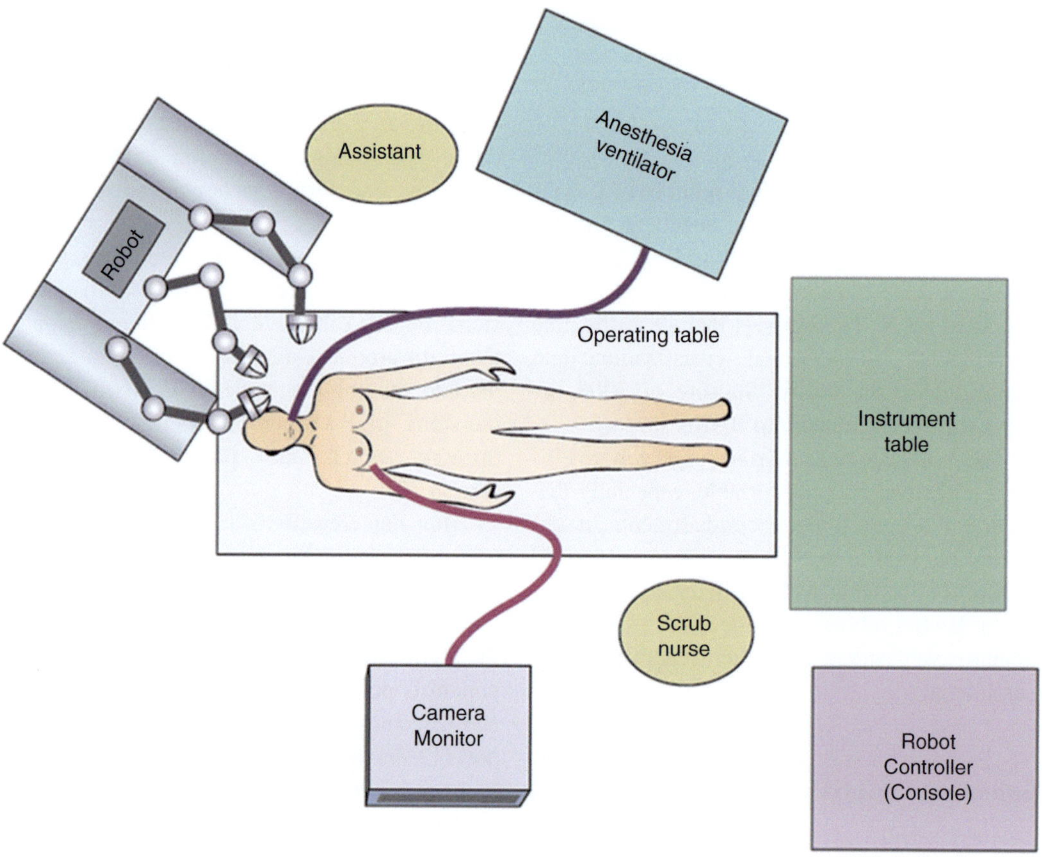

Fig. 8.11 Schematic layout of the operating room for BABA robotic thyroidectomy

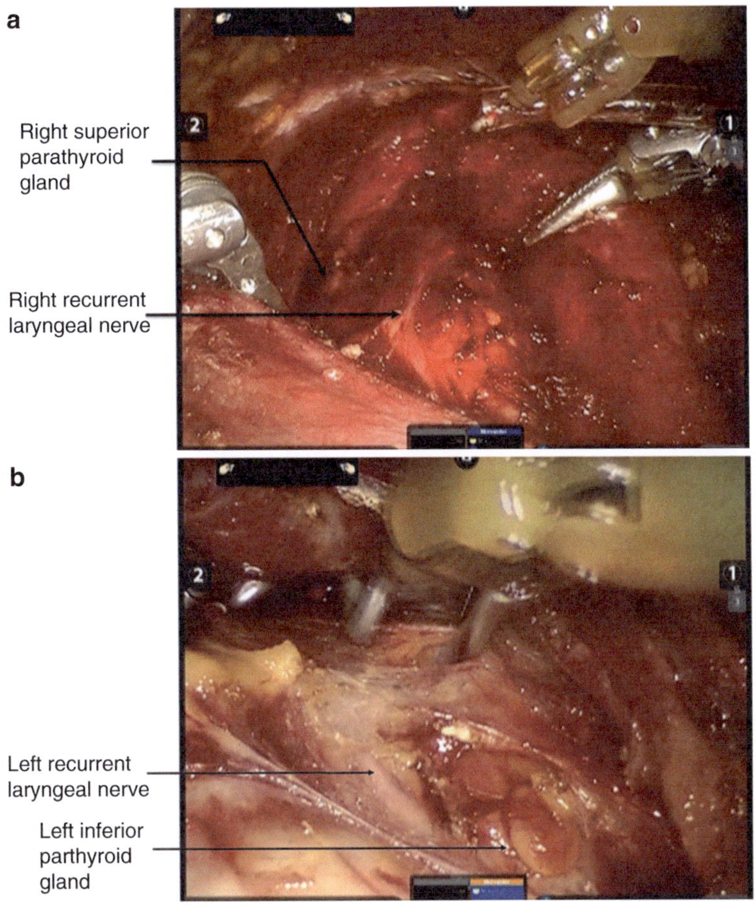

Fig. 8.12 (**a**) The results of a total thyroidectomy after exision of the gland are demonstrated. The right operative field. (**b**) The left side

In order to expose the lateral aspect of the gland, using a switching motion the instruments can retract the thyroid gland medially. The inferior parathyroid gland and recurrent laryngeal nerve are identified with dissection using the Maryland forceps. The harmonic shears, deployed through the left breast port, are used to retract the strap muscles at this moment. The dissection is continued cephalad to the point of the nerve entering underneath the inferior constrictor muscle.

After the inferior thyroid artery is divided, attention is turned to the superior aspect of the gland. With the Maryland forceps drawing the upper part of the strap muscles laterally, the thyroid upper pole is dissected with the harmonic shears. After the superior pedicle is divided, the thyroid gland is dissected away from the trachea. The specimen is then removed in the same fashion as endoscopic BABA, through the left axillary port. If the incision of the left axilla is not long enough to extract the specimen, the incision may be widened posteriorly.

Contralateral surgery can be completed in a similar fashion (Fig. 8.12a, b). Ipsilateral central neck dissection can also be performed if needed.

After achieving hemostasis, the strap muscles are sutured together with a continuous running suture. If a total thyroidectomy is performed, drains are placed into both thyroid pockets via the axillary incisions. The skin incisions are closed with buried stitches with an absorbable suture. Postoperative care is the same as with endoscopic BABA.

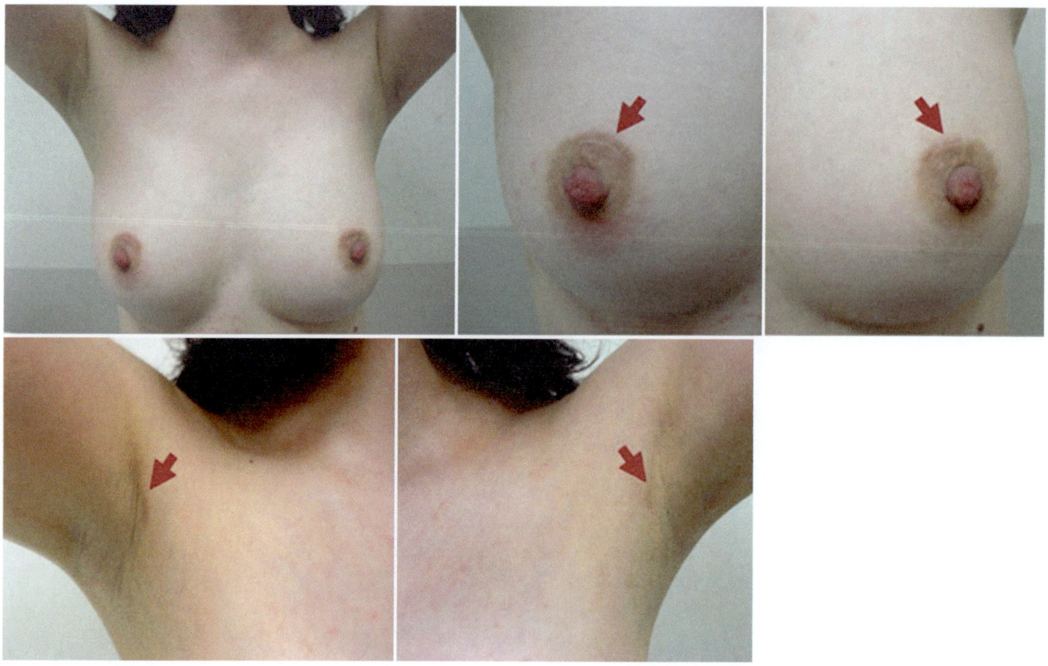

Fig. 8.13 Postoperative cosmetic results are shown. Incisions of BABA robotic surgery (*arrows*)

Outcomes

Results with BABA robotic have been excellent (Fig. 8.13). As with patients undergoing endoscopic BABA thyroidectomy, the rates of temporary hypocalcemia and transient vocal cord palsy are higher than with conventional thyroidectomy. However, permanent complication rates are the same as with open thyroidectomy. Studies have shown that for patients with low-risk thyroid malignancies, BABA robotic thyroidectomy provides excellent surgical results.

Conclusions

The BABA technique has been shown to be a safe and effective method for patients with a range of thyroid disorders. For patients interested in avoiding a cervical incision, BABA is an ideal option.

Recommended Reading

Brunt LM, Jones DB, Wu JS, Quasebarth MA, Meininger T, Soper NJ. Experimental development of an endoscopic approach to neck exploration and parathyroidectomy. Surgery. 1997;122:893–901.

Choe JH, Kim SW, Chung KW, Park KS, et al. Endoscopic thyroidectomy using a new bilateral axillo-breast approach. World J Surg. 2007;31:601–6.

Choi JY, Lee KE, Chung KW, et al. Endoscopic thyroidectomy via bilateral axillo-breast approach (BABA): review of 512 cases in a single institute. Surg Endosc. 2012;26(4):948–55.

Chung YS, Choe JH, Kang KH, Kim SW, et al. Endoscopic thyroidectomy for thyroid malignancies: comparison with conventional open thyroidectomy. World J Surg. 2007;31:2302–6.

Gagner M. Endoscopic subtotal parathyroidectomy in patients with primary hyperparathyroidism. Br J Surg. 1996;83:875.

Huscher CS, Chiodini S, Napolitano C, Recher A. Endoscopic right thyroid lobectomy. Surg Endosc. 1997;11:877.

Kim SJ, Lee KE, Choe JH, Lee J, et al. Endoscopic completion thyroidectomy by the bilateral axillo-breast approach. Surg Laparosc Endosc Percutan Tech. 2010; 20:312–6.

Lee KE, Rao J, Youn YK. Endoscopic thyroidectomy with the da Vinci robot system using the bilateral axillary breast approach (BABA) technique: our initial experience. Surg Laparosc Endosc Percutan Tech. 2009;19:e71–5.

Lee KE, Koo do H, Kim SJ, Lee J, et al. Outcomes of 109 patients with papillary thyroid carcinoma who underwent robotic total thyroidectomy with central node dissection via the bilateral axillo-breast approach. Surgery. 2010;148:1207–13.

Lee KE, Koo DH, Im HJ, et al. Surgical completeness of bilateral axillo-breast approach robotic thyroidectomy: Comparison with conventional open thyroidectomy after propensity score matching. Surgery. 2011a;150:1266–74.

Lee KE, Choi JY, Youn YK. Bilateral axillo-breast approach robotic thyroidectomy. Surg Laparosc Endosc Percutan Tech. 2011b;21:230–6.

Yeung GH. Endoscopic thyroid surgery today: a diversity of surgical strategies. Thyroid. 2002;12:703–6.

9 Robot-Assisted Transaxillary Thyroidectomy

Sohee Lee and Woong Youn Chung

Introduction

Since Theodor Kocher transformed thyroid surgery into a safe and reliable procedure, open thyroidectomy has been considered the standard operative approach to the thyroid gland. However, due to increased interest in patient quality of life during recent decades, there has been a need for advanced surgical techniques that minimize the unattractive, conspicuous scar in the neck area that results from a thyroidectomy. Accordingly, various endoscopic techniques have been developed using smaller cervical or remote access incisions.

In 2001 we introduced the gasless, endoscopic transaxillary thyroidectomy approach. Through 2007 more than 650 of these cases have been performed successfully. However, an endoscopic thyroidectomy has some limitations in obtaining adequate visualization. Additionally, precise, meticulous manipulation of the surgical tissues can be challenging due to certain shortcomings, including two-dimensional imaging, the absence of tactile sensation and the use of unsophisticated endoscopic instruments in the narrow working space.

S. Lee, MD (✉)
Division of Breast-Thyroid Surgery, Department of Surgery, Seoul St. Mary's Hospital, The Catholic University of Korea, 222 Banpo-daero, Seocho-gu, Seoul, Republic of Korea
e-mail: leesohee@catholic.ac.kr

W.Y. Chung, MD
Department of Surgery, Yonsei University College of Medicine, Seoul, Republic of Korea

With the innovation of robotic technology, application of surgical robotic systems has enabled surgeons to overcome the abovementioned shortcomings of endoscopic procedures by providing three-dimensional images in magnified view and more dexterous and accurate instrument movements. Since 2007, when we first introduced robot-assisted transaxillary thyroidectomy (RAT), many studies have been performed defining the technical safety, feasibility, and functional or surgical outcomes of robotic thyroid surgery. With greater experience, robotic thyroidectomy can be performed through a single incision, and the indication of the procedure extended to include thyroid carcinoma with lateral neck node metastasis or Graves' disease. In this chapter, the specific indications for and detailed method of robot-assisted transaxillary thyroidectomy for the management of thyroid disease are described.

Selection Criteria

Surgeon and Specialized Team

Surgeons should be experienced at conventional open thyroid gland surgery before conducting robotic procedures. They should be fully acquainted with the relevant anatomy because it may be unfamiliar to them due to a different access point and a lack of preexisting working space. Before conducting operations in patients, surgeons should also receive sufficient education

D.J. Terris, M.C. Singer (eds.), *Minimally Invasive and Robotic Thyroid and Parathyroid Surgery*, DOI 10.1007/978-1-4614-9011-1_9, and training (using animals or cadavers) both for developing the working space and in the use of the robot. Furthermore, a surgeon should perform incrementally more challenging cases, starting with straightforward cases and progressing to more advanced cases.

Moreover, robot-assisted transaxillary thyroidectomy is a complex procedure, which is best performed along with a specialized robotic team. The team should consist of an anesthesiologist, an operating room staff (bedside assistant and nurse), and a robotic technician. All team members should become familiar not only with the robot (including robotic devices, instrument assignments, setup, and operation and entry/exit) but also with the overall flow of the surgery. The robotic system should be tested for normal operation before usage, and a technician should troubleshoot the robot immediately when a system error occurs.

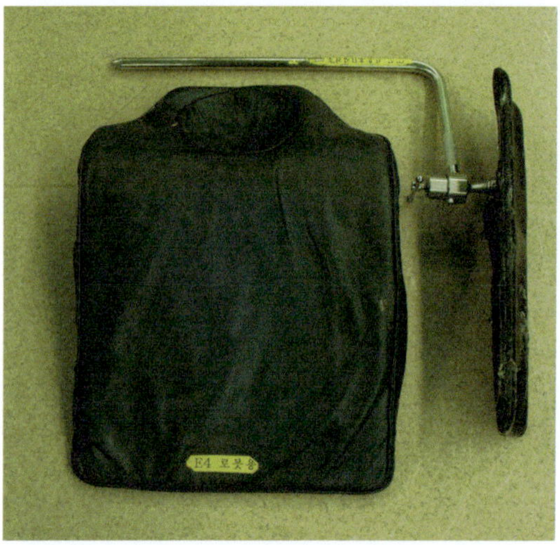

Fig. 9.1 Soft pillow and arm board for patient positioning

Special Equipment

In terms of patient positioning, a soft pillow (for neck extension) and an arm board (placed on the lesion side) attached to the operative table should be prepared (Fig. 9.1). During development of the working space, electrocautery, a vascular DeBakey forceps, and various retractors (army-navy retractors, right-angled retractors, and lighted breast retractors) are used for subcutaneous flap dissection and elevation (Fig. 9.2). For maintaining the working space, we use an external retractor we designed (Chung's retractor; Fig. 9.3).

For the robotic procedure, a da Vinci S or Si system (Intuitive, Inc., Sunnyvale, CA, USA) can be used. Three robotic instruments (5-mm Maryland dissector, 8-mm ProGrasp forceps, and 5-mm Harmonic curved shears) and a

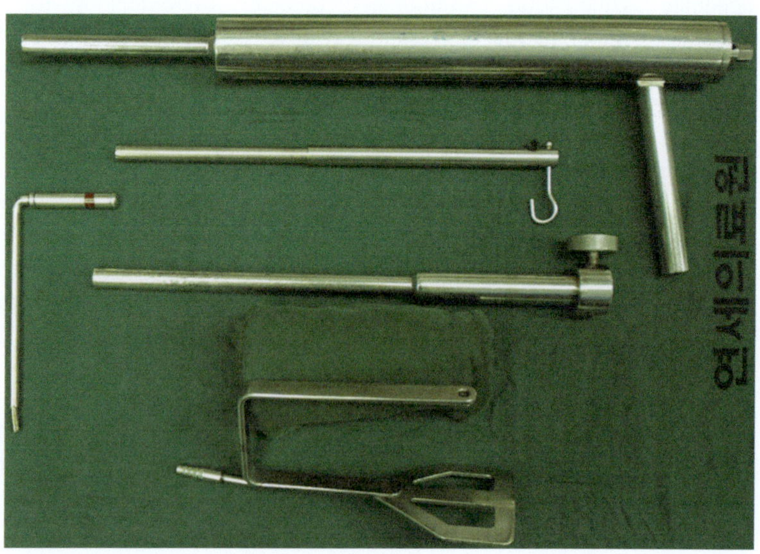

Fig. 9.2 External retractor for maintaining the working space

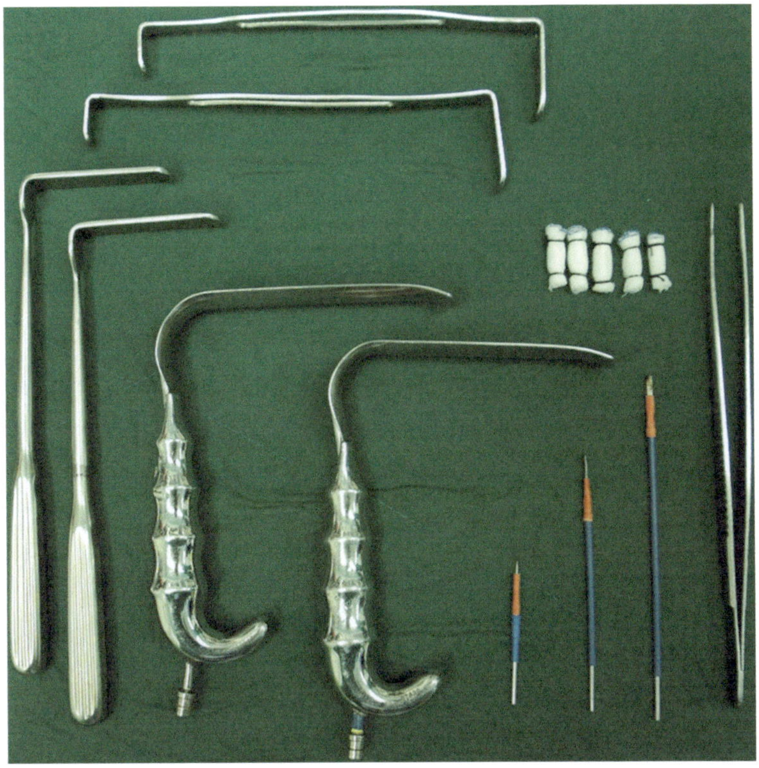

Fig. 9.3 Devices for developing the working space

dual-channel camera (30° down) are needed (Table 9.1). Small rolled-up gauzes are used for control of bleeding.

Surgical Indications

Based on the feasibility and safety of endoscopic transaxillary thyroidectomy for low-risk papillary thyroid microcarcinomas, the initial eligibility criteria for RAT were limited to well-differentiated thyroid carcinomas with a tumor size of ≤2 cm (without extrathyroidal tumor extension) or to benign tumors with a size of ≤5 cm. At that time, due to the possibility of injuring critical structures (trachea, esophagus, or recurrent laryngeal nerve [RLN]) during the procedure, lesions located deep in the thyroid bed, especially those adjacent to the tracheoesophageal groove, were considered ineligible. With greater experience the indications have expanded and now include advanced cancer cases, such as those with definite adjacent muscle invasion, RLN invasion, and lateral neck node metastasis.

Table 9.1 Special equipment for the robot-assisted transaxillary thyroidectomy

Patient positioning (Fig. 9.1)
Soft pillow
Arm board
Development of working space (Fig. 9.2)
Electrocautery with short, regular, and long tip
Vascular DeBakey
Army-navy retractor × 2
Right-angled retractors × 2
Breast lighted retractor × 2
Maintenance of working space (Fig. 9.3)
Chung's retractor
Table mount and suspension device (BioRobotics, Seoul, Korea, or Marina Medical, Sunrise, FL)
Robotic procedure
5-mm Maryland dissector
8-mm ProGrasp forceps
5-mm Harmonic curved shears
Dual-channel 30° endoscope (used in the rotated down position)
Assistant instruments
Ethicon Endopath graspers and forceps
Ethicon Endopath suction irrigator
Miscellaneous
Small rolled-up gauzes

Currently, the eligibility criteria for RAT are as follows: (1) benign tumor or follicular neoplasm with a size of ≤5 cm, (2) mild- to moderate-size Graves' goiters, and (3) well-differentiated thyroid carcinomas with a primary tumor size of ≤4 cm and minimal invasion by the primary tumor into the anterior thyroid capsule and strap muscles. The contraindications for RAT include (1) definite tumor invasion into an adjacent organ (RLN, esophagus, major vessels, or trachea), (2) metastasis to multiple lymph nodes in multiple levels of the lateral neck, and (3) perinodal infiltration around a metastatic lymph node. Prior to surgery, all patients should be evaluated by an ultrasonography-guided fine needle aspiration biopsy and the clinical stage should be checked by a staging neck ultrasonography or computed tomography scan.

Procedural Details

Patient Positioning

The patient is placed in the supine position with neck extension by inserting a soft pillow under the shoulders. The lesion-side arm is raised to shorten the distance between the axillary incision and the target area. To avoid brachial plexus paralysis, the arm is extended naturally within the range of shoulder motion and should not be fixed by force. A modified arm position or a laterally abducted position is helpful with a stiff shoulder.

Creating Working Space

The neck region is relatively narrow and encases many vital structures without a natural body cavity, therefore, making an artificial space for accessing the thyroid gland is demanding. Additionally, sufficient working space is essential for optimizing the use of the robot.

The working space consists of the outer and inner spaces. The outer space is the channel for approaching the target area and is bound by a subcutaneous skin flap and the pectoralis major muscle. The robotic dissection is performed in the inner space, which is surrounded by strap muscles and the sternal head of sternocleidomastoid (SCM) muscle ventrally and by the trachea, major blood vessels, and the clavicular head of SCM muscle dorsally (Fig. 9.4a).

The reference landmarks are (1) the sternal notch, (2) a transverse line from the sternal notch laterally to the axilla (inferior limit of the incision), (3) the upper limit of the lesion side of the thyroid gland, (4) a 70–80° oblique line from the upper pole of the thyroid to the axilla (superior limit of the incision), and (5) the medial border of the ipsilateral SCM muscle (Fig. 9.4b). A 5- to 6-cm vertical skin incision is made in the axillary area. The precise location of this incision (in a cephalad-caudad vector) should be based on the height of the upper limit of the thyroid gland. Additionally, it should be placed so that it is completely covered with the arm in the anatomic position. The subcutaneous skin flap from the axilla to the anterior neck area is dissected over the anterior surface of the pectoralis major muscle and clavicle. To develop sufficient working space without tension, the subcutaneous and subplatysmal flaps should be dissected up to level of the upper limit of thyroid gland and to the superior end of the incision. In addition, dissection should be carried to 2 cm inferior to the level of the sternal notch and to the lower edge of the incision. After the SCM muscle is exposed, the thyroid compartment is approached through the avascular space between the two heads of the SCM muscle and deep to the strap muscle. Dissection should continue until the contralateral side of the thyroid gland is exposed. The omohyoid muscle is fully mobilized and retracted ventrally and the clavicular head of the SCM muscle is dissected fully to the bottom of inner space so as not to block the surgeon's view. To assure sufficient inner working space, all soft tissues and the anterior surface of the thyroid gland are completely detached from the dorsal part of the strap muscles. The external retractor (Chung's retractor) is inserted through the skin incision to maintain the working space and placed between the thyroid gland and the strap muscles. Experience has shown that to achieve adequate working space, the height of incision entrance should be ≥4 cm and the space between the retractor blade and the

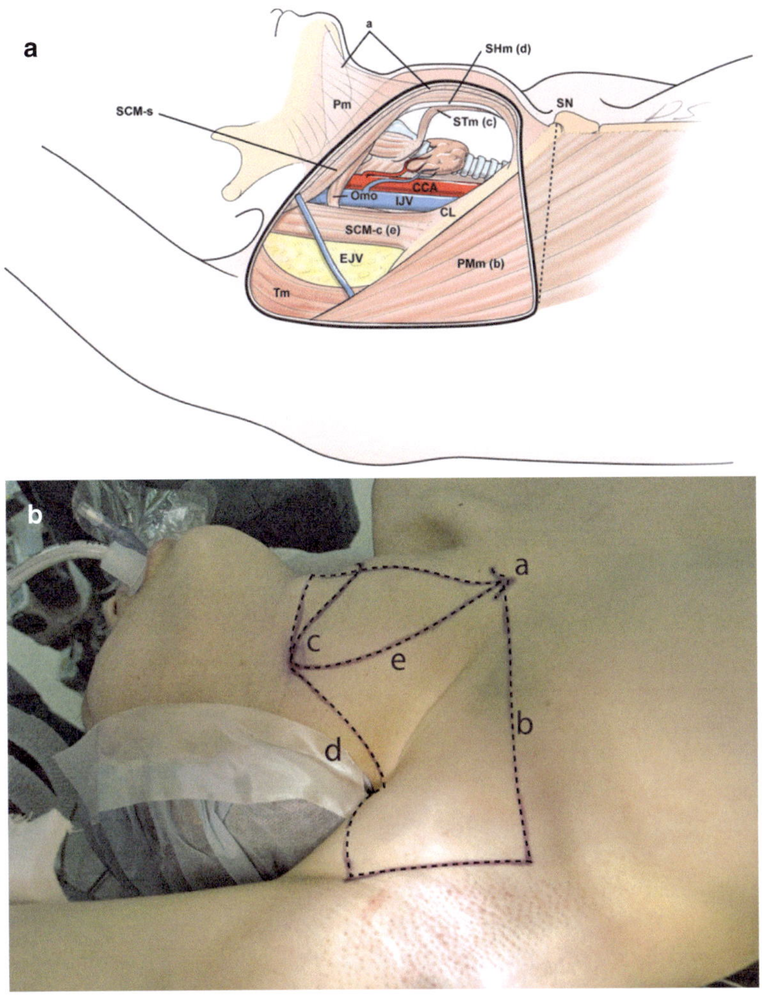

Fig. 9.4 (**a**) The working space of the robotic thyroidectomy consists of the outer and the inner spaces. The outer space is bound by a subcutaneous skin flap (*a*) and the pectoralis major muscle (*b*). The inner space is surrounded by strap muscles (*c*) and the sternal head of sternocleidomastoid (*SCM*) muscle (*d*) ventrally and by the trachea, major vessels, and the clavicular head of SCM muscle (*e*) dorsally. (**b**) The reference landmarks of robotic thyroidectomy: (*a*) the sternal notch, (*b*) a transverse line from the sternal notch laterally to the axilla (inferior limit of the incision), (*c*) the upper limit of the lesion side of the thyroid gland, (*d*) 70–80° oblique line from the thyroid upper pole laterally to the axilla (superior limit of the incision), and (*e*) the medial border of the ipsilateral SCM muscles. *Pm* platysma muscle, *STm* sternothyroid muscle, *SHm* sternohyoid muscle, *SN* sternal notch, *CCA* common arotid artery, *IJV* internal jugular vein, *CL* clavicle, *EJV* external jugular vein, *PMm* pectoralis major uscle, *Omo* omohyoid muscle, *Tm* trapezius muscle, *SCM-s* sternal head of SCM muscles, *SCM-c* clavicular head of SCM muscles

anterior surface of the thyroid gland should be ≥1 cm.

Robotic Docking

The patient cart is placed on the side contralateral to the axillary incision. To avoid inter-arm collisions, axis alignment is important. The operative table should be positioned slightly oblique, and the center column of patient cart should be aligned with the long axis of the external retractor.

Two-Incision Method

Robot-assisted transaxillary thyroidectomy was initially performed using a two-incision technique. The second incision is made on the anterior chest wall on the side of the thyroid pathology, 2–4 cm superior and 6–8 cm medial to the nipple, and away from the sternum. Of the four robotic arms, three arms are inserted through the axillary incision and the remaining arm is inserted through the anterior chest wall. The 30° down dual-channel endoscope is placed on the central arm and introduced in a downward to upward direction. It should be in line with both the center column of the patient cart and the long axis of the external retractor. The 8-mm Harmonic curved shears and the 5-mm Maryland dissector are placed on both sides of the scope and introduced in an upward to downward direction. The external third joints of these robotic arms should form an inverted triangle shape. The ProGrasp forceps, on the anterior chest arm, is inserted toward the targeted area and is placed laterally to the sternal head of the sternocleidomastoid (SCM) muscle.

Single-Incision Method

After performing more than 700 cases of the two-incision technique, we transitioned to using a single axillary incision. All four robotic arms are inserted through the axillary incision. As mentioned above, the dual-channel endoscope is placed at the center of the incision, aligned with the axis of the external retractor. To prevent interference between the robotic arms, the ProGrasp forceps are inserted caudal to the endoscope and positioned at the ceiling of the working space. The tip of the ProGrasp forceps is slid fully into the working space, and its external third joint moves backward and works in a different plane than the other three robotic arms. The 5-mm Maryland dissector and the 5-mm Harmonic curved shears are both inserted at the lateral border of the incision. From the outside, the arms form an inverted triangle with the external third joint of the endoscope.

Thyroidectomy (Dissection)

The surgical principles of robotic thyroidectomy and conventional open thyroidectomy are the same. Optimal dissection planes can be obtained by traction and countertraction using both a Maryland dissector and ProGrasp forceps, and all dissections and vascular ligations are performed using the Harmonic curved shears. The dissection proceeds in a superior to inferior direction. The upper pole of the thyroid gland is drawn in a medio-inferior direction using the ProGrasp forceps, and the superior thyroid vessels are ligated individually using the Harmonic curved shears (Fig. 9.5a). All vessels are identified and ligated close to the thyroid gland to avoid injuring the external branch of the superior laryngeal nerve. The thyroid gland is carefully detached from the cricopharyngeal and cricothyroid muscles by repeated re-grasping, which leads to gradual dissection of thyroid tissue. The upper pole dissection is continued until the superior parathyroid gland is exposed and released (Fig. 9.5b). The superior parathyroid gland is carefully preserved by avoiding lateral thermal spread from the Harmonic curved shears during dissection. For inferior pole dissection, the thyroid gland is pulled in a superior-medial direction. Before performing a central compartment neck dissection (CCND), the ipsilateral RLN is identified near the common carotid artery. After identifying the RLN, the ipsilateral CCND is started at the lateral side of the central compartment and is carried to the sternal notch inferiorly (Fig. 9.5c). All the soft tissues are removed from the paratracheal and pretracheal areas. The central neck contents and the inferior pole of thyroid gland are pulled upward and the whole course of the RLN is traced distally and preserved. The inferior thyroid artery is divided close to the thyroid gland using the Harmonic curved shears. Care is needed to avoid direct or indirect thermal injury to the RLN. The thyroid gland is meticulously peeled off the trachea using the Harmonic curved shears. In cases of total thyroidectomy, a contralateral lobectomy is performed by subcapsular dissection. The contralateral dissection is performed in the same order as that described for the ipsilateral side. The contralateral upper pole is drawn in an inferomedial direction using the ProGrasp forceps. The superior thyroid vessels are ligated close to the thyroid gland with subcapsular dissection (Fig. 9.5d). After detaching the upper

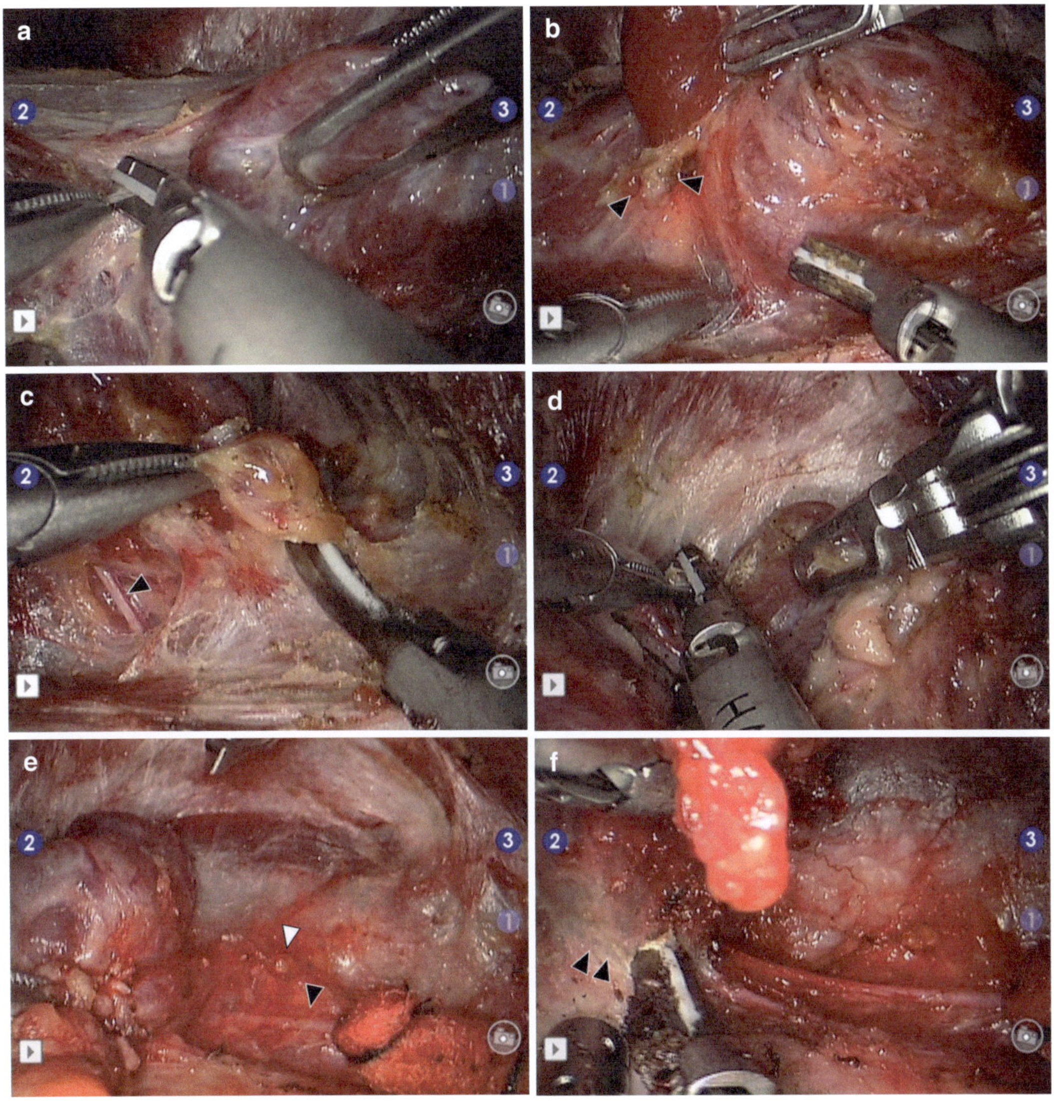

Fig. 9.5 The robotic view of a total thyroidectomy. The right side is completed first (**a–c**) and then the left (**d–f**). The patient's head is to the left and the feet to the right. (**a**) As the right thyroid lobe is retracted inferiorly, the ipsilateral superior thyroid vessels are ligated. (**b**) The right thyroid lobe is retracted medially and the superior parathyroid gland (*arrow heads*) is identified and preserved. (**c**) As the central neck is dissected, the ipsilateral RLN (*arrow head*) is clearly seen. (**d**) The contralateral (*left*) superior thyroid vessels are ligated. (**e**) The contralateral inferior parathyroid gland (*white arrow head*) and RLN (*black arrow head*) are seen during the contralateral inferior pole dissection. The lobe is being retracted superiorly. The trachea is seen at the bottom of the figure. (**f**) The dissection of the contralateral Berry's ligament area (*arrow heads*) is shown

pole from the cricothyroid muscle and preserving the superior parathyroid gland, the inferior pole dissection is completed. At the inferior pole, the inferior parathyroid gland and the contralateral RLN are preserved by subcapsular dissection (Fig. 9.5e). The contralateral RLN usually runs parallel to the dissection plane and is safe with subscapular dissection. After the inferior pole dissection, the thyroid gland is retracted medially using the ProGrasp forceps, and the lateral portion of the thyroid gland is detached until Berry's ligament is exposed. The thyroid gland is then retracted ventrally and the dissection proceeds in a medial-to-lateral direction, following the RLN until its insertion site (Fig. 9.5f). The specimen is extracted through the axillary incision, and a 3-mm closed suction drain is inserted into the surgical bed.

The single-incision method is performed in the same manner as the two-incision technique except for the use of the ProGrasp forceps. Because all four robotic arms are inserted through a single axillary incision, inter-arm collisions are prevented by using a slightly modified method. The ProGrasp forceps is placed as described above and its instrument arm is positioned in a different plane. The console surgeon uses only the wristed motions of the ProGrasp forceps, minimizing the movement of the instrument arm and its external joints.

Outcomes

Overall, outcomes have been excellent. However, complications can occur. Complications of RAT are classified as those that can occur with conventional thyroidectomy and CCND and those that are related to the robotic method itself. The prevalence of complications related to thyroidectomy and CCND (hypoparathyroidism (transient or permanent), RLN injury (transient or permanent), hematoma, and seroma formation) is similar with that of conventional open thyroidectomy. The complications specific to the RAT method include lesion-side brachial plexus paralysis, skin flap injury, and tracheal wall injury. The brachial plexus paralysis is a troublesome complication regarded as a stretch-induced neuropathy and is related to the patient's positioning. The symptoms are characterized by arm weakness and paresthesia, and these typically improve gradually over several weeks with conservative management. As mentioned previously, to prevent this type of injury, the arm ipsilateral to the lesion should be extended without tension. In cases of a patient with a stiff shoulder, a modified arm position is recommended. For patients with a frozen shoulder or limited shoulder motion, in order to avoid interference between the arm and the robotic instruments, the laterally abducted position is recommended. The monitoring of somatosensory-evoked potential responses for radial, ulnar, and median nerves can be helpful in high-risk patients. A skin injury during flap dissection can occur, particularly when the surgery is being performed by an inexperienced surgeon. The cosmetic expectation of a patient undergoing robotic thyroidectomy is very high; therefore, this complication can undermine the rationale for employing this technique. Therefore, a careful subplatysmal flap dissection should be performed with full understanding of the anatomy, particularly in the lateral neck area where the flap is thinnest. The prevalence of tracheal injury requiring primary repair in this approach is reported to be 0.3 %. A tracheal injury usually occurs during the process of peeling the thyroid gland off the trachea, from the vibration and heat produced by the Harmonic curved shears. Lifting the gland off the trachea helps to prevent this complication and the active blade of the Harmonic curved shears should be not applied directly to the tracheal wall for an extended period of time. Tracheal wall injury can be managed by primary suture or placement of a muscle flap using the robotic instruments.

Conclusions

The application of robotic technology to thyroid disease enables meticulous surgical treatment and frees the patient from a conspicuous neck scar. With instrumental advances and more experience, RAT will expand its indications and may replace the conventional open maneuver in more advanced cases.

Recommended Reading

Chang L, Satava RM, Pellegrini CA, Sinanan MN. Robotic surgery: identifying the learning curve through objective measurement of skill. Surg Endosc. 2003;17(11):1744–8. Epub 2003/09/06.

Duncan TD, Ejeh IA, Speights F, Rashid QN, Ideis M. Endoscopic transaxillary near total thyroidectomy. JSLS. 2006;10(2):206–11. Epub 2006/08/03.

Gagner M. Endoscopic subtotal parathyroidectomy in patients with primary hyperparathyroidism. Br J Surg. 1996;83(6):875. Epub 1996/06/01.

Herrell SD, Smith Jr JA. Robotic-assisted laparoscopic prostatectomy: what is the learning curve? Urology. 2005;66(5 Suppl):105–7. Epub 2005/10/01.

Holsinger FC, Terris DJ, Kuppersmith RB. Robotic thyroidectomy: operative technique using a transaxillary endoscopic approach without CO_2 insufflation. Otolaryngol Clin N Am. 2010;43(2):381–8, ix–x. Epub 2010/06/01.

Ikeda Y, Takami H, Sasaki Y, Takayama J, Niimi M, Kan S. Comparative study of thyroidectomies. Endoscopic surgery versus conventional open surgery. Surg Endosc. 2002;16(12):1741–5. Epub 2002/07/26.

Ikeda Y, Takami H, Sasaki Y, Takayama J, Niimi M, Kan S. Clinical benefits in endoscopic thyroidectomy by the axillary approach. J Am Coll Surg. 2003; 196(2):189–95. Epub 2003/02/22.

Inukai M, Usui Y. Clinical evaluation of gasless endoscopic thyroid surgery. Surg Today. 2005;35(3): 199–204. Epub 2005/03/18.

Jeong JJ, Kang SW, Yun JS, Sung TY, Lee SC, Lee YS, et al. Comparative study of endoscopic thyroidectomy versus conventional open thyroidectomy in papillary thyroid microcarcinoma (PTMC) patients. J Surg Oncol. 2009;100(6):477–80. Epub 2009/08/05.

Kandil EH, Noureldine SI, Yao L, Slakey DP. Robotic transaxillary thyroidectomy: an examination of the first one hundred cases. J Am Coll Surg. 2012;214: 558–64. Epub 2012/03/01.

Kang SW, Jeong JJ, Yun JS, Sung TY, Lee SC, Lee YS, et al. Gasless endoscopic thyroidectomy using transaxillary approach; surgical outcome of 581 patients. Endocr J. 2009a;56(3):361–9. Epub 2009/01/14.

Kang SW, Jeong JJ, Nam KH, Chang HS, Chung WY, Park CS. Robot-assisted endoscopic thyroidectomy for thyroid malignancies using a gasless transaxillary approach. J Am Coll Surg. 2009b;209(2):e1–7. Epub 2009/07/28.

Kang SW, Jeong JJ, Yun JS, Sung TY, Lee SC, Lee YS, et al. Robot-assisted endoscopic surgery for thyroid cancer: experience with the first 100 patients. Surg Endosc. 2009c;23(11):2399–406. Epub 2009/03/06.

Kang SW, Lee SC, Lee SH, Lee KY, Jeong JJ, Lee YS, et al. Robotic thyroid surgery using a gasless, transaxillary approach and the da Vinci S system: the operative outcomes of 338 consecutive patients. Surgery. 2009d;146(6):1048–55. Epub 2009/11/03.

Kang SW, Lee SH, Ryu HR, Lee KY, Jeong JJ, Nam KH, et al. Initial experience with robot-assisted modified radical neck dissection for the management of thyroid carcinoma with lateral neck node metastasis. Surgery. 2010;148(6):1214–21. Epub 2010/12/08.

Kang SW, Lee SH, Park JH, Jeong JS, Park S, Lee CR, et al. A comparative study of the surgical outcomes of robotic and conventional open modified radical neck dissection for papillary thyroid carcinoma with lateral neck node metastasis. Surg Endosc. 2012;26:3251–7. Epub 2012/06/01.

Kuppersmith RB, Holsinger FC. Robotic thyroid surgery: an initial experience with North American patients. Laryngoscope. 2011;121(3):521–6. Epub 2011/02/24.

Lee J, Chung WY. Current status of robotic thyroidectomy and neck dissection using a gasless transaxillary approach. Curr Opin Oncol. 2012;24(1):7–15. Epub 2011/11/15.

Lee J, Nah KY, Kim RM, Ahn YH, Soh EY, Chung WY. Differences in postoperative outcomes, function, and cosmesis: open versus robotic thyroidectomy. Surg Endosc. 2010;24(12):3186–94. Epub 2010/05/22.

Lee S, Ryu HR, Park JH, Kim KH, Kang SW, Jeong JJ, et al. Excellence in robotic thyroid surgery: a comparative study of robot-assisted versus conventional endoscopic thyroidectomy in papillary thyroid microcarcinoma patients. Ann Surg. 2011a;253(6): 1060–6. Epub 2011/05/19.

Lee J, Kang SW, Jung JJ, Choi UJ, Yun JH, Nam KH, et al. Multicenter study of robotic thyroidectomy: short-term postoperative outcomes and surgeon ergonomic considerations. Ann Surg Oncol. 2011b;18(9): 2538–47. Epub 2011/03/05.

Lee J, Lee JH, Nah KY, Soh EY, Chung WY. Comparison of endoscopic and robotic thyroidectomy. Ann Surg Oncol. 2011c;18(5):1439–46. Epub 2010/12/25.

Lee J, Yun JH, Nam KH, Choi UJ, Chung WY, Soh EY. Perioperative clinical outcomes after robotic thyroidectomy for thyroid carcinoma: a multicenter study. Surg Endosc. 2011d;25(3):906–12. Epub 2010/08/25.

Lee J, Yun JH, Nam KH, Soh EY, Chung WY. The learning curve for robotic thyroidectomy: a multicenter study. Ann Surg Oncol. 2011e;18(1):226–32. Epub 2010/08/04.

Lee J, Na KY, Kim RM, Oh Y, Lee JH, Lee JS, et al. Postoperative functional voice changes after conventional open or robotic thyroidectomy: a prospective trial. Ann Surg Oncol. 2012a;19(9):2963–70. Epub 2012/04/27.

Lee S, Ryu HR, Park JH, Kim KH, Kang SW, Jeong JJ, et al. Early surgical outcomes comparison between robotic and conventional open thyroid surgery for papillary thyroid microcarcinoma. Surgery. 2012b; 151(5):724–30. Epub 2012/01/31.

Miccoli P, Berti P, Raffaelli M, Conte M, Materazzi G, Galleri D. Minimally invasive video-assisted thyroidectomy. Am J Surg. 2001;181(6):567–70. Epub 2001/08/22.

Nam KH, Owen R, Inabnet WB. Prevention of complications in transaxillary single-incision robotic thyroidectomy. Thyroid. 2012;22:1266–74. Epub 2012/08/08.

Ryu HR, Kang SW, Lee SH, Rhee KY, Jeong JJ, Nam KH, et al. Feasibility and safety of a new robotic thyroidectomy through a gasless, transaxillary single-incision approach. J Am Coll Surg. 2010;211(3):e13–9. Epub 2010/08/31.

Shimizu K, Kitagawa W, Akasu H, Tanaka S. Endoscopic hemithyroidectomy and prophylactic lymph node dissection for micropapillary carcinoma of the thyroid by using a totally gasless anterior neck skin lifting method. J Surg Oncol. 2001;77(3):217–20. Epub 2001/07/17.

Tae K, Ji YB, Cho SH, Lee SH, Kim DS, Kim TW. Early surgical outcomes of robotic thyroidectomy by a gasless unilateral axillo-breast or axillary approach for papillary thyroid carcinoma: 2 years' experience. Head Neck. 2012a;34(5):617–25.

Tae K, Kim KY, Yun BR, Ji YB, Park CW, Kim DS, et al. Functional voice and swallowing outcomes after robotic thyroidectomy by a gasless unilateral axillo-breast approach: comparison with open thyroidectomy. Surg Endosc. 2012b;26(7):1871–7.

Tan CT, Cheah WK, Delbridge L. "Scarless" (in the neck) endoscopic thyroidectomy (SET): an evidence-based review of published techniques. World J Surg. 2008;32(7):1349–57. Epub 2008/03/25.

Welbourn RB. Highlights from endocrine surgical history. World J Surg. 1996;20(5):603–12. Epub 1996/06/01.

Yoon JH, Park CH, Chung WY. Gasless endoscopic thyroidectomy via an axillary approach: experience of 30 cases. Surg Laparosc Endosc Percutan Tech. 2006; 16(4):226–31. Epub 2006/08/22.

10 Robotic Facelift Thyroidectomy

Michael C. Singer

Background

Due to particular cultural attitudes and a predilection for hypertrophic scarring, avoidance of cervical incisions has been particularly sought after in Asia. Initially, remote access endoscopic procedures were utilized. These tended to be technically challenging and protracted procedures.

Over the last several years, Woong Youn Chung and his colleagues have advanced remote access thyroid surgery with two critical innovations. The first was introduction of a fixed retractor system, which eliminated the need for gas insufflation to maintain the operative pocket. Following this, Dr. Chung further enhanced the field by introducing the use of the surgical robot into his robot-assisted, gasless transaxillary thyroidectomy technique (RAT). The robot's ability to perform delicate maneuvers in constrained spaces is ideally suited for the restricted operative pocket created in RAT and other remote access techniques. This group of surgeons has now demonstrated that these procedures could be done in a high-volume, safe, and efficient manner in a Korean population. This operation generated tremendous enthusiasm in other parts of Asia, and eventually in North America.

M.C. Singer, MD
Division of Thyroid and Parathyroid Surgery,
Department of Otolaryngology – Head and Neck Surgery,
Henry Ford Hospital, 2799 West Grand Boulevard,
Detroit, MI 48202, USA
e-mail: msinger1@hfhs.org

However, the introduction of RAT in the United States was accompanied by a number of significant complications, including brachial plexus injury, large volume blood loss, and persistent pain. It became clear that performance of the transaxillary thyroidectomy technique in American patients posed significant challenges. Many surgeons have suggested that the difficulties lie in the substantial differences in body habitus and morphology that exist between American and Korean patients. American patients are typically heavier and taller, with larger necks. In addition to patient differences, the size and type of disease encountered in the United States versus Korea is another possible obstacle to smooth implementation of RAT in the United States. Many of the nodules and cancers operated on in Korea represent disease which would not even be likely biopsied in the United States.

In an effort to overcome these barriers and to develop a remote access technique that is less challenging and easier to learn, RFT was conceptualized. Development of RFT benefitted from several factors. All previous remote access techniques were designed as endoscopic procedures and only later was use of the robot incorporated into them. RFT was the first remote access technique conceived with use of the robot in mind, so that the surgery was designed to optimize its abilities. Additionally, RFT was implemented with lessons drawn from the development and evolution of other remote access techniques. RFT consequently is a hybrid approach, which integrates important

D.J. Terris, M.C. Singer (eds.), *Minimally Invasive and Robotic Thyroid and Parathyroid Surgery*,
DOI 10.1007/978-1-4614-9011-1_10, © Springer Science+Business Media New York 2014

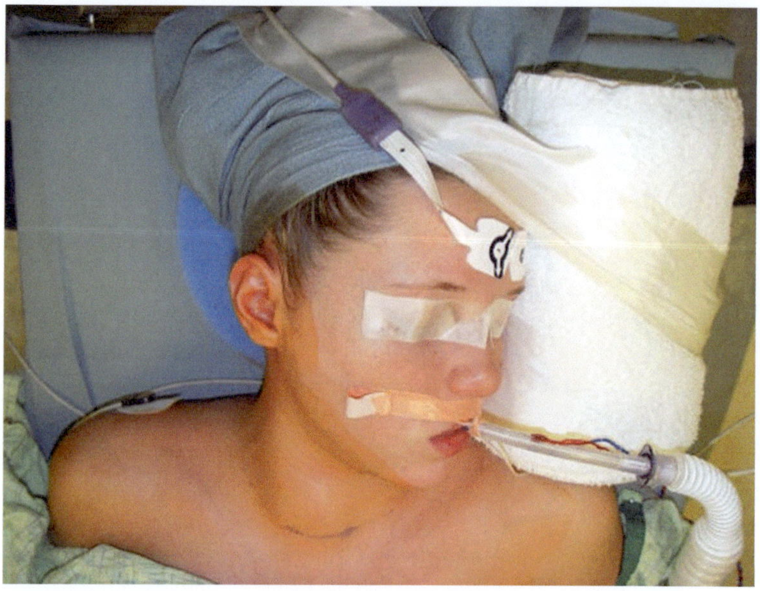

Fig. 10.1 Positioning of the patient for RFT is straightforward. While lying supine on the operating table, the head is turned 30° away from the side of surgery. A cushion is then used to prevent excessive rotation of the head

components of traditional thyroid surgery with several innovative principles. These include use of the modified facelift incision, the integration of the da Vinci robot (Intuitive Surgical Inc., Sunnyvale, CA), and the use of a fixed retractor system as described by Chung.

The rational development of RFT imparts it with several potential advantages over other remote acess techniques. The modified facelift incision, the value of which is demonstrated by its widespread adoption in parotid surgery, results in a completely concealed incision after surgery. Additionally, this incision requires significantly less tissue dissection to approach the thyroid compartment compared to RAT. Furthermore, this dissection occurs along the anterior aspect of the sternocleidomastoid muscle and adjacent structures, surgical planes that are more familiar to many head and neck surgeons. This is likely partially responsible for the faster learning curve associated with RFT. Avoiding the need for special positioning of the arm, as is used in RAT, eliminates the possibility of brachial plexus injury (Fig. 10.1). Finally, as RFT does not require placement of a drain and can be performed as an outpatient procedure, fewer of the tremendous benefits achieved with "minimally invasive" thyroidectomy techniques have to be surrendered.

Selection Criteria

As with all surgical procedures, careful patient selection is fundamental for successful outcomes with RFT. Both disease and patient characteristics determine eligibility for the procedure.

Patients with presumed benign disease, with nodules not exceeding 4 cm in greatest dimension and with no substernal extension, are candidates for RFT. In order to ease the dissection during the procedure, the absence of thyroiditis is preferred. At this time, RFT should be limited to unilateral surgery. Due to anatomical constraints and the current state of robotic technology, visualization and dissection of the contralateral recurrent laryngeal nerve cannot be adequately achieved in order to perform a true total thyroidectomy.

Patient criteria must also be considered when assessing suitability for RFT. Patients should not be morbidly obese. Additionally, patients should be sufficiently healthy to tolerate a longer anesthetic exposure than is required for conventional thyroid surgery. Perhaps the most important factor is that the patient should be motivated to completely eliminate a neck scar, as this represents the principal advantage of remote access surgery. The patient should be fully informed of the risks of the procedure, including the expectation of hypesthesia in the region of the greater auricular nerve.

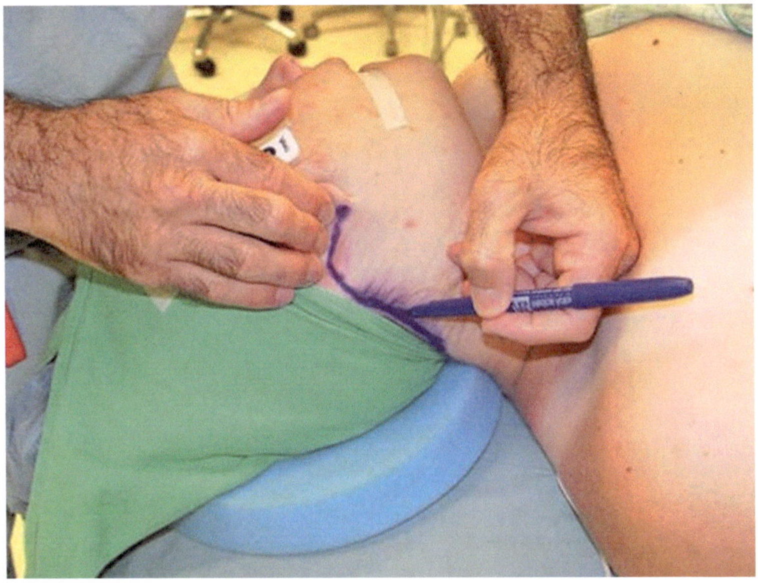

Fig. 10.2 The incision is placed in the postauricular crease and then crosses into the occipital hairline

Procedural Details

Preoperative

Safe and successful performance of RFT requires contributions from the entire surgical team—nurses, anesthesiologists, and surgeons. All members of the robotic team should be well versed in the principle steps of the procedure. This will ensure efficiency of the operation.

The anesthesiologist should use circuit extenders to facilitate a 180° turn of the operative table. Laryngeal nerve monitoring is typically utilized, and intubation using a video laryngoscope device helps to ensure proper positioning of the laryngeal electromyographic endotracheal tube. Given the nerve monitoring, paralytic agents should be avoided.

Preoperatively, the surgeon should mark the incision both for RFT and for a cervical approach (Fig. 10.2). This would be used only in the rare case in which conversion to an open approach is needed. Both of these marks should be placed with the patient in the upright position in the holding area, in order to identify the most cosmetically pleasing sites. The postauricular incision begins just behind the ear lobule and runs in the postauricular crease. It crosses into the occipital hairline at a point above where the incision will be hidden by the auricle, and then extends down within the occipital hairline (this hair is clipped after intubation and positioning).

Intraoperative

One of the benefits of RFT is that positioning of the patient is straightforward. The patient is placed on the operating table in the supine position. After intubation, the endotracheal tube is secured in position and the table is turned 180° away from the anesthesia cart. The patient's head is turned 30° away from the side of the surgery. In order to prevent excessive rotation of the neck during the procedure, a cushion is placed next to the head on the side contralateral to the side of surgery. No urinary catheter is needed.

Approximately 1 cm of hair is clipped along the descending limb of the incision. Quarter percent bupivacaine with 1:200,000 of epinephrine is then injected along the length of the incision. After sterile prepping and draping, the table is placed in reverse Trendelenburg position and airplaned away from the side of surgery to improve ergonomics for the operative surgeon.

After the incision is made, dissection is performed down to the level of the sternocleidomastoid muscle. Flap elevation is achieved first in the subcutaneous and then the subplatysmal plane.

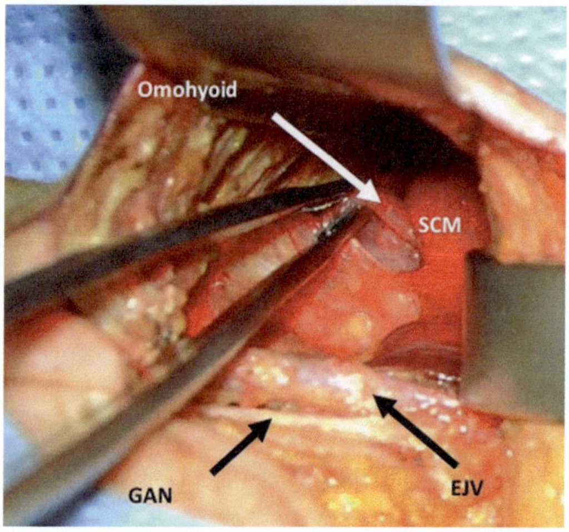

Fig. 10.3 A view of a right-sided operative pocket, with critical landmarks highlighted. The great auricular nerve (*GAN*), external jugular vein (*EJV*), sternocleidomastoid muscle (*SCM*), and the omohyoid muscle are indicated

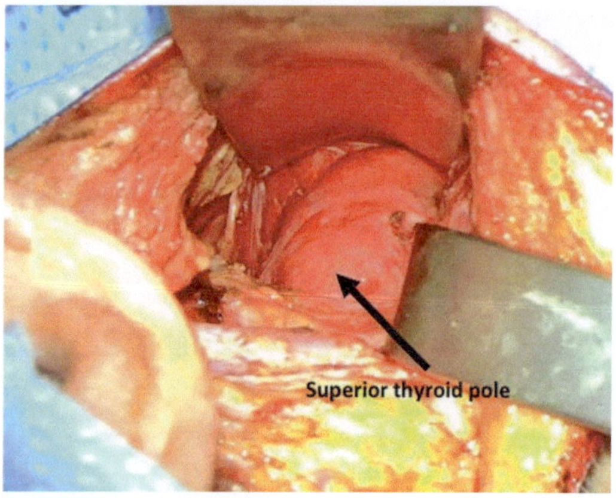

Fig. 10.4 After the strap muscles are elevated off of the underlying thyroid gland, the superior pole of the gland is well visualized (Reprinted with permission from Terris DJ, Singer MC, Seybt MW. Robotic facelift thyroidectomy: II. Clinical feasibility and safety. Laryngoscope. 2011;121(8):1636–41)

Particularly in thinner patients with less subcutaneous fat, care must be taken to avoid creating a buttonhole through the flap and skin. After identifying the sternocleidomastoid muscle, the great auricular nerve and then the external jugular vein are encountered. Dissection should be maintained ventral to these structures. The entire length of the sternocleidomastoid muscle is then exposed, with particular attention paid to releasing the anterior border of the muscle.

Identification of the omohyoid muscle is the next critical step. By dissecting and then retracting this muscle ventrally, the sternohyoid and sternothyroid muscles are exposed (Fig. 10.3). These muscles are then reflected from lateral to medial, exposing the upper pole of the thyroid gland.

The omohyoid muscle is most readily seen by rolling the anterior border of the sternocleidomastoid muscle laterally, a maneuver performed well with a malleable retractor. Cadaver dissections and intraoperative assessments have revealed that the omohyoid muscle can be consistently identified just inferior to an axial line drawn through the inferior aspect of the thyroid notch (Singer MC, 2012). The sternohyoid and sternothyroid muscles are elevated off the underlying thyroid gland down to the level of the sternum and then retracted ventrally with a modified version of the Chung retractor blade (Marina Medical, Sunrise, Florida) (Fig. 10.4). This maintains the operative pocket. Additional exposure is achieved by retracting the sternocleidomastoid muscle laterally using a retractor fixed to the operating table.

After the retractors are positioned, the da Vinci surgical robot is deployed. The pedestal of the patient side cart is positioned on the side contralateral to the surgery, with the arms extended parallel to the long axis of the fixed retractor. Three arms are utilized: the camera arm is positioned first, holding a 30° down endoscope parallel to the retractor system, or angled slightly upward. A Maryland grasper is placed in the nondominant arm, and a Harmonic device (Ethicon Endo-Surgery Inc., Cincinnati, Ohio) is placed in the dominant arm. These are positioned on either side of the endoscope. In order to minimize collisions of the robotic arms, the working arms should be angled in such a way that they create a "V" in the axial plane.

For excision of the gland, the operative surgeon is seated at the robotic console. A bedside assistant supports performance of the surgery by

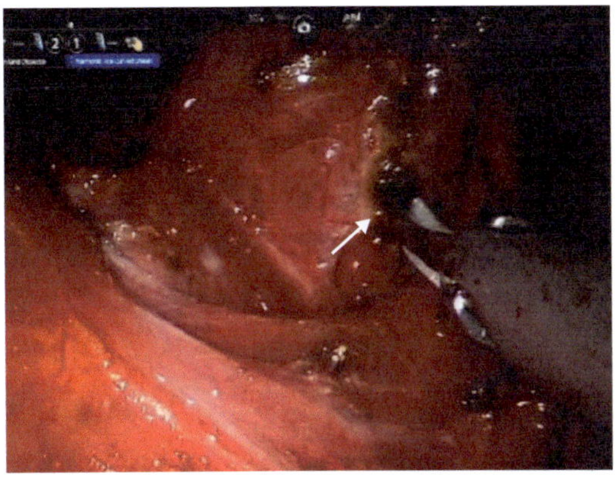

Fig. 10.5 After the superior pedicle is ligated, the superior parathyroid gland (*white arrow*) can often be identified on the posterior aspect of the thyroid gland. Releasing it posteriorly preserves the parathyroid gland

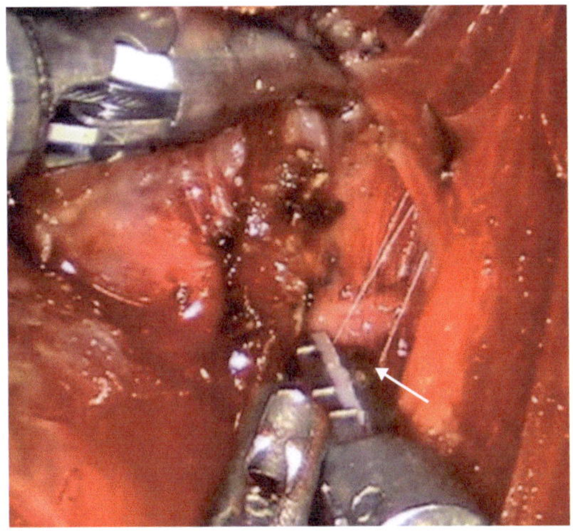

Fig. 10.6 The recurrent laryngeal nerve (*white arrow*) is sought just inferior to its entry deep to the inferior constrictor muscle, its most constant location. Here, a right-sided nerve is seen after dissection

suctioning and retracting as necessary. At this point, the upper pedicle of the gland, exposed during the open phase of the case, is further mobilized. Once isolated the pedicle is ligated in a single bundle using the Harmonic device. The superior aspect of the thyroid lobe is then reflected inferiorly, exposing the inferior constrictor muscle. Frequently, the superior parathyroid gland is visualized in this area. This gland is preserved by dissecting it posterolaterally (Fig. 10.5). Medially, the superior laryngeal nerve can be observed running on the inferior constrictor muscle. At this point, the recurrent laryngeal nerve is sought and clearly delineated. Using blunt dissection to demarcate the inferior border of the inferior constrictor muscle, the nerve can be recognized laterally, just prior to its entry deep to the muscle. Often the origin of the inferior constrictor muscle from the cricoid cartilage can be visualized. If observed, this oblique line can be used as a landmark for identifying the recurrent nerve, as the entry point of the nerve is approximately 1 cm lateral to this line. After initial recognition the recurrent nerve is dissected inferiorly for a short distance (Fig. 10.6). To confirm proper function of the nerve monitoring system, the recurrent nerve can be stimulated at this time. As the nerve is now exposed laterally, the tissue medial to this, including the ligament of Berry, may be safely divided using the Harmonic device. The thyroid isthmus is then divided and the middle thyroid vein ligated. Attention is then turned to the inferior aspect of the gland. The inferior parathyroid gland is mobilized with its blood supply intact and released. The remaining attachments inferiorly, including the inferior thyroid artery and vein, are then transected. Final attachments of the gland to the trachea are lysed, completing release of the lobe. The specimen can now be delivered through the wound. The surgeon can elect to stimulate the recurrent nerve a final time at this point. The robotic arms and patient cart are then withdrawn.

Following irrigation, the operative bed should be examined for the presence of any bleeding. Typically, bleeding is minimal but absolute hemostasis should be assured. Surgicel (Ethicon Inc., Somerville, New Jersey) is placed in the wound and the subcutaneous tissues are closed with interrupted sutures of 4-0 Vicryl. The incision is then closed as per the surgeon's preference (cyanoacrylate glue is used in our practice, with an overlying dressing). No drain is placed. A deep extubation, which may help prevent oozing, is recommended.

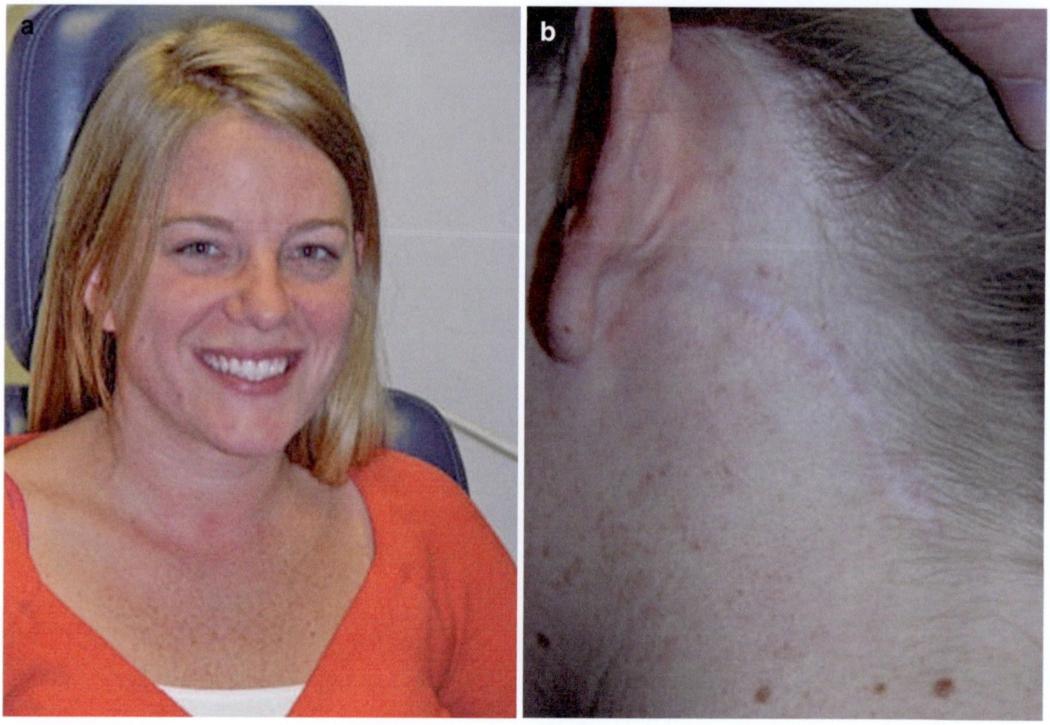

Fig. 10.7 Frontal view of patient 1 year after undergoing robotic facelift thyroidectomy (**a**). Note that from a frontal view, the scar is completely hidden. The resulting scar is shown (**b**)

Postoperative

Patients are managed on an outpatient basis. They are observed in the recovery room and discharged home as per the hospital's routine.

Patients are prescribed antiemetic and pain medications. They are instructed to limit activities for 14 days postoperatively. As per routine, patients who have undergone bilateral or completion surgery are prescribed a 3-week course of oral calcium supplementation beginning on the evening of surgery and are counseled regarding the signs and symptoms of hypocalcemia.

Outcomes

Clinical outcomes have been excellent. Risk of permanent recurrent nerve injury or hypocalcemia is low. Due to dissection during development of the operative pocket, patients do experience hyperesthesia in the distribution of great auricular nerve. This resolves over the course of several months. However, patients should be alerted preoperatively to the possibility of this periauricular discomfort, in addition to other complications that are the same as with traditional thyroid surgery. As the postauricular wound is completely hidden (particularly in women with longer hair), cosmetic results are superb (Fig. 10.7).

Future Directions

RFT is early in its clinical evolution. As noted earlier, due to anatomical and technological constraints, RFT currently should be limited to unilateral surgery. Improvements in robotic technology will likely in the near future allow for improved visualization and dissection of the contralateral thyroid compartment. These advances will allow for total thyroidectomy to be performed safely from a single incision. Additionally, the access obtained through the RFT incision exposes other critical anatomy and this approach could be used to perform other procedures. Surgeons have already begun to utilize this approach to perform lateral neck dissections. As experience with the RFT technique expands, the indications for the procedure will likely widen.

Recommended Reading

Kang SW, Jeong JJ, Nam KH, Chang HS, Chung WY, Park CS. Robot-assisted endoscopic thyroidectomy for thyroid malignancies using a gasless transaxillary approach. J Am Coll Surg. 2009;209(2):e1–7.

Kuppersmith RB, Holsinger FC. Robotic thyroid surgery: an initial experience with North American patients. Laryngoscope. 2011;121(3):521–6.

Landry CS, Grubbs EG, Morris GS, Turner NS, Holsinger FC, Lee JE, Perrier ND. Robot assisted transaxillary surgery (RATS) for the removal of thyroid and parathyroid glands. Surgery. 2011;149(4):549–55.

Miccoli P, Berti P, Materazzi G, Massi M, Picone A, Minuto MN. Results of video-assisted parathyroidectomy: single institution's six-year experience. World J Surg. 2004;28(12):1216–8.

Singer MC, Seybt MW, Terris DJ. Robotic facelift thyroidectomy: I. Pre-clinical simulation and morphometric assessment. Laryngoscope. 2011;121(8):1631–5.

Singer MC, Bhakta D, Seybt MW, Terris DJ. Calcium management after thyroidectomy: a simple and cost-effective method. Otolaryngol Head Neck Surg. 2012;146(3):362–5.

Terris DJ, Singer MC. Qualitative and quantitative differences between 2 robotic thyroidectomy techniques. Otolaryngol Head Neck Surg. 2012;147(1):20–5.

Terris DJ, Tuffo KM, Fee Jr WE. Modified facelift incision for parotidectomy. J Laryngol Otol. 1994;108(7):574–8.

Terris DJ, Singer MC, Seybt MW. Robotic facelift thyroidectomy: patient selection and technical considerations. Surg Laparosc Endosc Percutan Tech. 2011a;21(4):237–42.

Terris DJ, Singer MC, Seybt MW. Robotic facelift thyroidectomy: II. Clinical feasibility and safety. Laryngoscope. 2011b;121(8):1636–41.

Conservative Central Neck Dissection

11

Salem I. Noureldine and Ralph P. Tufano

Introduction

Cervical lymph node metastasis has been reported to occur in up to 90 % of patients with papillary thyroid cancer (PTC) and in a smaller proportion in patients with other histotypes. Metastatic thyroid cancer to the lymph nodes of the neck has long been recognized to significantly correlate with both persistence and recurrence of disease, and potentially survival. In the early 1800s, complete removal of cervical metastatic disease was considered impossible, although some surgeons attempted to remove involved cervical lymph nodes at the time of primary tumor resection. In January 1888, Jawdynski first described, in detail, a systematic approach to en bloc resection of cervical lymph node disease. This approach was later popularized and illustrated, based on anatomical principles, by Crile, providing a consistent and more effective treatment that forms the basis of our current techniques. The radical en bloc resection was intended to control metastatic lymph nodes by completely resecting involved lymph nodes between the superficial and deep cervical fascias together with neck structures in close proximity to the disease, from the base of the skull to the level of the clavicle. The greatest boost to the popularity of radical neck dissection, based on the principles developed by Jawdynski and Crile, came from Hayes Martin. Martin's technical principles include the removal of all the lymph nodes from levels I to V together with the spinal accessory nerve, internal jugular vein, sternocleidomastoid muscle, and various other structures in a single block of resected tissue. His technique of radical neck dissection was followed until the late twentieth century when technical modifications to neck dissection procedures began to find general acceptance, due to the significant long-term morbidity and deformity produced by this aggressive technique.

The concept of conservative neck dissection was first introduced in the early 1900s, with the goal of decreasing morbidity while achieving equivalent oncological outcomes to radical neck dissection. Suarez proposed an effective technique and achieved satisfactory results with a modified radical neck dissection, where important structures, such as muscles, vessels, and nerves were preserved without adversely affecting regional control. This technique allowed complete elimination of the nodal tissue in the neck along with the primary tumor while carefully preserving important structures such as the

S.I. Noureldine, MD
R.P. Tufano, MD, MBA, FACS (✉)
Division of Head and Neck Endocrine Surgery, Department of Otolaryngology – Head and Neck Surgery, Johns Hopkins University
School of Medicine, Baltimore, MD, USA
e-mail: snourel1@jhmi.edu; rtufano@jhmi.edu

D.J. Terris, M.C. Singer (eds.), *Minimally Invasive and Robotic Thyroid and Parathyroid Surgery*,
DOI 10.1007/978-1-4614-9011-1_11,

sternocleidomastoid muscle, omohyoid muscle, submandibular gland, internal jugular vein, and in some cases the spinal accessory nerve. This modified neck dissection technique was later refined and popularized by various authors in the English literature. However, still hindering its widespread adoption was the basic misperception that this type of dissection was not radical enough for cancer control, and therefore thought to be unacceptable.

In the 1930s, using a labeling system to describe the levels of a neck dissection developed at the Memorial Sloan-Kettering Cancer Center, the locations of cervical lymph node groups were delineated. This system not only defined the anatomical locations of lymph node groups but also reflected the path of tumor extension through the neck and indicated which levels are at greatest risk for early metastasis. By the late twentieth century, with a better understanding of lymphatic spread and cancer behavior, the concept of selective neck dissection, consisting of resection of only the nodal groups at greatest risk for containing metastases from a given primary site, was developed. These selective dissections are now widely employed for therapeutic treatment and staging of the neck. The development of contemporary concepts of neck dissection clearly represents an important development in the management of patients with head and neck cancer. A better understanding of the biology and behavior of the disease permits the use of procedures that result in both local control and better functional outcomes.

Other modifications related to cervical lymph node metastasis to the central neck include a revised system for classification of neck dissections in 2002, the use of molecular techniques for identification of lymph node metastases not detectable by microscopy, and the possibility of endoscopic and robotic cervical lymph node dissections. Central neck dissection (CND), in its various forms, continues to evolve as a fundamental tool in managing patients with cervical lymph node metastases from thyroid cancer.

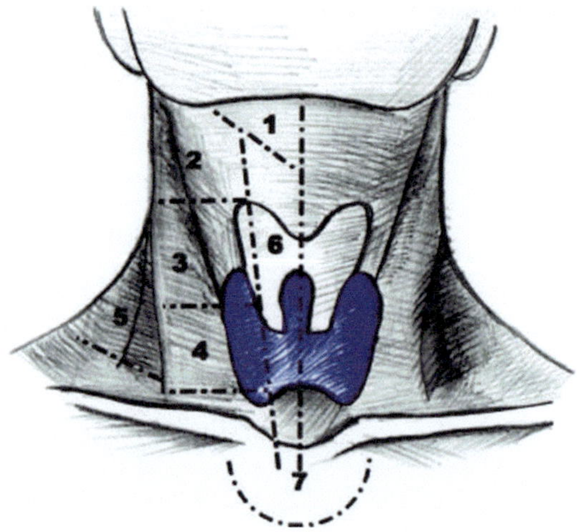

Fig. 11.1 The lymph node groups are divided into six cervical levels (levels 1-6) and one upper mediastinal (level 7), comprising seven levels each bounded by distinct anatomical borders (From Kharchenko VP, Kotlyarov PM, Mogutoy MS, Alexandrov YK, Sencha AN, Patrunoy YN, Belyaev DV, editors. Ultrasound diagnostics of thyroid diseases. Berlin/Heidelberg: Springer; 2010. With permission)

Central Compartment Lymph Node Metastasis

Anatomy and Nomenclature

The classification system of cervical lymph node compartments is well defined and is important not only in identifying the location of pathologic lymph nodes but also in providing an anatomical roadmap for surgical treatment as outlined in the recent American Thyroid Association (ATA) guidelines. The lymph node groups are divided into six cervical levels and one upper mediastinal, comprising seven levels each bounded by distinct anatomical borders (Fig. 11.1). Level VI contains the thyroid gland and consists of pretracheal and paratracheal nodes, the precricoid (Delphian) node, and the perithyroidal nodes, including nodes along the recurrent laryngeal nerves. Level VII contains the upper mediastinal nodes. The central compartment group includes levels VI and VII. The structures defining the anatomical boundaries of the neck levels and sublevels are summarized in Table 11.1.

Table 11.1 Anatomical landmarks for the neck and upper mediastinum levels and sublevels

Level	Superior	Inferior	Medial	Lateral
IA	Symphysis of mandible	Hyoid bone	Anterior belly of contralateral digastric muscle	Anterior belly of ipsilateral digastric muscle
IB	Mandibular body	Posterior belly of digastric muscle	Anterior belly of digastric muscle	Stylohyoid muscle
IIA	Skull base	Horizontal plane – inferior body of the hyoid bone	Stylohyoid muscle	Vertical plane – spinal accessory nerve
IIB	Skull base	Horizontal plane – inferior border of the hyoid bone	Vertical plane – spinal accessory nerve	Lateral border of the SCM muscle
III	Horizontal plane – inferior border of the hyoid bone	Horizontal plane – inferior border of the cricoid cartilage	Lateral border of the sternohyoid muscle	Lateral border of the SCM muscle
IV	Horizontal plane – inferior border of the cricoid cartilage	Clavicle	Lateral border of the sternohyoid muscle	Lateral border of the SCM muscle
VA	Convergence of the SCM and trapezius muscles	Horizontal plane – inferior border of the cricoid cartilage	Posterior border of the SCM muscle	Anterior border of the trapezius muscle
VB	Horizontal plane – inferior border of the cricoid cartilage	Clavicle	Posterior border of the SCM muscle	Anterior border of the trapezius muscle
VI	Hyoid bone	Suprasternal notch	Carotid sheath	Carotid sheath
VII	Upper border of the sternum	Aortic arch	Carotid sheath	Carotid sheath

Key: *SCM* sternocleidomastoid

A therapeutic central compartment neck dissection implies that lymph node metastases are clinically apparent (preoperatively or intraoperatively) or radiographically identified (clinically N1a). A prophylactic or elective compartment dissection implies lymph node metastases are not detected clinically or by imaging (clinically N0). Lymph node "berry picking" implies removal only of the clinically involved nodes rather than a complete nodal group within the compartment and is not synonymous with a selective compartment-oriented dissection. There is a general agreement that therapeutic node dissection should be performed in patients with PTC who have visibly involved nodes. This should include a systemic or en bloc compartment-oriented neck dissection. Isolated removal of only grossly involved lymph nodes ("berry picking") violates the nodal compartment and may be associated with higher recurrence rates and morbidity from reoperative surgery. Although cervical lymph node metastases are rare in patients with FTC, patients with the Hurthle cell variant may have nodal disease or soft tissue metastases and should undergo a therapeutic CND if metastatic lymph nodes are identified.

The recent ATA consensus statement on CND emphasizes that it is important to define the terminology used to classify the procedure. It defines CND as all perithyroidal and paratracheal soft tissue and lymph nodes with borders extending superiorly to the hyoid bone, inferiorly to the innominate artery, and laterally to the common carotid arteries. The goal of defining the terminology and classification scheme for CND is to allow investigators to communicate without uncertainty and compare the efficacy of these interventions. For the first time, this consensus statement defined the extent of CND as unilateral or bilateral. Bilateral CND is preferred as the initial management of clinically involved central nodes with therapeutic intention. Nonetheless, operative reports should clearly describe the extent (unilateral vs. bilateral) and the intent (elective vs. therapeutic) of CND. Lack of standardized reporting has been somewhat responsible for the debate regarding the role of elective or prophylactic CND in PTC. The inclusion of the level VII nodes in the superior mediastinum with the CND should be noted as this is often a site of persistent disease following CND.

Detection of Metastasis

The management of a patient with suspected thyroid cancer should include a detailed examination of the thyroid gland and the cervical lymph node compartments. Patients with PTC occasionally present with cervical lymphadenopathy, which is most often located in the central neck compartment or levels III and IV of the lateral neck, usually in conjunction with an ipsilateral thyroid nodule. Cervical ultrasound (US) is often the initial imaging modality employed in the assessment since it is readily accessible, inexpensive, and noninvasive. High-resolution ultrasonography can detect cervical nodal metastasis in up to 20 % of patients with PTC. These US findings may alter the planned surgical procedure in up to 39 % of thyroid cancer patients. Pathologic lymph nodes have sonographic features that include round shape, absent hilus, calcification, intranodal necrosis, reticulation, matting, soft tissue edema, and peripheral vascularity. However, many nodal metastases demonstrate a wide variety of nondiagnostic features. To detect nonpalpable lymph node metastases in patients undergoing surgical evaluation for any thyroid cancer, a dedicated cervical ultrasound (including levels II–VI) should be performed, ideally by a dedicated clinician such as a thyroid endocrinologist, the operating surgeon, or a radiologist. However, US can miss as many as 50 % of involved lymph nodes in the central neck as the overlying thyroid gland hinders adequate visualization. In patients with suspected mediastinal disease or with bulky cervical lymphadenopathy, cross-sectional imaging with computed tomography (CT), magnetic resonance imaging (MRI), or positron emission tomography (PET) should be considered. These often identify pathologic level VI and VII lymph nodes within the superior mediastinum that are not detected on cervical US or physical examination. This consideration for additional anatomical imaging is made despite the relatively low sensitivities of CT, MRI, and PET for the screening and detection of cervical lymph node metastases (30–40 %).

A CT with iodinated contrast is considered extremely helpful to evaluate the extent of cervical lymphadenopathy when there is gross nodal disease present, as it can help define the extent of surgery necessary to clear all gross disease in the neck. CT with contrast can delay postoperative thyroid scanning and radioactive iodine (RAI) administration for 4–8 weeks. However, this delay would seem justified in cases of bulky lymphadenopathy or locally invasive disease since complete surgical resection of gross disease is of paramount importance for disease control.

Conservative Central Neck Dissection

Therapeutic Central Neck Dissection

Therapeutic CND should be performed in patients with differentiated thyroid cancer (DTC) and pathologic lymph node involvement identified preoperatively, on clinical exam or imaging, or intraoperatively. The goal of removing these lymph nodes is to aid in local control, prevent recurrences, and perhaps, improve survival. Standard therapeutic CND should include a systemic or en block neck dissection of both the ipsilateral and the contralateral central compartments. However, there is controversy regarding whether the extent of central dissection needs to be ipsilateral to the thyroid tumor alone or bilateral. Moo et al. compared ipsilateral vs. bilateral CND for PTC and concluded that an ipsilateral dissection was sufficient in tumors smaller than 1 cm, while larger tumors required bilateral CND based on the high incidence of contralateral central compartment neck disease. Liberal parathyroid autotransplantation during CND should be employed to prevent postoperative hypoparathyroidism.

The management in patients with medullary thyroid cancer (MTC) deserves special mentioning. MTC is a more aggressive tumor with a high incidence of lymph node metastasis and there is no role for radioiodine treatment in this type of disease. Lymph node metastasis can occur in up to 81 % of patients. Patients with MTC can only be cured with surgical intervention, which should at least include a total thyroidectomy with meticulous CND.

Prophylactic Central Neck Dissection

The role of prophylactic CND remains a contentious issue. The American Thyroid Association (ATA) guidelines suggest that prophylactic CND may be performed for advanced primary tumors (>4 cm and/or with extrathyroidal invasion) but is not necessary for small, noninvasive papillary and most follicular thyroid cancers. An essential component of any discussion on the extent of lymphadenectomy is whether patients derive any additional benefit from having a lymphadenectomy and whether this can be done without significantly increasing the morbidity of the operation. Because microscopic nodal disease is rarely of clinical importance, many authors argue that prophylactic CND of microscopic lymph node metastases may not improve long-term outcome and could subject patients to more risk than benefit. However, the precise role of prophylactic CND for DTC remains controversial because in experienced hands, this procedure can be done with minimal additional risk and may in some patients provide a survival benefit.

Proponents of prophylactic CND argue that the incidence of central neck metastases is high and the sensitivity of preoperative US to detect pathologic lymph nodes in PTC patients is higher in the lateral neck (94 %) than in the central neck compartments (53–55 %). Furthermore, prophylactic CND advocates argue that clearing the central neck at the initial operation removes potential sources of recurrence, increases the accuracy of staging for RAI ablation, permits accurate long-term surveillance, and avoids the potential morbidity of a reoperation. An additional benefit of reduced postoperative Tg levels after CND was also cited. We and others have suggested that prophylactic CND be considered in patients with thyroid cancer harboring the BRAF mutation, since they have the potential to be more clinically aggressive and less responsive to RAI therapy. The BRAF mutation has been widely found in PTC, with a prevalence of approximately 45 %. Recent studies have established a strong association between the presence of the BRAF mutation and aggressive clinicopathologic characteristics of PTC. However, additional studies are needed to demonstrate the clinical benefit of this approach.

Conservative Surgery for Persistent/Recurrent Disease

Regardless of the initial treatment paradigm utilized for thyroid cancer, some patients will manifest persistent or recurrent disease. Much of persistent or recurrent disease is detected subclinically by surveillance strategies advocated by the ATA guidelines. High-resolution US and serum thyroglobulin (Tg) assays, with or without thyrotropin stimulation, have led to a new category of patients with persistent or recurrent small volume disease of uncertain clinical significance. Many authors have demonstrated that reoperative surgery for this disease, especially in the central compartment, is safe. Definitions of microscopic and macroscopic nodal recurrences should help to define which groups of patients could be observed versus those that should be offered surgery. Reasonable and realistic expectations should be set for the practitioners and patients involved. When surgery is chosen, a compartmental dissection of the neck nodal region involved should be performed to reduce the risk of locoregional recurrence and the morbidity of further reoperation. Many of these patients with persistent disease have undergone multiple surgeries in the central or lateral compartments. Further attempts at formal compartmental dissection must be conducted with a thoughtful assessment of the risks and benefits to the patient. Perhaps the realistic goal of all reoperative surgery should not be to render the serum Tg level undetectable but rather to prevent local disease progression in critical areas of the neck. Long-term follow-up of these patients is warranted to determine the optimal surveillance and treatment paradigm.

Preoperative laryngoscopy should be performed before all reoperative procedures to determine the presence of vocal fold paralysis. Intraoperative RLN identification and dissection significantly reduces the risk of its injury and is superior to limited nerve exposure. Recognition of the extralaryngeal branching of the RLN is also crucial during the operation. The motor fibers of RLN are located in the anterior branch while the posterior branch is only sensory in function. Therefore, great caution is required after the presumed identification of the RLN to ensure there is no unidentified anterior branch, which may lead to increased risk of postoperative nerve injury. The surgeon can expect to encounter difficulty in identifying and preserving the RLNs due to the fibrotic tissue that distorts the anatomy of the central neck area. Given the challenging nature of reoperative neck dissection, consideration of the use of RLN monitoring to help map out the location of the nerve and special care to preserve the parathyroid vasculature or parathyroid autotransplantation are important.

Conclusion

A long path has been crossed since the initial radical neck dissections performed for cervical nodal metastases to the development of effective conservative surgical techniques for the management of cervical lymph node metastasis from thyroid cancer. A greater understanding of the clinical significance of lymph node metastases in thyroid cancer will promote continued refinements in the approach to CND.

Recommended Reading

Ahn JE, Lee JH, Yi JS, Shong YK, Hong SJ, Lee DH, et al. Diagnostic accuracy of CT and ultrasonography for evaluating metastatic cervical lymph nodes in patients with thyroid cancer. World J Surg. 2008;32(7):1552–8.

Arturi F, Russo D, Giuffrida D, Ippolito A, Perrotti N, Vigneri R, et al. Early diagnosis by genetic analysis of differentiated thyroid cancer metastases in small lymph nodes. J Clin Endocrinol Metab. 1997;82(5):1638–41.

Bishop JA, Wu G, Tufano RP, Westra WH. Histological patterns of locoregional recurrence in Hurthle cell carcinoma of the thyroid gland. Thyroid. 2012;22(7):690–4.

Bonnet S, Hartl D, Leboulleux S, Baudin E, Lumbroso JD, Al Ghuzlan A, et al. Prophylactic lymph node dissection for papillary thyroid cancer less than 2 cm: implications for radioiodine treatment. J Clin Endocrinol Metab. 2009;94:1162–7. United States.

Carty SE, Cooper DS, Doherty GM, Duh QY, Kloos RT, Mandel SJ, et al. Consensus statement on the terminology and classification of central neck dissection for thyroid cancer. Thyroid. 2009;19(11):1153–8.

Chisholm EJ, Kulinskaya E, Tolley NS. Systematic review and meta-analysis of the adverse effects of thyroidectomy combined with central neck dissection as compared with thyroidectomy alone. Laryngoscope. 2009;119(6):1135–9.

Clayman GL, Shellenberger TD, Ginsberg LE, Edeiken BS, El-Naggar AK, Sellin RV, et al. Approach and safety of comprehensive central compartment dissection in patients with recurrent papillary thyroid carcinoma. Head Neck. 2009;31(9):1152–63.

Coatesworth AP, MacLennan K. Cervical metastasis in papillary carcinoma of the thyroid: a histopathological study. Int J Clin Pract. 2002;56(4):241–2.

Cohen Y, Rosenbaum E, Clark DP, Zeiger MA, Umbricht CB, Tufano RP, et al. Mutational analysis of BRAF in fine needle aspiration biopsies of the thyroid: a potential application for the preoperative assessment of thyroid nodules. Clin Cancer Res. 2004;10(8):2761–5.

Cooper DS, Doherty GM, Haugen BR, Kloos RT, Lee SL, Mandel SJ, et al. Management guidelines for patients with thyroid nodules and differentiated thyroid cancer. Thyroid. 2006;16(2):109–42.

Cooper DS, Doherty GM, Haugen BR, Kloos RT, Lee SL, Mandel SJ, et al. Revised American Thyroid Association management guidelines for patients with thyroid nodules and differentiated thyroid cancer. Thyroid. 2009;19(11):1167–214.

Crile G. Landmark article Dec 1, 1906: excision of cancer of the head and neck. With special reference to the plan of dissection based on one hundred and thirty-two operations. By George Crile. JAMA. 1987;258(22):3286–93.

Ducci M, Appetecchia M, Marzetti M. Neck dissection for surgical treatment of lymphnode metastasis in papillary thyroid carcinoma. J Exp Clin Cancer Res. 1997;16(3):333–5.

Ellenhorn JD, Shah JP, Brennan MF. Impact of therapeutic regional lymph node dissection for medullary carcinoma of the thyroid gland. Surgery. 1993;114:1078–81; discussion 81–2 United States.

Farrag TY, Agrawal N, Sheth S, Bettegowda C, Ewertz M, Kim M, et al. Algorithm for safe and effective reoperative thyroid bed surgery for recurrent/persistent papillary thyroid carcinoma. Head Neck. 2007;29(12):1069–74.

Gilliland FD, Hunt WC, Morris DM, Key CR. Prognostic factors for thyroid carcinoma. A population-based study of 15,698 cases from the Surveillance, Epidemiology and End Results (SEER) program 1973–1991. Cancer. 1997;79:564–73. United States.

Gimm O, Rath FW, Dralle H. Pattern of lymph node metastases in papillary thyroid carcinoma. Br J Surg. 1998;85(2):252–4.

Grebe SK, Hay ID. Thyroid cancer nodal metastases: biologic significance and therapeutic considerations. Surg Oncol Clin N Am. 1996;5(1):43–63.

Henry JF, Gramatica L, Denizot A, Kvachenyuk A, Puccini M, Defechereux T. Morbidity of prophylactic lymph node dissection in the central neck area in patients with papillary thyroid carcinoma. Langenbecks Arch Surg. 1998;383(2):167–9.

Hughes DT, Doherty GM. Central neck dissection for papillary thyroid cancer. Cancer Control. 2011;18(2): 83–8.

Hughes DT, White ML, Miller BS, Gauger PG, Burney RE, Doherty GM. Influence of prophylactic central lymph node dissection on postoperative thyroglobulin levels and radioiodine treatment in papillary thyroid cancer. Surgery. 2010;148:1100–6; discussion 006–7.

Kim MK, Mandel SH, Baloch Z, Livolsi VA, Langer JE, Didonato L, et al. Morbidity following central compartment reoperation for recurrent or persistent thyroid cancer. Arch Otolaryngol Head Neck Surg. 2004;130:1214–6. United States.

Kloos RT, Eng C, Evans DB, Francis GL, Gagel RF, Gharib H, et al. Medullary thyroid cancer: management guidelines of the American Thyroid Association. Thyroid. 2009;19(6):565–612.

Koo BS, Choi EC, Yoon YH, Kim DH, Kim EH, Lim YC. Predictive factors for ipsilateral or contralateral central lymph node metastasis in unilateral papillary thyroid carcinoma. Ann Surg. 2009;249(5):840–4.

Kouvaraki MA, Shapiro SE, Fornage BD, Edeiken-Monro BS, Sherman SI, Vassilopoulou-Sellin R, et al. Role of preoperative ultrasonography in the surgical management of patients with thyroid cancer. Surgery. 2003;134:946–54; discussion 54–5.

Machens A, Hinze R, Thomusch O, Dralle H. Pattern of nodal metastasis for primary and reoperative thyroid cancer. World J Surg. 2002;26(1):22–8.

Machens A, Holzhausen HJ, Dralle H. Skip metastases in thyroid cancer leaping the central lymph node compartment. Arch Surg. 2004;139:43–5. United States.

Martin H, Del Valle B, Ehrlich H, Cahan WG. Neck dissection. Cancer. 1951;4(3):441–99.

Mazzaferri EL. What is the optimal initial treatment of low-risk papillary thyroid cancer (and why is it controversial)? Oncology (Williston Park). 2009;23(7):579–88.

Mazzaferri EL, Jhiang SM. Long-term impact of initial surgical and medical therapy on papillary and follicular thyroid cancer. Am J Med. 1994;97:418–28. United States.

Mazzaferri EL, Doherty GM, Steward DL. The pros and cons of prophylactic central compartment lymph node dissection for papillary thyroid carcinoma. Thyroid. 2009;19(7):683–9.

Moley JF, DeBenedetti MK. Patterns of nodal metastases in palpable medullary thyroid carcinoma: recommendations for extent of node dissection. Ann Surg. 1999;229(6):880–7; discussion 7–8.

Moo TA, Umunna B, Kato M, Butriago D, Kundel A, Lee JA, et al. Ipsilateral versus bilateral central neck lymph node dissection in papillary thyroid carcinoma. Ann Surg. 2009;250(3):403–8.

Pereira JA, Jimeno J, Miquel J, Iglesias M, Munne A, Sancho JJ, et al. Nodal yield, morbidity, and recurrence after central neck dissection for papillary thyroid carcinoma. Surgery. 2005;138:1095–100; discussion 100–1 United States.

Roh JL, Park JY, Park CI. Total thyroidectomy plus neck dissection in differentiated papillary thyroid carcinoma patients: pattern of nodal metastasis, morbidity, recurrence, and postoperative levels of serum parathyroid hormone. Ann Surg. 2007;245:604–10. United States.

Roman S, Lin R, Sosa JA. Prognosis of medullary thyroid carcinoma: demographic, clinical, and pathologic predictors of survival in 1252 cases. Cancer. 2006; 107(9):2134–42.

Scheumann GF, Gimm O, Wegener G, Hundeshagen H, Dralle H. Prognostic significance and surgical management of locoregional lymph node metastases in papillary thyroid cancer. World J Surg. 1994;18(4):559–67; discussion 67–8.

Schuff KG, Weber SM, Givi B, Samuels MH, Andersen PE, Cohen JI. Efficacy of nodal dissection for treatment of persistent/recurrent papillary thyroid cancer. Laryngoscope. 2008;118(5):768–75.

Shindo M, Stern A. Total thyroidectomy with and without selective central compartment dissection: a comparison of complication rates. Arch Otolaryngol Head Neck Surg. 2010;136:584–7. United States.

Son YI, Jeong HS, Baek CH, Chung MK, Ryu J, Chung JH, et al. Extent of prophylactic lymph node dissection in the central neck area of the patients with papillary thyroid carcinoma: comparison of limited versus comprehensive lymph node dissection in a 2-year safety study. Ann Surg Oncol. 2008;15(7):2020–6.

Stulak JM, Grant CS, Farley DR, Thompson GB, van Heerden JA, Hay ID, et al. Value of preoperative ultrasonography in the surgical management of initial and reoperative papillary thyroid cancer. Arch Surg. 2006;141:489–94; discussion 94–6 United States.

Suarez O. El problema de las metastasis linfaticas y alejadas del cancer de laringe e hipofaringe. Rev Otorrinolaringol; 1963;23:83–99.

Sugitani I, Fujimoto Y, Yamada K, Yamamoto N. Prospective outcomes of selective lymph node dissection for papillary thyroid carcinoma based on preoperative ultrasonography. World J Surg. 2008;32(11): 2494–502.

Sywak M, Cornford L, Roach P, Stalberg P, Sidhu S, Delbridge L. Routine ipsilateral level VI lymphadenectomy reduces postoperative thyroglobulin levels in papillary thyroid cancer. Surgery. 2006;140:1000–5; discussion 5–7 United States.

Tisell LE, Nilsson B, Molne J, Hansson G, Fjalling M, Jansson S, et al. Improved survival of patients with papillary thyroid cancer after surgical microdissection. World J Surg. 1996;20(7):854–9.

Tufano RP, Kandil E. Considerations for personalized surgery in patients with papillary thyroid cancer. Thyroid. 2010;20(7):771–6.

Tufano RP, Bishop J, Wu G. Reoperative central compartment dissection for patients with recurrent/persistent papillary thyroid cancer: efficacy, safety, and the association of the BRAF mutation. Laryngoscope. 2012;122(7):1634–40.

Tuttle RM, Fagin JA. Can risk-adapted treatment recommendations replace the 'one size fits all' approach for early-stage thyroid cancer patients? Oncology (Williston Park). 2009;23(7):592, 600, 3.

White ML, Gauger PG, Doherty GM. Central lymph node dissection in differentiated thyroid cancer. World J Surg. 2007;31(5):895–904.

Zetoune T, Keutgen X, Buitrago D, Aldailami H, Shao H, Mazumdar M, et al. Prophylactic central neck dissection and local recurrence in papillary thyroid cancer: a meta-analysis. Ann Surg Oncol. 2010;17(12):3287–93.

12 Minimal Access Neck Dissection

C. Arturo Solares, J. Drew Prosser, Lana Jackson, and Carrie Bush

Introduction

Since the description of the systematic en bloc neck dissection by Crile in 1906, neck dissections have evolved to include functional and minimally invasive techniques. Evidence-based medicine has allowed for the adoption of the selective neck dissection in a number of circumstances. Furthermore, as the primary disease becomes better understood and life expectancies increase, cosmetic outcomes have become an increasing concern in patient care. While this remains secondary to oncologic outcomes, reducing the morbidity of neck dissections has become of great interest. When the primary operative purpose is as a staging procedure, the minimally invasive approach is particularly desirable.

In the 1990s Paolo Miccoli first described the minimally invasive video-assisted thyroidectomy (MIVAT), which represented one of the first successful attempts to bring minimally invasive surgery to the head and neck. Although this has become a mainstay in thyroid and parathyroid surgery, the minimally invasive neck dissection is still controversial.

C.A. Solares, MD (✉)
Department of Otolaryngology,
Department of Neurosurgery, Georgia Skull Base Center,
Georgia Health Sciences University, 1120 15th Street,
BP 4109, Augusta, GA 30912, USA
e-mail: CSOLARES@georgiahealth.edu

J.D. Prosser • L. Jackson, MD, PharmD • C. Bush, MD
Department of Otolaryngology, Georgia Regents
University, Augusta, GA, USA

Of interest, the endoscopic neck dissection has also become a source of much research, with successful small series presented in the literature. In 1996, the first use of endoscopes in head and neck surgery, for parathyroidectomy, was reported. Adoption of endoscopes in head and neck surgery has been slow, which is attributed to the number of vital structures, as well as the relatively confined space of the neck. However, there are now a number of reports that site success with endoscopic removal of the submandibular gland and branchial cleft cyst and with lateral neck dissections. At our institution we use a small (6 cm) incision for neck dissections that allows for equal access to all levels of the neck with appropriate retraction. This provides an optimal cosmetic outcome for the patient with equal oncologic outcomes.

In this chapter, we will highlight both our technique of the minimally invasive neck dissection (via a small incision) as well as some of the documented endoscopic techniques that are present in the literature. Of note, most recently, endoscopic techniques have been described using the robot to complete neck dissections.

Procedural Details

Minimal Access Neck Dissection

A 6-cm horizontal incision is marked on the neck, appropriately placed within a neck crease (Fig. 12.1). The incision is made and carried through the level of the platysma muscle.

D.J. Terris, M.C. Singer (eds.), *Minimally Invasive and Robotic Thyroid and Parathyroid Surgery*, DOI 10.1007/978-1-4614-9011-1_12, © Springer Science+Business Media New York 2014

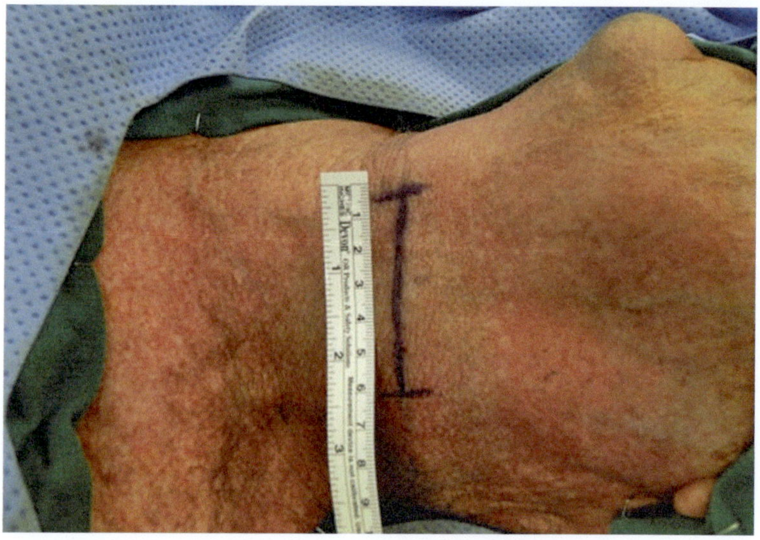

Fig. 12.1 A 6-cm incision site is marked within a horizontal neck crease

Subplatysmal flaps are then elevated. Inferiorly the flap is carried to the level of the clavicle. Superiorly the flap is elevated to the level of the submandibular gland. As the incision is limited, in order to obtain adequate exposure, flaps must be developed laterally beyond the border of the sternocleidomastoid muscle (SCM) and medially to the midline of the neck.

At this point the fascia overlying the submandibular gland is incised at the most inferior aspect of the gland. The fascia is then bluntly elevated from the underlying submandibular gland to allow for preservation of the marginal mandibular nerve. If level I of the neck warrants dissection based on pathology, then the submandibular gland and remainder of the level I contents of the neck are excised. If level I does not warrant dissection, then the submandibular gland is elevated and lifted with the superior flap to allow for identification of the digastric muscle and hypoglossal nerve.

This "minimal access" form of neck dissection commences in the traditional fashion of selective neck dissection. However, as the incision is small and typically at the inferior aspect of the dissection, focus is placed on sequential retraction to allow for adequate visualization of all aspects of the neck. Initially, static retraction is placed at four points with the use of tapered hooks or silk sutures. Dynamic retraction is then applied as needed throughout the case to visualize the borders of the neck dissection. This may be accomplished with use of Army-Navy retractors, as well as appendiceal retractors in the deeper portions of the neck.

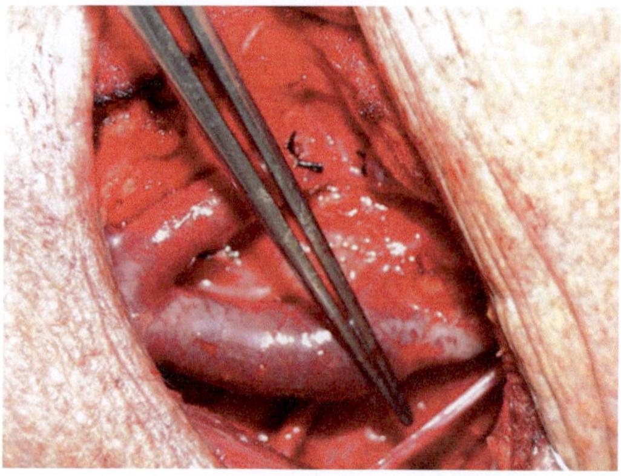

Fig. 12.2 With use of retraction, a left-sided accessory nerve is easily identified and preserved. The forceps indicate the nerve. Dynamic retraction allows for visualization of the neck from the level of the digastric muscle to the clavicle

Once the digastric muscle has been identified, it is traced laterally to the medial border of the SCM. The fascia overlying the SCM is then excised, and the SCM is rotated laterally. The omohyoid is identified and retracted inferiorly to allow for visualization of the level 4 contents of the neck. The accessory nerve is identified to allow for careful preservation (Fig. 12.2). The level IIb through V contents of the neck may then be unrolled from the muscular floor of the neck and carotid sheath in the standard surgical fashion.

Other Techniques

Endoscopic Neck Dissection

As the endoscopic neck dissection is still a matter of study, there has yet to be an established standard. Methods include both gas insufflation techniques and endoscopic-assisted techniques that rely on retraction to maintain the operative space. A few of the described methods will be highlighted in this section.

Gas Insufflation Technique

The gas insufflation technique has been described for performing selective neck dissections and submandibular gland resections. This approach is in the development phase, but the central components of this technique have been defined. The incisions for the camera and operative ports are marked and injected with local anesthetic. A 14 mm incision for the operative port is then made. With use of a blunt trocar, a subplatysmal tunnel is created. A surgical balloon is then inserted through this tunnel and inflated to 300–500 ml while monitoring the patient's heart rate and blood pressure. The surgical balloon bluntly creates space for the gas insufflation. The balloon is then removed and a 10–12 mm trocar is inserted. This serves as the port for a 10 mm, 0° endoscope. CO_2 insufflation at 4 mmHg is then provided. The operative ports are then established by making 7 mm incisions and placing spring-loaded, bladed trocars under endoscopic visualization.

Once visualization is achieved with the endoscope, the steps of the procedure follow those of conventional, open surgery (Fig. 12.3). Grasping instruments are used in the nondominant hand and cutting instruments are controlled by the dominant hand. An assistant holds the camera. Advanced energy devices or clips may be used for ligation of blood vessels. Once the tissue has

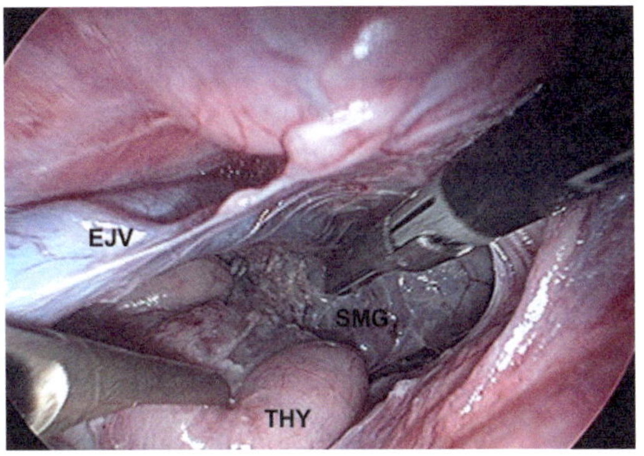

Fig. 12.3 Endoscopic view of the porcine neck immediately after insufflation. (*EJV*) external jugular vein, (*THY*) thymus, (*SMG*) submandibular gland

been dissected, it is retrieved through the larger camera port incision. This retrieval is completed under direct visualization provided by a 5 mm endoscope placed through an operative port.

Minimal Access Video-Assisted Functional Lateral Neck Dissection

The video-assisted approach to lateral neck dissection was described by Lombardi et al. in 2007 and applied to patients with metastatic papillary thyroid carcinoma. This approach is an extended version of MIVAT. In order to facilitate the extended dissection, a 4-cm central incision is made. In these patients a total thyroidectomy and central compartment dissection was completed utilizing the standard MIVAT technique. The endoscope is then used to aid in dissection of levels II–IV, as well as part as level V of the neck.

Outcomes

At our institution we performed a quality control study to assure adequate oncologic outcome with the minimal access neck dissection. In this study we compared results of lateral neck dissections (levels II–IV) performed by two different surgeons, one who uses the minimal access technique and a second who uses the conventional hockey-stick incision. A total of 58 patients were included. No statistical difference was found in the number of nodes removed by the two techniques. An average of 27 nodes were removed by the minimal access technique and an average of 26 with the conventional technique ($p = 0.34$) (Solares et al.). No complications occurred in either group.

With the video-assisted technique, Lombardi et al. achieved comparable oncologic outcomes, with a total of 25 lymph nodes removed on average. They also experienced no major complications. There is also data supporting the safety and efficacy of the video-assisted approach for central neck dissection in patients with thyroid carcinoma.

Conclusion

The goal of minimal access neck dissection is to achieve the same oncologic outcomes of conventional neck dissection while minimizing morbidity and improving the cosmetic outcomes of the procedure. There continues to be a lack of literature devoted to the topic. Use of these techniques clearly allows for smaller incisions. Theoretically, decreased tissue trauma and manipulation could also result in less postoperative pain and faster recovery times. Initial efforts with minimally invasive neck dissections have been promising, and continued efforts should be made to further refine these techniques.

Recommended Reading

Dulguerov P, Leuchter I, Szalay-Quinodoz I, Allal AS, Marchal F, Lehmann W, Fasel JH. Endoscopic neck dissection in human cadavers. Laryngoscope. 2001;111(12):2135–9.

Gagner M. Endoscopic subtotal parathyroidectomy in patients with primary hyperparathyroidism. Br J Surg. 1996;83(6):875.

Guerrissi JO. Innovation and surgical techniques: endoscopic resection of cervical branchiogenic cysts. J Craniofac Surg. 2002;13(3):478–82.

Kang SW, Lee SH, Ryu HR, Lee KY, Jeong JJ, Nam KH, Chung WY, Park CS. Initial experience with robot-assisted modified radical neck dissection for the management of thyroid carcinoma with lateral neck node metastasis. Surgery. 2010;148(6):1214–21.

Kang SW, Lee SH, Park JH, Jeong JS, Park S, Lee CR, Jeong JJ, Nam KH, Chung WY, Park CS. A comparative study of the surgical outcomes of robotic and conventional open modified radical neck dissection for papillary thyroid carcinoma with lateral neck node metastasis. Surg Endosc. 2012;26(11):3251–7.

Lombardi CP, Raffaelli M, Princi P, De Crea C, Bellantone R. Minimally invasive video-assisted functional lateral neck dissection for metastatic papillary thyroid carcinoma. Am J Surg. 2007;193(1):114–8.

Miccoli P, Berti P, Ambrosini CE. Perspectives and lessons learned after a decade of minimally invasive video-assisted thyroidectomy. ORL J Otorhinolaryngol Relat Spec. 2008;70(5):282–6.

Neidich MJ, Steward DL. Safety and feasibility of elective minimally invasive video-assisted central neck dissection for thyroid carcinoma. Head Neck. 2012;34(3):354–8.

Terris DJ, Monfared A, Thomas A, Kambham N, Sáenz Y. Endoscopic selective neck dissection in a porcine model. Arch Otolaryngol Head Neck Surg. 2003;129(6):613–7.

Terris DJ, Haus BM, Gourin CG. Endoscopic neck surgery: resection of the submandibular gland in a cadaver model. Laryngoscope. 2004;114(3):407–10.

Terris DJ, Haus BM, Gourin CG, Lilagan PE. Endo-robotic resection of the submandibular gland in a cadaver model. Head Neck. 2005;27(11):946–51.

Werner JA, Sapundzhiev NR, Teymoortash A, Dünne AA, Behr T, Folz BJ. Endoscopic sentinel lymphadenectomy as a new diagnostic approach in the N0 neck. Eur Arch Otorhinolaryngol. 2004;261(9):463–8.

Robot-Assisted Neck Dissection in Papillary Thyroid Carcinoma

13

Yoon Woo Koh and Eun Chang Choi

Introduction

Cervical lymph node metastases outside the central compartment are not uncommon in the management of papillary thyroid carcinoma (PTC). The papillary thyroid carcinoma (PTC) with lateral neck metastasis (LNM) has been treated with total thyroidectomy and lateral neck dissection through the anterior transverse or J-shaped incision to secure an enough surgical field. Since the advent of robotic surgical systems, some have adopted the concept of remote access surgery into developing various robotic thyroidectomy techniques. The more former and widely acknowledged robotic thyroidectomy technique uses a transaxillary (TA) approach which has been developed by Chung et al. in Korea. This particular technique though has some limitations in the sense that accessing the lymph nodes of the central compartment is troublesome. Terris et al. realized some shortcomings of robotic TA thyroidectomy especially in their patients in the United States and developed and reported the feasibility of robotic facelift thyroidectomy.

In cases of thyroid carcinomas with lateral neck node metastases, most abandoned the concept of minimally invasive or remote access surgery and safely adopted conventional open surgical methods to remove the tumor burden. However, Chung et al. have attempted to perform concomitant modified radical neck dissection (MRND) after robotic thyroidectomy through the same TA port. This type of robot-assisted neck dissection (RAND), however, had some inherent limitations due to fact that lymph nodes of the upper neck were difficult to remove. We previously assessed the difficulty of dissecting level II via the TA approach in a cadaveric study. According to studies examining the pattern of nodal metastasis in PTC, the incidence of metastatic disease in level II ranges from 52 to 72.2 %. These sizeable figures prompted us to devise a modified approach called the transaxillary and retroauricular (TARA) approach, which was shown to be feasible for the management of nodal metastasis in head and neck cancer (HNC). With the accumulation of experience with the TARA approach, we realized that the retroauricular (RA) or modified facelift (MFL) approach is sufficient for RAND in HNC. Over the past few years, we have developed a RAND via RA or MFL approach and reported the feasibility and safety of this technique. Based on our surgical experiences, we could eventually adopt this particular technique to robotic total thyroidectomy and also MRND where needed. This chapter introduces the specific operative technique, simultaneous robotic

Y.W. Koh, MD, PhD (✉) • E.C. Choi
Department of Otorhinolaryngology,
Yonsei University College of Medicine,
Severance Hospital, Yonsei University Health System,
50 Yonsei-ro, Seodaemun-gu, Seoul
120-752, Republic of Korea
e-mail: ywkohent@yuhs.ac

D.J. Terris, M.C. Singer (eds.), *Minimally Invasive and Robotic Thyroid and Parathyroid Surgery*,
DOI 10.1007/978-1-4614-9011-1_13, © Springer Science+Business Media New York 2014

total thyroidectomy, and RAND via TARA or RA approach in detail.

Indications

1. Patients with biopsy-proven lateral lymph node metastasis of the papillary thyroid carcinoma
2. Lymph node metastasis with residual nodal architecture (extracapsular extension (ECE) under grade 3 in the grading system of Lewis et al.)
3. Patients eligible for robotic surgery and who are willing to receive the operation after having been informed of certain disadvantages including high medical costs

Contraindications

1. Recurrent thyroid papillary carcinoma
2. Suspicious severe extracapsular spread of the metastatic lymph node (e.g., carotid encasement) on preoperative imaging
3. Thyroid carcinomas with gross invasion to local structures or extrathyroidal capsular
4. Patients with past history of neck surgery of any kind

Surgical Anatomy

The surgical anatomy which the surgeon needs to be familiar of is similar to all other endoscopic or robotic neck surgeries utilizing the TA and RA approach.

To elevate the skin flap from the axillary skin incision, surgeon should be well informed of the anatomy of platysma muscle and sternocleidomastoid muscle and the structures of level V area (external jugular vein, brachial plexus) located just below the muscle. Knowledge of the surgical anatomy required for RAND via TA approach is quite different from that of conventional technique. After skin incision is made in the axilla, the axilla to the anterior neck area is dissected over the anterior surface of the pectoralis major muscle and clavicle under direct vision. At that time, great care should be taken not to injure the brachial plexus, which lies deep in the axillary fossa. After exposing the medial border of the sternocleidomastoid muscle, the avascular space between the sternal and clavicular heads should be identified and dissection should be continued through the space.

To elevate the skin flap from the retroauricular skin incision, the operator would encounter the sternocleidomastoid (SCM) muscle first when elevating the skin flap and continuing the flap elevation through the subplatysmal plane just as in conventional thyroidectomy or neck dissection, the great auricular nerve and the external jugular vein would come into view. On the contrary to the TA approach, the operation is executed from superior to inferior direction, so try to picture in mind the local anatomical structures which would be encountered according to this fashion. Remember that the upper portion of the larynx would be found first before localizing the superior portion of the thyroid and that the great vessels of the carotid sheath would be brought into view first before localizing the lateral border of the ipsilateral thyroid gland and the recurrent laryngeal nerve (RLN). If the RAND is performed as well, bear in mind also that the neck dissection is being progressed from the posterior direction. The parotid tail, the retromandibular vein, the posterior belly of digastric muscle, and the spinal accessory nerve can be sequentially visualized, and the contour of the submandibular gland can be identified at the anterior portion of the working space.

Instrumentations

Retractors to Secure the Skin Flap

- Army-Navy retractor
- Right angle "breast" retractor
- Self-retaining retractor: original Chung's retractor and new one modified from Chung's retractor which was originally made for transaxillary robotic thyroidectomy (Sangdosa Inc., Seoul, Korea) (Fig. 13.1a)
- Codman® GREENBERG Universal Retractor

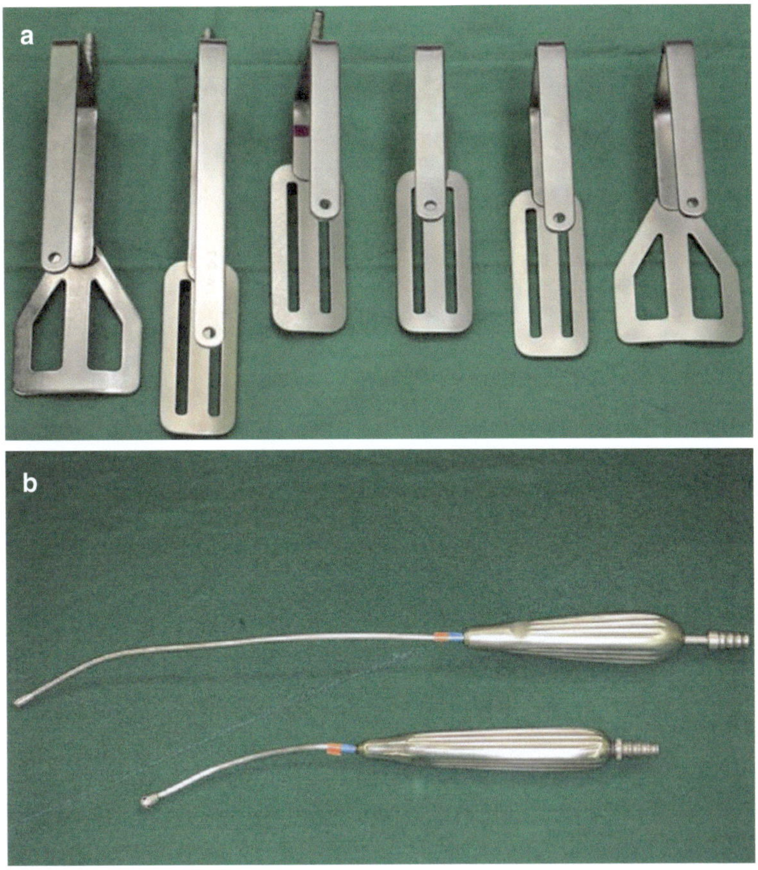

Fig. 13.1 Self-retaining retractors and Yankauer suctions. (**a**) Two retractors which are located on the left side had already been developed by Professor Chung for robotic thyroidectomy via a transaxillary approach. Remaining four retractors were invented by Professor Koh for robot-assisted neck dissection via a modified facelift or retroauricular approaches. (**b**) A long Yankauer suction which is located on the superior side devised for robot-assisted neck dissection

Robotic Instruments (da Vinci Robotic System – Intuitive Surgical Inc., Sunnyvale, CA)

- 12 mm, 30° face-down dual-channel endoscope (Intuitive Surgical Inc., Sunnyvale, CA)
- 5 mm, Maryland forceps (Intuitive Surgical Inc., Sunnyvale, CA)
- 5 mm, Harmonic curved shears (Intuitive Surgical Inc., Sunnyvale, CA)
- 8 mm, ProGrasp forceps (Intuitive Surgical Inc., Sunnyvale, CA)

Other Instruments to Facilitate Surgical Process

- Bovie tip (electrocautery tip): conventional size of spatula type and also additional tips which progressively lengthens
- Hemoclip or Hem-o-lok® (Teleflex Inc., NC, USA): for ligating uncontrollable vessels such as branches of the internal jugular vein
- Yankauer suction (Fig. 13.1b)

Operative Technique

Robot-Assisted Modified Radical Neck Dissection of Levels II–V via Transaxillary and Retroauricular (TARA) Approach

Step 1. Positioning of the Patient and Skin Flap Elevation

After general anesthesia, the patient is positioned supine with the head rotated to the contralateral side of the dissection. The operation can be greatly facilitated if the neck is relaxed by natural placement and not extended. A retroauricular

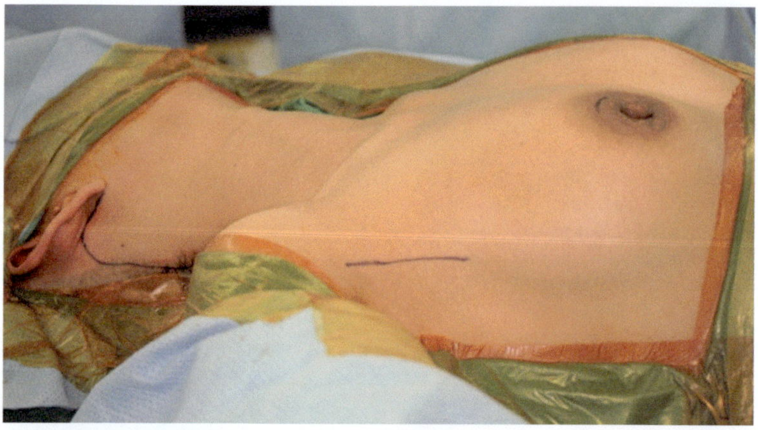

Fig. 13.2 Patient's position and skin incision design. The patient is placed in the supine position without neck extension and the patient's head is slightly rotated to contralateral side. A retroauricular incision is made around the retroauricular sulcus and along the hairline

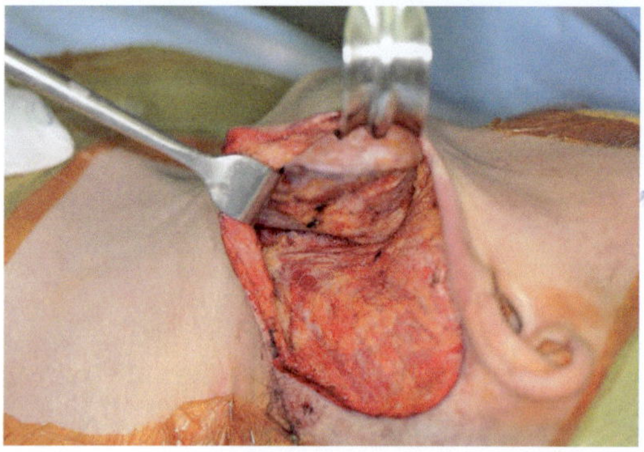

Fig. 13.3 Creating a working space. Then subplatysmal flap is elevated medially over the midline, inferiorly to the clavicle, and laterally to the anterior border of the trapezius muscle. The external jugular vein and greater auricular nerve are landmarks for subplatysmal flap elevation

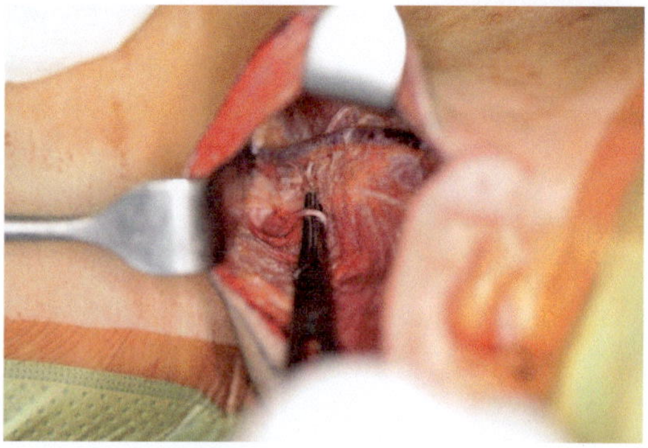

Fig. 13.4 Identification of the spinal accessory nerve. The trapezius branch of the spinal accessory nerve is identified about 1 cm lower than the point where the greater auricular nerve crosses the posterior border of the sternocleidomastoid muscle

incision is made around the retroauricular sulcus and along the hairline. The design for the skin incision is similar to the MFL incision for parotidectomy, but without the preauricular limb (Fig. 13.2). Sufficient skin flap elevation is mandatory for adequate working space creation. After skin incision, subplatysmal flaps are elevated above the SCM muscle preserving the external jugular vein and great auricular nerve (Fig. 13.3). The sub-SMAS (superficial musculoaponeurotic system) flap elevation should be performed until the platysma muscle is met. Then the subplatysmal flap is elevated medially over the midline, inferiorly to the clavicle, and laterally to the anterior border of the trapezius muscle (Fig. 13.3). After the flap elevation is performed, modified Chung's retractor (Sangdosa Inc., Seoul, Korea) is placed to maintain the working space.

Step 2. Upper Neck Dissection Using Conventional Technique Under Direct Vision via Retroauricular Approach (Level IIA, IIB, and VA Dissection)

For the management of the papillary thyroid carcinoma with lateral neck metastasis, level II–V dissection is performed sparing level I. The inferior border of the submandibular gland is dissected and the posterior belly of the digastric muscle is identified. The inferior border of the parotid gland is dissected and retracted superiorly. The spinal accessory nerve (SAN) is sought near the internal jugular vein (IJV) using the transverse process of the second cervical spine as a landmark. The trapezius branch of the SAN is identified about 1 cm lower than the point where the greater auricular nerve crosses the posterior border of the sternocleidomastoid (SCM)

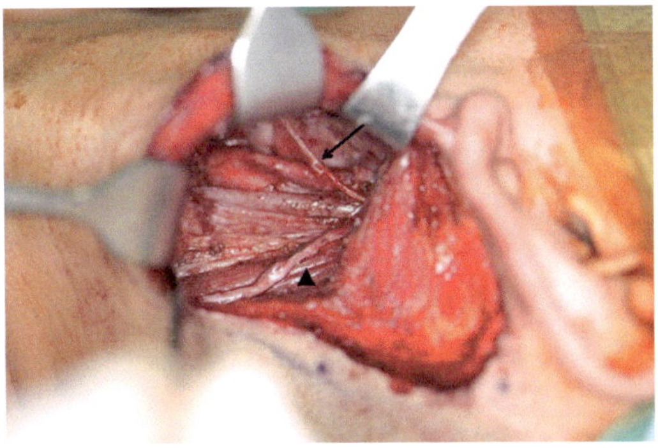

Fig. 13.5 Elevation of the sternocleidomastoid (SCM) muscle. The SCM is skeletonized and elevated using Army-Navy retractors. With the preservation of both the SCM muscle branch (*arrow*) and the trapezius branch (*arrowhead*), the whole course of the spinal accessory nerve is identified

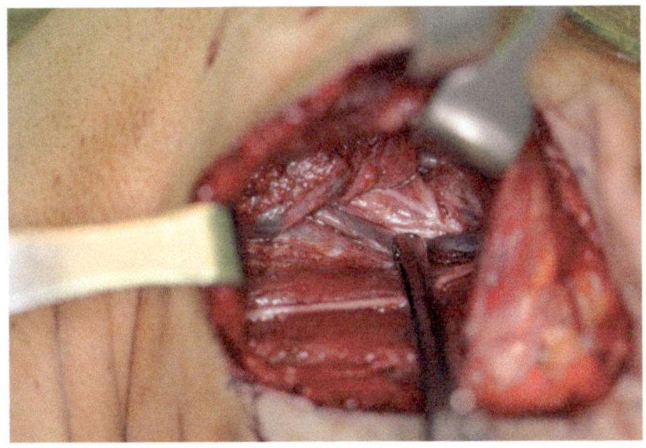

Fig. 13.6 The completion of upper neck dissection. The lymphofatty tissues in level II and upper III are then dissected carefully not to damage the internal jugular vein or the carotid artery

muscle (Fig. 13.4). With the preservation of both the sternocleidomastoid (SCM) muscle branch and the trapezius branch, the whole course of the SAN is identified (Fig. 13.5). The SCM is skeletonized and elevated using Army-Navy retractors. The adipose tissues in levels IIB and VA are dissected and passed underneath the SAN, and the lymphofatty tissues in level IIA are then dissected carefully not to damage the IJV or the carotid artery (Fig. 13.6). The upper portion of level III can be also done under direct vision using conventional technique.

Step 3. Lower Neck Dissection Using Robotic Surgical System (Level III, IV, and VB Dissection) via Transaxillary Approach

The approach from the axilla may be unfamiliar with most of head and neck surgeon. The operator will see the fat tissues immediately after incision in the anterior axillary line. With no guidance of plane, the operator may have hard times to find the pectoralis major fascia. After that, the dissection for the transaxillary flap elevation can be proceeded relatively quickly over the fascia of the pectoralis major muscle. The next obstacle is the clavicle. From the view point of axilla to neck, the clavicular head of the SCM muscle can be met after crossing over the clavicular eminence. Previously formed working space from the retroauricular approach can be reached from the

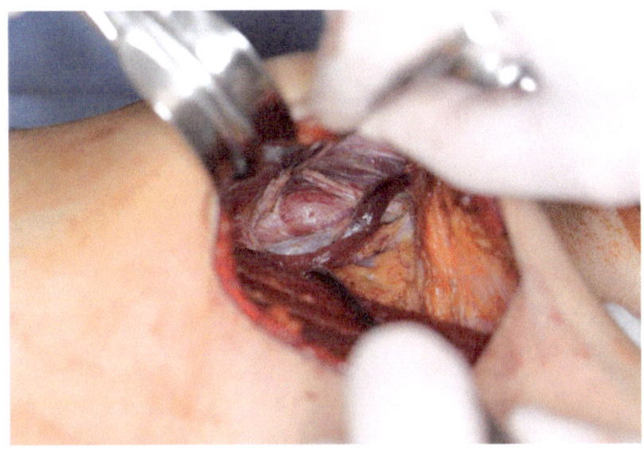

Fig. 13.7 Making a working space from the transaxillary incision. Previously formed working space from the retroauricular approach can be reached also from the transaxillary approach. The thyroid gland can be visualized after the elevation of the strap muscles

transaxillary approach (Fig. 13.7). After finishing the flap elevation, self-retaining retractor (Chung's retractor) is inserted through the axillary incision and is fixed firmly to the operation table. A face-down 30° endoscope is used for visualization of the surgical field. A 5 mm Maryland forceps and 5 mm Harmonic curved shears are equipped on either side of the endoscope (Fig. 13.8). The lower neck dissection procedure is started at levels IV and VB. With the preservation of the SAN, the inferior margin of the adipose tissues at level VB is dissected (Fig. 13.9). The omohyoid muscle is identified and cut using Harmonic curved shears. The brachial plexus and the phrenic nerve are identified beneath the fascial carpet and the transverse cervical vessels (Fig. 13.10). In level IV dissection, the transverse cervical artery and

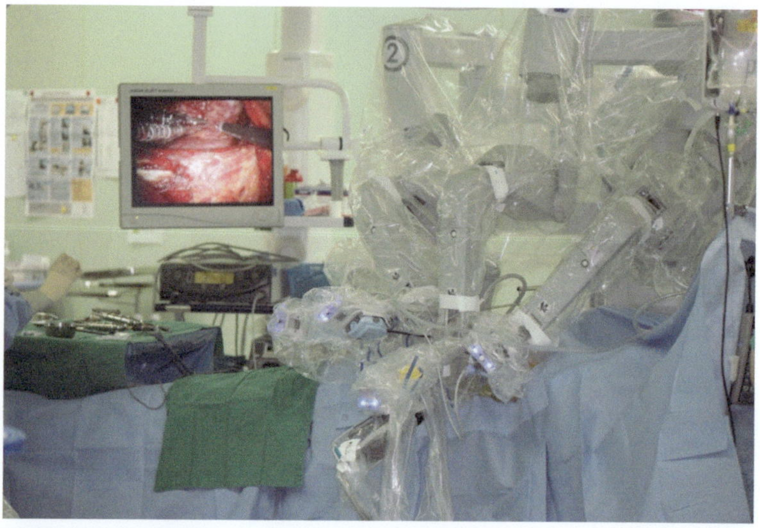

Fig. 13.8 Docking of robotic surgical system. A face-down 30° endoscope is used for visualization of the surgical field. A 5 mm Maryland forceps and 5 mm Harmonic curved shears are equipped on either side of the endoscope

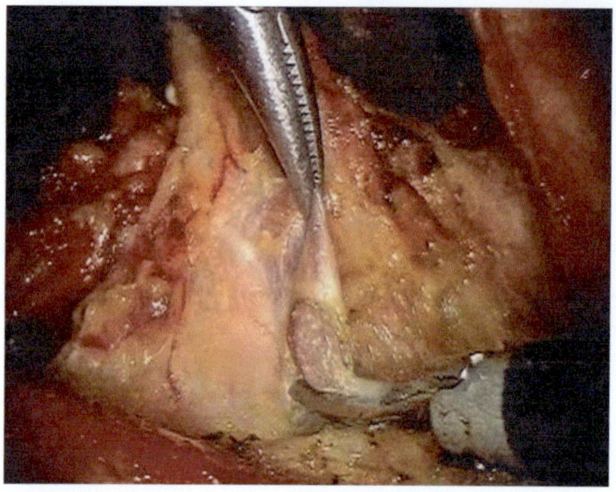

Fig. 13.9 Robot-assisted lower neck dissection. With the preservation of the pre-identified spinal accessory nerve, the inferior margin of the adipose tissues at level VB is dissected

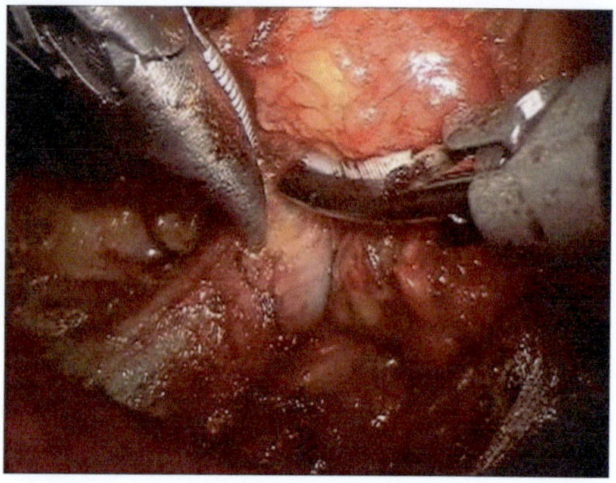

Fig. 13.11 Level IV dissection. Carotid sheath dissection is carried out using Harmonic curved shears with great caution, and the vagus nerve, carotid artery, and internal jugular vein are exposed in level IV

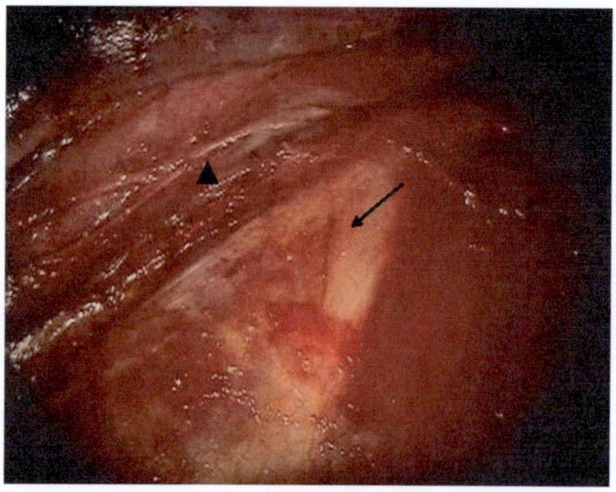

Fig. 13.10 Brachial plexus and phrenic nerve. The brachial plexus (*arrow*) and the phrenic nerve (*arrowhead*) are identified beneath the fascial carpet and the transverse cervical vessels

vein are verified and the phrenic nerve is preserved. Carotid sheath dissection is carried out using Harmonic curved shears with great caution, and the vagus nerve, carotid artery, and IJV are exposed in level IV (Fig. 13.11). The management of the thoracic or lymphatic duct is very important. For the prevention of chyle leakage, the sealing of the thoracic or lymphatic duct with the Harmonic curved shears is not enough. Those structures should be ligated with vessel clips or Hem-o-lok ligation system. Lymphofatty tissue in level Vb is dissected with the previously dissected level Va. Cervical plexus is ligated with the Harmonic curved shears (Fig. 13.12). The inferior-to-superior dissection over level III can be performed along the carotid sheath and internal

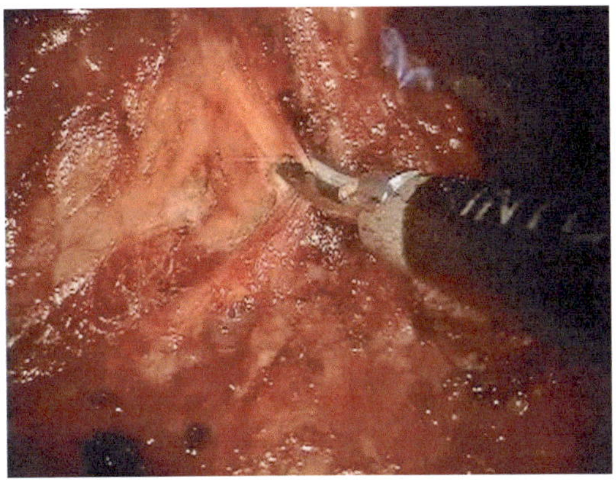

Fig. 13.12 Cervical plexus ligation. Cervical plexus is ligated with the Harmonic curved shears

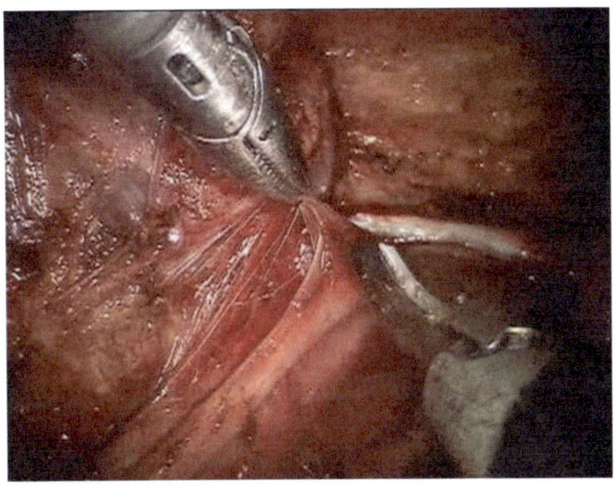

Fig. 13.13 The dissections over levels III and IIa. The inferior-to-superior dissection over level III can be performed along the carotid sheath and internal jugular chain. The previously dissected specimen of level IIb is positioned medially, and the level IIa node dissection is performed in an inferior-to-superior fashion

jugular chain. The superior thyroid artery anterior to the carotid sheath is identified and preserved. After level III dissection, the axis of the robotic arms is realigned upward for level II dissection. The previously dissected specimen of level IIb is positioned medially, and the level IIa node dissection is performed in an inferior-to-superior fashion (Fig. 13.13). Careful dissection should be performed to identify the hypoglossal nerve in the area of the carotid artery bifurcation. The superior thyroid artery is identified close to the external carotid artery. With previously dissected upper neck dissection specimen, the whole neck dissection specimen is pulled out through the transaxillary incision (Figs. 13.14 and 13.15).

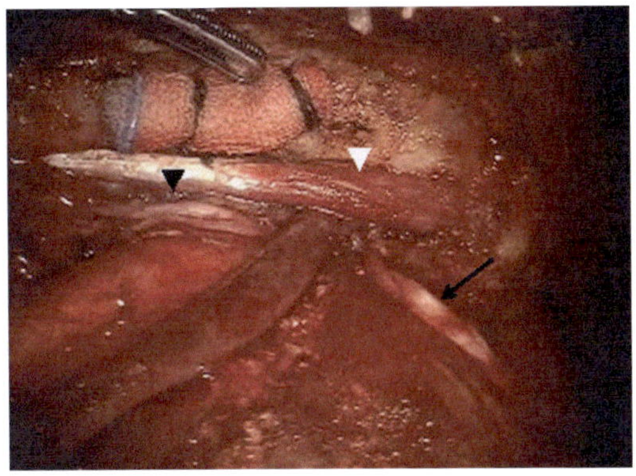

Fig. 13.14 Surgical field after specimen extraction. The posterior belly of digastric muscle (*white arrowhead*) was identified. The spinal accessory nerve (*arrow*) and the hypoglossal nerve (*black arrowhead*) were also preserved

Step 4. Robotic Total Thyroidectomy
Robotic modified neck dissection via TARA approach is followed by ipsilateral thyroidectomy with central compartment neck dissection (CCND) via the same approach. Finally, contralateral thyroidectomy with CCND is carried out via TARA approach.

Robot-Assisted Modified Radical Neck Dissection of Levels II–V via Retroauricular Approach

Step 1. Positioning of the Patient
Under general anesthesia, patient is placed in supine position on the surgical bed. The operation can be greatly facilitated if the neck is relaxed by natural placement and not extended. When RAND is performed simultaneously, the patient's neck can be extended at times to aid the process of lower neck dissection (Fig. 13.16).

Step 2. Skin Incision Design
A retroauricular incision is designed to perform level II–V dissection through single skin incision (Fig. 13.16). The design for the skin incision is similar to the MFL incision for parotidectomy, but without the preauricular limb. The RA incision is designed around the origin of the earlobe and along the RA sulcus and the hairline. At about the level of the tragus, it is extended posteriorly and then curved towards occipital direction

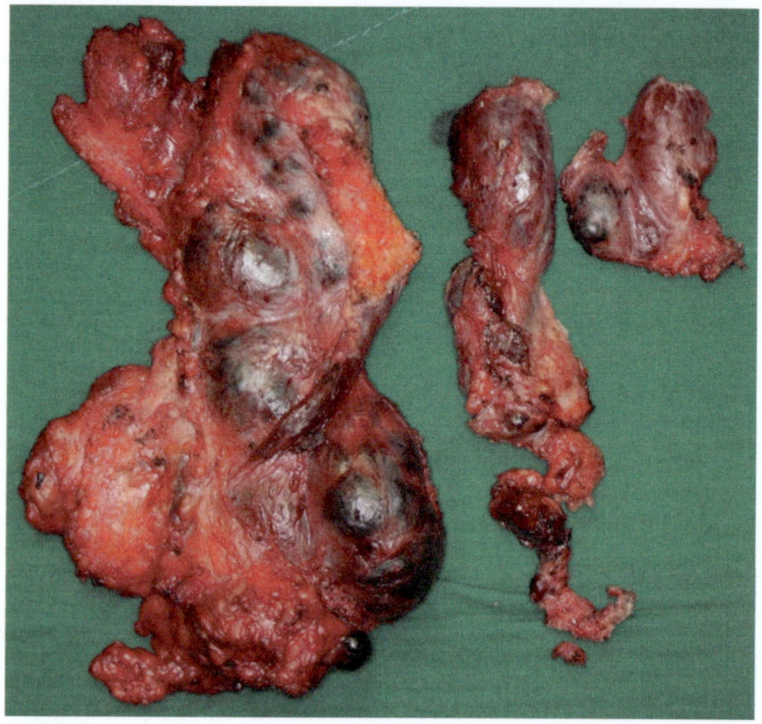

Fig. 13.15 Specimen. The neck specimen has multiple gross metastases. Both lobes of the thyroid gland and the lymph nodes in the central compartment have gross lesions

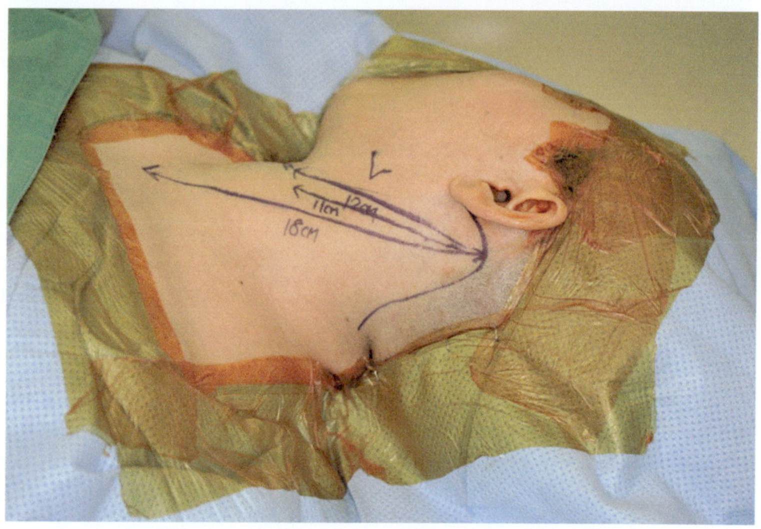

Fig. 13.16 Patient's position and skin incision. The actual distances from the entry of the retroauricular port to the ipsilateral thyroid gland and the sternal notch (the lowest limit of the modified radical neck dissection procedure) have been each shown for reference

below the hairline. Local anesthetic material is injected on the skin incision line. To make the exact and easy approximation of skin incision after the completion of operation, ink tattooing can be used.

Step 3. Skin Flap Elevation

Sufficient skin flap elevation is mandatory for adequate working space creation. After skin incision, subplatysmal flaps are elevated above the SCM muscle preserving the external jugular vein

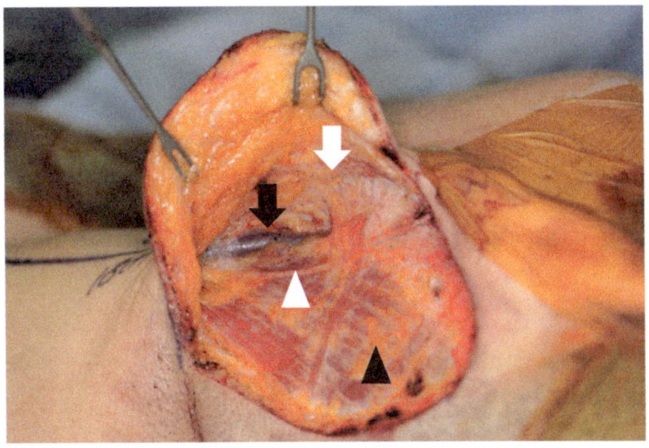

Fig. 13.17 Skin flap elevation. The skin flap is elevated along the subplatysmal plane preserving the external jugular vein and great auricular nerve (platysma muscle, *white arrow*; external jugular vein, *black arrow*; greater auricular nerve, *white arrowhead*; sternocleidomastoid muscle, *black arrowhead*)

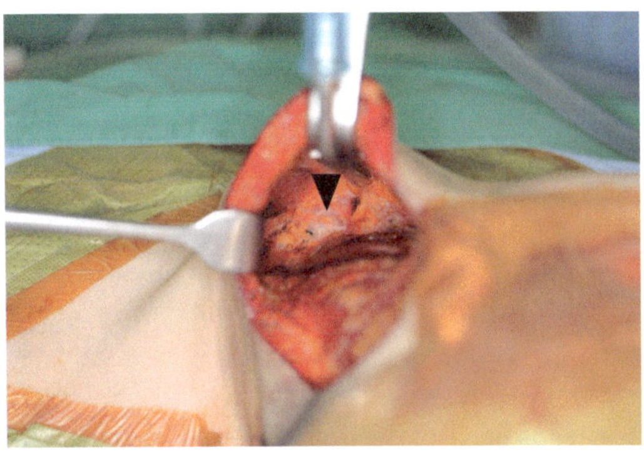

Fig. 13.18 Setting up the self-retaining retractor. The skin flap is elevated to create adequate working space so that the lowest extent reaches the sternal notch. When sufficient working space is acquired, a self-retaining retractor is applied (clavicle: *black arrowhead*)

and great auricular nerve (Fig. 13.17). After reaching the anterior portion of the neck, the skin flap is elevated along the subplatysmal plane to the midline anteriorly, to the inferior border of the mandible superiorly, and to the clavicle inferiorly (Fig. 13.18). During this step, the procedure can be aided with the retractors held by an assistant surgeon. Assistants pull the skin flap upward using Army-Navy retractor and right-angled retractor and the surgeon pushes the sternocleidomastoid muscle (SCM) downward using Yankauer

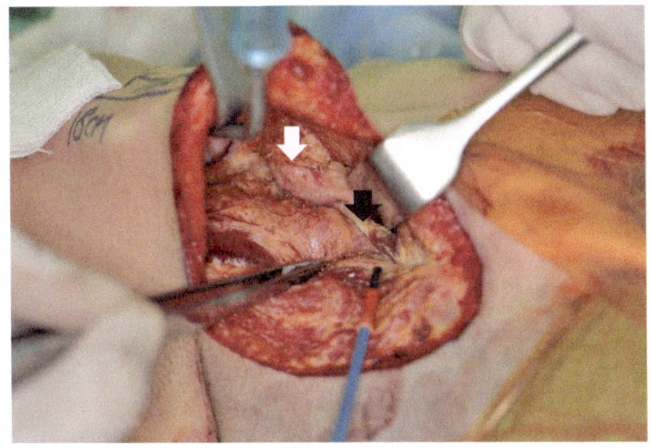

Fig. 13.19 Identifying of the proximal portion of the spinal accessory nerve (submandibular gland, *white arrowhead*; posterior belly of digastric muscle, *black arrowhead*)

suction and Cushing forceps. Subplatysmal skin flap is elevated inferiorly to the level of clavicle. When sufficient working space is acquired, a self-retaining retractor (Sangdosa Inc., Seoul, Korea) is applied (Fig. 13.18).

Step 4. Upper Neck Dissection Using Conventional Technique Under Direct Vision via Retroauricular Approach (Level IIA, IIB, and VA Dissection)

Upper neck levels such as IIB, IIA, or VA can be dissected under direct vision using conventional instruments according to a kind of neck dissection. Dissection proceeds along the inferior border of the submandibular gland using standard surgical instruments under naked eye. After identifying the posterior belly of the digastric muscle and internal jugular vein, the proximal portion of the spinal accessory nerve is identified near the IJV with the transverse process of atlas as a landmark (Fig. 13.19). As we approach level IIb through retroauricular approach, the exposure of level IIb can be obtained easily. Then, the fascia is opened along the posterior border of SCM and the SCM is pulled upwardly by using Army-Navy retractor. Fibrofatty tissues are dissected from the medial side of SCM (Fig. 13.20).

Step 5. Docking of the Robotic Arms

A dual-channel 30° endoscope was placed on the central camera arm of the robotic system and inserted in an upward direction. Maryland forceps and Harmonic curved shears were placed on either side of the camera (Fig. 13.21). Lower skin flap can be easily retracted laterally using GREENBERG Universal Retractor. One assistant surgeon and one nurse are located beside the patient's head. The assistant surgeon sucks out the blood from the operative field during the operation and ligates vessels using Hemoclip or Hem-o-lok®.

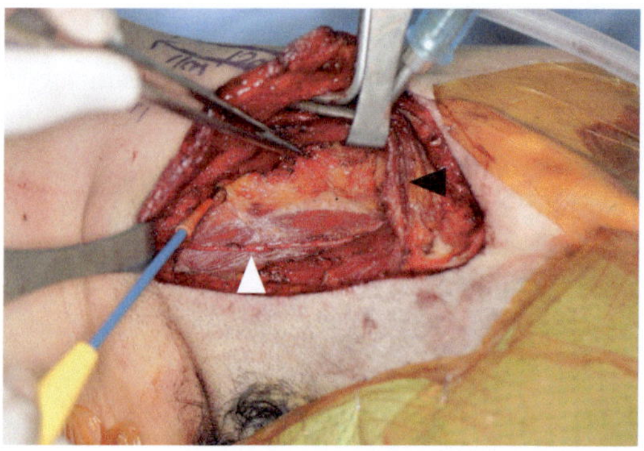

Fig. 13.20 Opening the fascia along the posterior border of SCM. SCM is pulled upwardly by using Army-Navy retractor. Fibrofatty tissues are dissected from the medial side of SCM (sternocleidomastoid muscle, *black arrowhead*; spinal accessory nerve, *white arrowhead*)

Step 6. Lower Neck Dissection Using Robotic System via Retroauricular Approach (Level IIII, IV, and VB Dissection)

Level III is dissected in the direction of superior to inferior by using robotic system. The dissection was performed over the carotid sheath and extended to levels IV and VB. During the level III and IV dissection, fibrofatty tissue is dissected from internal jugular vein by using Harmonic curved shear (Fig. 13.22). The small branches of the IJV are ligated with Harmonic curved shears, whereas the large ones are ligated with a Hem-o-lok ligation system by an assistant. It is easy to dissect level V area because the subplatysmal flap and sternocleidomastoid muscle are elevated upwardly. Dissection proceeds from posterior portion to anterior portion, identifying and preserving the transcervical artery, the brachial plexus, and the phrenic nerve located on the floor of level V (Figs. 13.23 and 13.24). Then, level IV dissection is conducted after medial retraction of the specimen (Fig. 13.25). The lymphatic or thoracic duct should be ligated by using Hemoclip or Hem-o-lok® (Fig. 13.26).

Step 7. Robotic Total Thyroidectomy

First, RAND through the RA incision is followed by ipsilateral thyroidectomy with central compartment neck dissection (CCND) via the same approach. Finally, contralateral thyroidectomy with CCND is carried out via the single RA port.

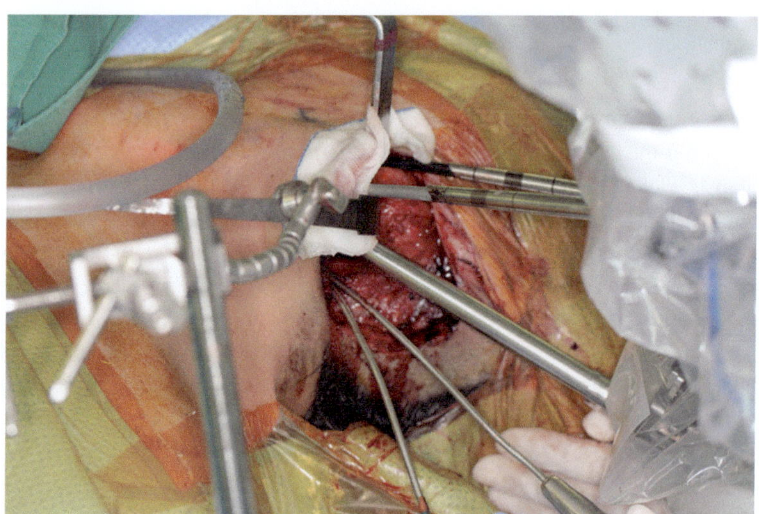

Fig. 13.21 Docking of robotic arms. Lower skin flap can be easily retracted laterally using GREENBERG Universal Retractor

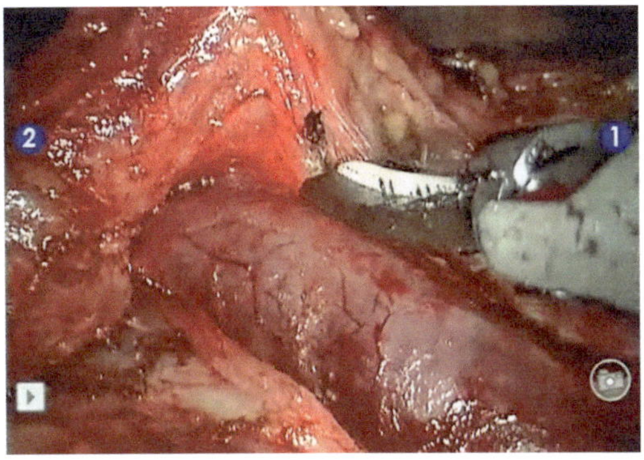

Fig. 13.22 Level III dissection

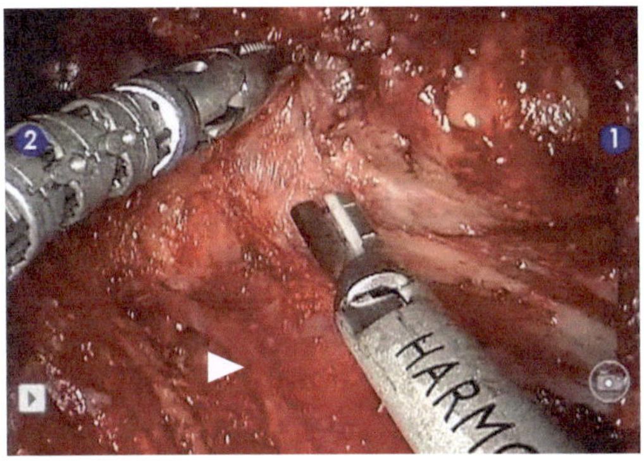

Fig. 13.23 Level V dissection. Spinal accessory nerve: *white arrowhead*

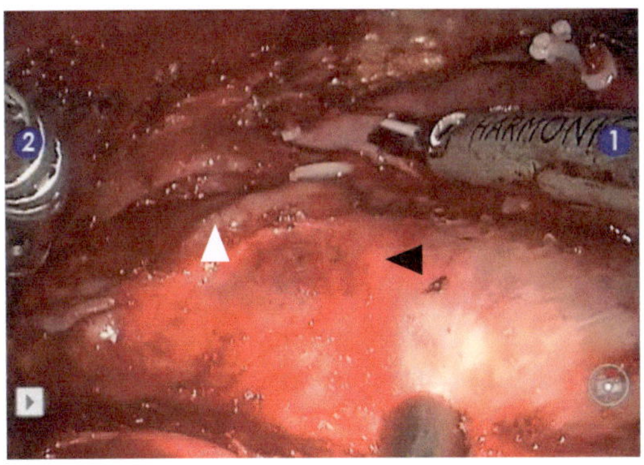

Fig. 13.24 Surgical field. Transverse cervical artery, *white arrowhead*; phrenic nerve, *black arrowhead*

Step 8. Finishing the Operation

After the completion of neck dissection, the specimen is taken out through RA incision (Fig. 13.27). After removal of the final specimen, the surgical bed is irrigated with warm saline and thorough observation and meticulous bleeding control is performed under endoscopic visualization. The surgical bed is placed with a closed suction drain which is inserted from behind the hairline and skin wound closure with simple, interrupted sutures is done.

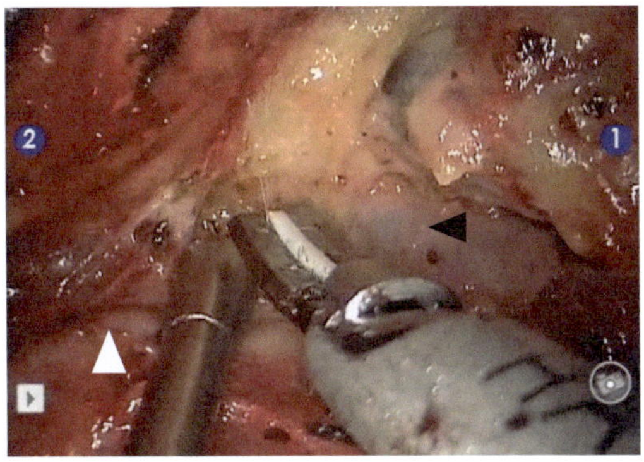

Fig. 13.25 Level IV dissection. Transverse cervical artery, *white arrowhead*; internal jugular vein, *black arrowhead*

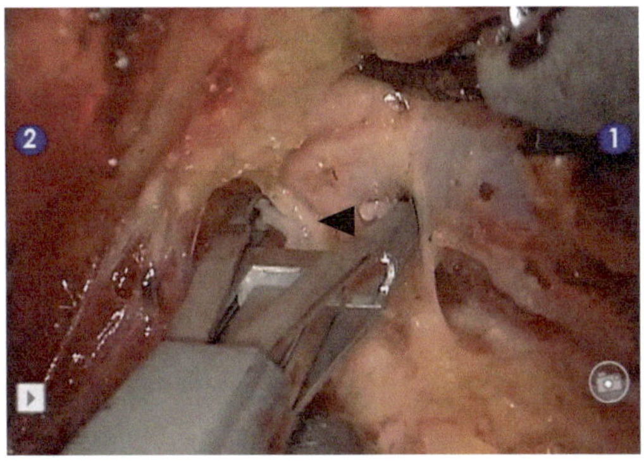

Fig. 13.26 Thoracic duct ligation. Thoracic duct: *black arrowhead*

Postoperative Care

The postoperative management is similar to that of the conventional total thyroidectomy with neck dissection. Cranial nerves such as the hypoglossal nerve, vagus nerve, spinal accessory nerve, and lingual nerve should be identified and preserved during the operation. Lymphoadipose tissue

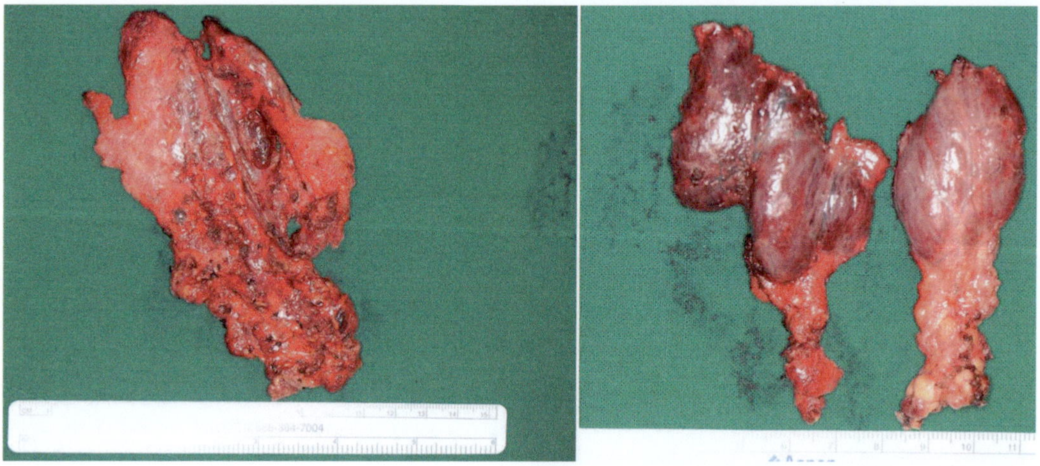

Fig. 13.27 Surgical specimen

should be cautiously dissected from the internal jugular vein to prevent significant bleeding from great vessels. The closed suction drain should be carefully monitored whether there are any signs of bleeding. The most common source of postoperative bleeding is the vessels of the skin flap. A meticulous hemostasis before the wound closure is important in preventing the bleeding event. The major bleeding should be handled in the operating room immediately after the detection of the event. The retroauricular and transaxillary skin wound should be cared with daily dressing. Routine checkup for any local signs of wound dehiscence or infection should be closely monitored daily. The chyle leakage can be managed with needle aspiration, local compression, and fat-suppressed diet. The indication for reoperation to ligate the thoracic or the lymphatic duct is the same as the conventional neck dissection. The ionized calcium and the serum parathyroid hormone level should be checked and the calcium and the vitamin D should be replaced on demand.

Complications

Some possible postoperative complications are listed below. In uncomplicated situations, the retroauricular or transaxillary skin incisions are healed well without any wound dehiscence. Massive hemorrhage or hematoma can rarely occur from rupture or loosening of the previously ligated or clipped vessels or the nearby carotid artery. Minor, trivial bleeding or hematoma can be managed locally with compression, but in such uncontrollable or massive bleeding situations, do not hesitate to open the wound in the operating room.

Possible Postoperative Complications from Therapeutic RAND

- Nerve-related injury
  - Recurrent laryngeal nerve and vagus nerve injury (vocal cord palsy)
  - Spinal accessory nerve injury (shoulder syndrome)
  - Hypoglossal nerve injury
  - Phrenic nerve injury
  - Sympathetic nerve injury (Horner's syndrome)
  - Marginal mandibular branch of facial nerve
- Hematoma/hemorrhage
- Seroma
- Chyle leakage
- Hypoparathyroidism
- Wound problems
  - Hair loss along incision line
  - Wound infection, dehiscence

- Skin flap necrosis, discoloration
- Hypertrophic scar, keloid formation

Discussion

Robotic total thyroidectomy with or without concomitant MRND via TARA or unilateral RA approach without axillary incision is technically feasible. According to studies documenting nodal metastasis patterns in PTC, the incidence of level II lymph nodes cannot be disregarded, suggesting a need for a modified approach to completely remove upper-neck-level nodes. Following our report on the feasibility of the TARA approach in HNC, we applied the TARA approach in the management of PTC with LNM, expecting competent extirpation of level II lymph nodes. There were no significant differences between the TARA group and the conventional ND group regarding the number of retrieved lymph nodes by neck level (unpublished data). Inclusion of level IIB in our study may be one of the factors leading to a higher retrieval of level II lymph nodes, though we cannot compare our results statistically with these earlier studies. However, we speculate that good accessibility under direct vision for level II dissection and less concern regarding injury to the SAN and the hypoglossal nerve in the TARA approach may have helped with competent clearance of lymph nodes in that area.

RAND in conjunction with thyroidectomy via RA approach integrates the surgical technique of robotic facelift thyroidectomy as reported by Terris et al. and the surgical technique of RAND via a MFL or RA approach as reported by our institution. Appropriate positioning of the patient and configuration of the robotic arms are essential elements to successful operation. The surgical procedure would be more manageable to conduct if the patient's neck is relaxed. What is more during contralateral thyroidectomy, the patient should be tilted or rotated towards the surgeon at the patient's table for optimal exposure. The patient's head could be supported and secured from the contralateral side with soft pad and sand bag. It is essentially important that sufficient working space must be created for comfortable movements of the robotic arms through the RA port during both total thyroidectomy and neck dissection. The greatest advantage offered by this operative procedure would be an excellent cosmetic outcome (Fig. 13.28). In comparison with conventional transcervical open methods, by placing the surgical incision behind the auricle and within the hairline, an obvious cervical incision would be completely eliminated, however, at the cost of more extensive dissections just like any other remote access surgical techniques. However, according to the findings of Terris et al., the area of dissection required would be 38 % lesser for the RA approach compared with the TA approach. Additionally, the operation would be relatively more comfortable for the surgeon due to familiar local anatomical structures, and the thyroid gland and lymph node tissues at the neck could be easily reached due to the decreased area of dissection when compared with the TA approach. Another advantage with respect to the TA thyroidectomy would be that the central compartment lymph nodes would be easier to address. The risk of intraoperative brachial plexus injury or any other physical sequelae resulting from the specific positioning of the patient for TA approach would be eliminated. This operative procedure, however, has a disadvantage of relatively longer operation times. Another important disadvantage of this operation is that it requires a considerable experience for the surgeon before he/she feels comfortable and is familiar with it. It is recommended that for optimal treatment outcomes, careful selection of clinically node negative patients must be carried out.

In conclusion, we successfully performed RAND via TARA or RA approach in PTC patients with LNM. The surgical outcomes of this approach were comparable with those of conventional ND. These approaches are an alternative option with an excellent aesthetic result for the management of LNM in PTC patients. The long-term outcomes of RAND via TARA or

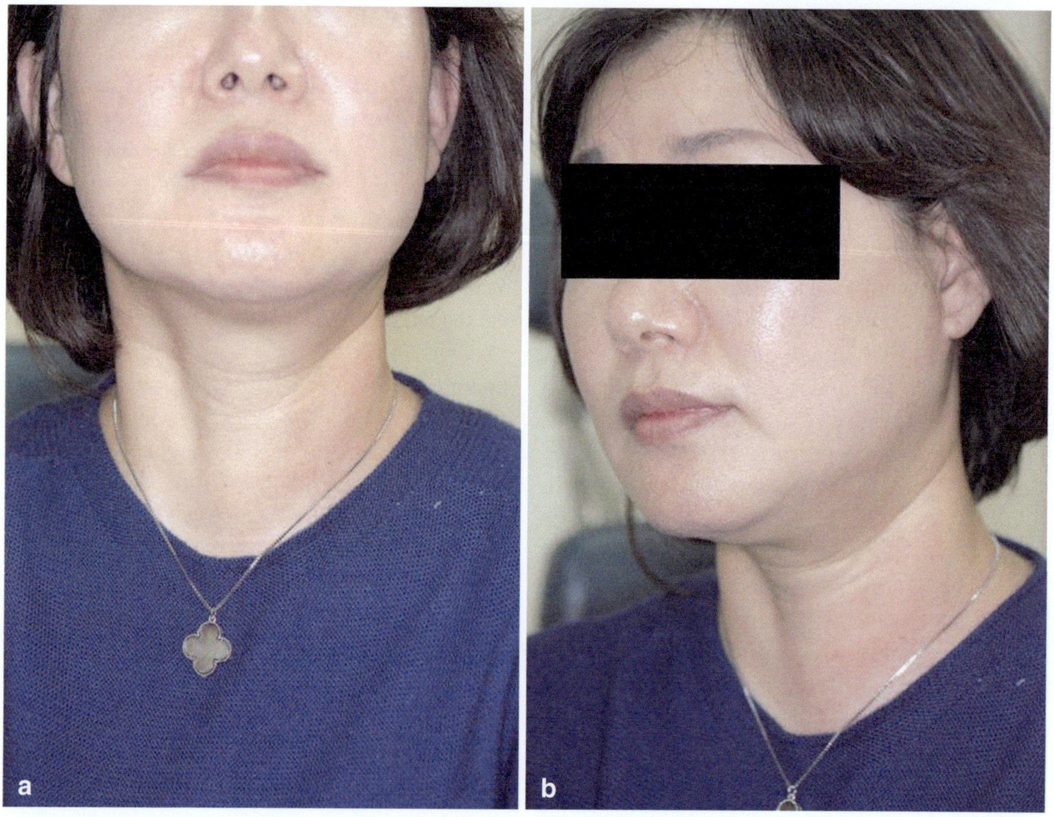

Fig. 13.28 Postoperative photo of a patient who has undergone RAND via RA approach. (**a** and **b**) RA approach. The operative wound is completely hidden behind the ear and within the hairline

RA approach should be further assessed to determine its oncologic safety.

Recommended Reading

Kang SW, Lee SC, Lee SH, et al. Robotic thyroid surgery using a gasless, transaxillary approach and the da Vinci S system: the operative outcomes of 338 consecutive patients. Surgery. 2009;146:1048–55.

Kang SW, Lee SH, Ryu HR, et al. Initial experience with robot-assisted modified radical neck dissection for the management of thyroid carcinoma with lateral neck node metastasis. Surgery. 2010;148:1214–21.

Kim WS, Lee HS, Kang SM, et al. Feasibility of robot-assisted neck dissections via a transaxillary and retroauricular ("TARA") approach in head and neck cancer: preliminary results. Ann Surg Oncol. 2012;19:1009–17.

Kim CH, Koh YW, Kim D, Chang JW, Choi EC, Shin YS. Robotic-assisted neck dissection in submandibular gland cancer: preliminary report. J Oral Maxillofac Surg. 2013;71(8):1450–57.

Kim CH, Chang JW, Choi EC, Shin YS, Koh YW. Robotically assisted selective neck dissection in parotid gland cancer: preliminary report. Laryngoscope. 2013b;123(3):646–50.

Kupferman ME, Patterson M, Mandel SJ, et al. Patterns of lateral neck metastasis in papillary thyroid carcinoma. Arch Otolaryngol Head Neck Surg. 2004;130: 857–60.

Lee S, Ryu HR, Park JH, et al. Excellence in robotic thyroid surgery: a comparative study of robot-assisted versus conventional endoscopic thyroidectomy in papillary thyroid microcarcinoma patients. Ann Surg. 2011;253:1060–6.

Lee HS, Kim WS, Hong HJ, Ban MJ, Lee D, Koh YW, Choi EC. Robot-assisted supraomohyoid neck dissection via a modified face-lift or retroauricular approach in early-stage cN0 squamous cell carcinoma of the oral cavity: a comparative study with conventional technique. Ann Surg Oncol. 2012;19(12):3871–8.

Lewis Jr JS, Carpenter DH, Thorstad WL, Zhang Q, Haughey BH. Extracapsular extension is a poor predictor of disease recurrence in surgically treated oropharyngeal squamous cell carcinoma. Mod Pathol. 2011;24:1413–20.

Park YM, Holsinger FC, Kim WS, Park SC, Lee EJ, Choi EC, Koh YW. Robot-assisted selective neck dissection of levels II to V via a modified facelift or retroauricular approach. Otolaryngol Head Neck Surg. 2013;148(5):778–85.

Roh J, Kim J, Park CI. Lateral cervical lymph node metastases from papillary thyroid carcinoma: pattern of nodal metastases and optimal strategy for neck dissection. Ann Surg Oncol. 2008;15:1177–82.

Shaha AR, Shah JP, Loree TR. Patterns of nodal and distant metastasis based on histologic varieties in differentiated carcinoma of the thyroid. Am J Surg. 1996;172:692–4.

Shin YS, Hong HJ, Koh YW, et al. Gasless transaxillary robot-assisted neck dissection: a preclinical feasibility study in four cadavers. Yonsei Med J. 2012;53:193–7.

Singer MC, Seybt MW, Terris DJ. Robotic facelift thyroidectomy: I. Preclinical simulation and morphometric assessment. Laryngoscope. 2011;121:1631–5.

Terris DJ, Singer MC. Qualitative and quantitative differences between 2 robotic thyroidectomy techniques. Otolaryngol Head Neck Surg. 2012a;147:20–5.

Terris DJ, Singer MC. Robotic facelift thyroidectomy: facilitating remote access surgery. Head Neck. 2012b;34:746–7.

Terris DJ, Singer MC, Seybt MW. Robotic facelift thyroidectomy: II. Clinical feasibility and safety. Laryngoscope. 2011a;121:1636–41.

Terris DJ, Singer MC, Seybt MW. Robotic facelift thyroidectomy: patient selection and technical considerations. Surg Laparosc Endosc Percutan Tech. 2011b;21:237–42.

14 Imaging for Parathyroid Surgery

Neelima Tummala and Lisa A. Orloff

Introduction

Preoperative parathyroid localization is the sine qua non of minimally invasive parathyroidectomy. Fortunately, there are several effective imaging modalities available today for precise localization of parathyroid disease. While the normal parathyroid gland still eludes visualization other than by open surgical identification, the enlarged parathyroid gland can be identified by noninvasive imaging techniques in the great majority of patients. Prior to the advent of these imaging modalities, bilateral cervical exploration was considered the gold standard. Ironically, some of the most ardent former critics of localizing studies, who defended routine bilateral parathyroid exploration, are the very same surgeons who currently market and practice a focused approach to parathyroidectomy that is dependent on accurate preoperative localization. Over the past several decades, with the use of imaging methods that enable mapping of disease, a minimally invasive surgical approach to treating parathyroid disease has come to represent the most common practice. Limited exploration, with a focal (single gland) or unilateral (single side) approach, is now the most frequent approach.

N. Tummala, MD • L.A. Orloff, MD (✉)
Department of Otolaryngology/Head and Neck Surgery, University of California, San Francisco, 2380 Sutter Street, Second Floor, San Francisco, CA 94115, USA
e-mail: lorloff@ohns.ucsf.edu

Approximately 83 % of patients have four parathyroid glands: two inferior glands and two superior glands. Another 13 % have more than four glands (supernumerary parathyroids), and 3 % of patients have fewer than four glands. The superior glands arise from the fourth brachial pouch, along with the thyroid gland. They descend during embryonic development into the neck alongside the thyroid gland and are rarely ectopic. They are typically located posterior to the upper-mid pole of the thyroid gland. They are more rarely located posterior to the esophagus or pharynx, in a deep, descended location.

The inferior glands arise from the third brachial pouch, along with the thymus. These glands have a longer descent and are more variable in position, with 35 % present at ectopic locations along the thymopharyngeal duct course. They are found at the inferior pole of the thyroid gland about two-thirds of the time and are at an ectopic location, anywhere from the angle of the mandible to the lower mediastinum, in the remaining cases. Due to their close proximity to the thyroid gland, the parathyroid glands may be covered by or attached to the thyroid capsule, resulting in intracapsular or intrathyroid location.

Primary hyperparathyroidism is due to idiopathic enlargement and hypersecretion of one or more parathyroid glands. The majority (about 85 %) of patients with primary hyperparathyroidism have a single adenoma, namely, a benign neoplasm of any one of the parathyroid glands. A smaller subset (about 15 %) of patients has multigland disease, including hyperplasia of all of

D.J. Terris, M.C. Singer (eds.), *Minimally Invasive and Robotic Thyroid and Parathyroid Surgery*, DOI 10.1007/978-1-4614-9011-1_14, © Springer Science+Business Media New York 2014

their parathyroid glands or hyperfunction due to two or more simultaneous parathyroid adenomas. A typical parathyroid adenoma is about 10–30 mm in length, while a normal gland usually measures about 5×3×1 mm. Hence, on imaging, a parathyroid adenoma is often identified as a round or oval mass that is well circumscribed, solid, and hypervascular. Likewise on imaging, lymph nodes, thyroid nodules, parathyroid cysts, the esophagus, and (rarely) parathyroid cancers may be mistaken for adenomas.

Preoperative localization of parathyroid disease is essential for a minimally invasive parathyroidectomy. It reduces operating room time and limits dissection while aiding in identification of multigland or ectopic disease, particularly in the mediastinum, that may not be amenable to a minimally invasive approach. Although imaging is very useful for identifying disease, it must be remembered that a positive finding on imaging does not confirm diagnosis, while a negative finding cannot rule out the existence of disease. In addition, the use of imaging modalities for parathyroid disease should be limited to patients who have a biochemical diagnosis of primary hyperparathyroidism.

There are a variety of noninvasive and invasive imaging studies that are available both for initial evaluation of patients and for patients with persistent or recurrent disease. The most common noninvasive studies include ultrasonography, nuclear scintigraphy scans that utilize sestamibi, computed tomography (CT), and magnetic resonance imaging (MRI), with variations of each type of study available. Invasive studies include fine-needle aspiration (which can be guided by ultrasound or CT), parathyroid angiography, and selective venous sampling for parathyroid hormone gradient.

Ultrasound

Ultrasonography is a highly useful tool in the preoperative evaluation of patients with parathyroid disease. It is cost effective and noninvasive, performed efficiently, does not require any preparation, and does not introduce the patient to any radiation exposure. High-frequency (7 MHz or greater), high-resolution ultrasonography provides detailed anatomic information on enlarged parathyroid glands as well as concomitant thyroid disease, if present. Ultrasonography also reveals dynamic as well as three-dimensional detail regarding parathyroid position. Ultrasonography has demonstrated sensitivities of 77–96 % and positive predictive values of 74–98 % in identifying parathyroid adenomas. Ultrasonography has been shown to be more sensitive than nuclear medicine imaging for multigland parathyroid disease, and accuracy rates for surgeon-performed ultrasonography have been some of the highest cited (up to 91 %).

On ultrasound, as with other imaging modalities, normal parathyroid glands are not visualized due to their small size and similarity to surrounding tissues. The sonographic appearance of a typical parathyroid adenoma is a solid, homogenous, hypoechoic mass, which is in distinction to the more hyperechoic thyroid tissue (Fig. 14.1). The adenoma is typically adjacent to the thyroid gland and medial to the carotid artery. It is often bean or oval shaped but can also be multilobulated, depending on its size. It is highly vascular, and if color Doppler is used, an extrathyroidal peripheral feeding vessel with a rim of vascularity around the adenoma may be visualized (Fig. 14.2).

Limitations of ultrasound include its area of coverage, as it is limited to the neck region, and the fact that it is highly operator dependent. Surgeon-performed ultrasound has been shown to be equal or superior to non-clinician-performed ultrasound for parathyroid localization, a fact that makes intuitive sense since the surgeon is ultimately responsible for the success or failure of the operation and cure of the disease. In addition, ultrasound offers real-time imaging with greater anatomic detail, as compared to scintigraphy. However, there is limited identification of retrosternal and retrotracheal disease. Another shortcoming is its use in obese patients and in patients with short necks or limited neck extension, as well as those with nodular thyroid disease, in whom it is much more difficult to obtain an adequate view to identify adenomas.

It can be difficult to distinguish small lymph nodes from diseased glands based solely on

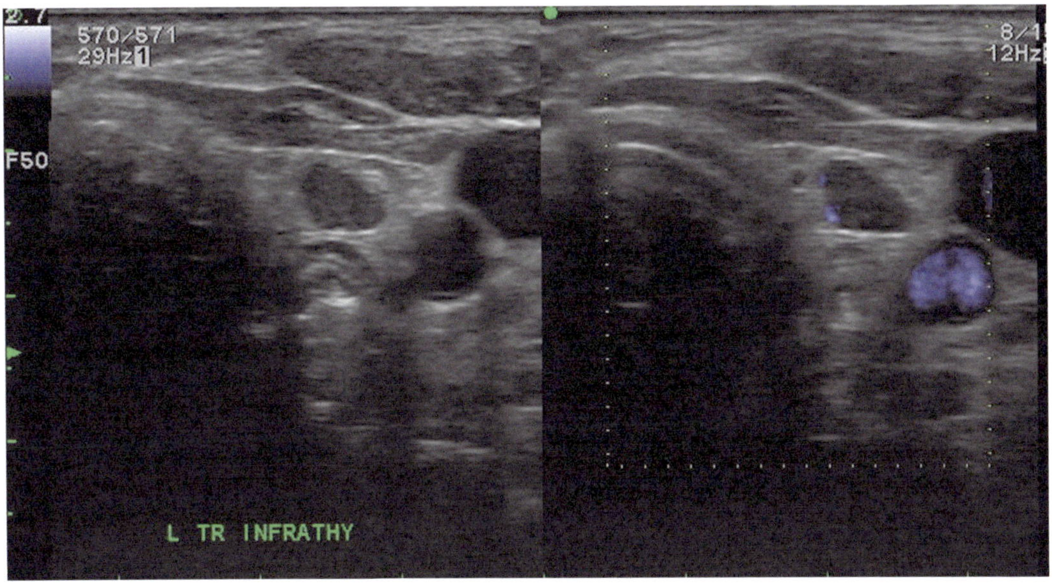

Fig. 14.1 Gray-scale ultrasound (*left*) and color Doppler ultrasound (*right*), both showing transverse view of a left inferior parathyroid adenoma, situated between the trachea and the carotid artery. A typical parathyroid adenoma is a solid, homogenous, hypoechoic mass

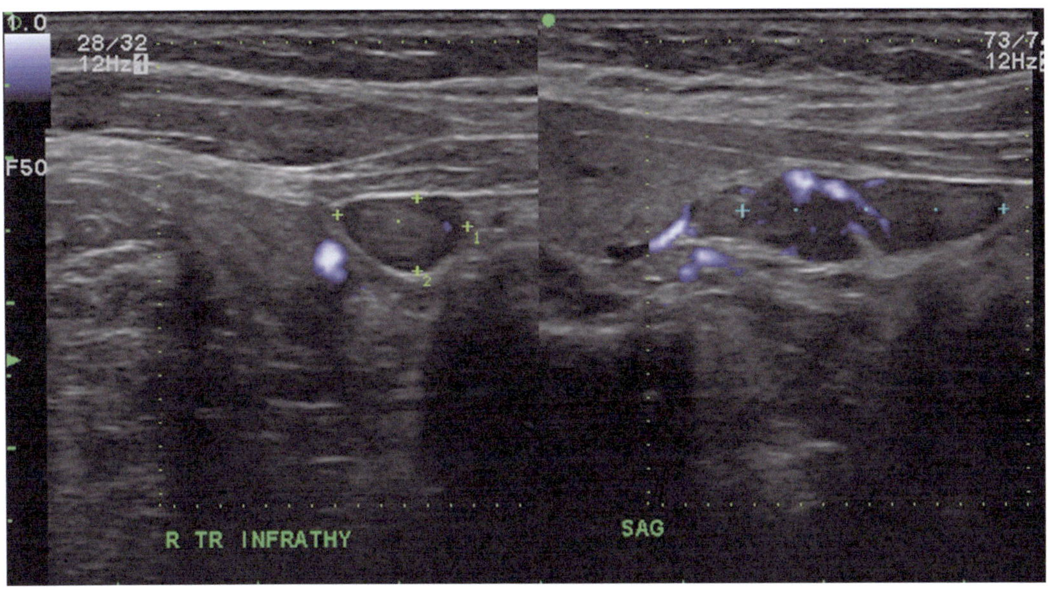

Fig. 14.2 On color Doppler ultrasound, an extrathyroidal peripheral feeding vessel and a rim of vascularity around the adenoma are typically seen (transverse and sagittal views)

ultrasound. The use of ultrasound in combination with other imaging modalities, especially the sestamibi scan, is common and in fact preferred by many surgeons. A parathyroid adenoma identified both on sestamibi scan and on ultrasound imaging is highly specific. Combining the two modalities, a false-negative rate as low as 2 % has been found, as compared to 23 % with ultrasound alone and 12 % for sestamibi alone. Ultrasound is also useful for guiding fine-needle aspiration (FNA) of a lesion, as described below.

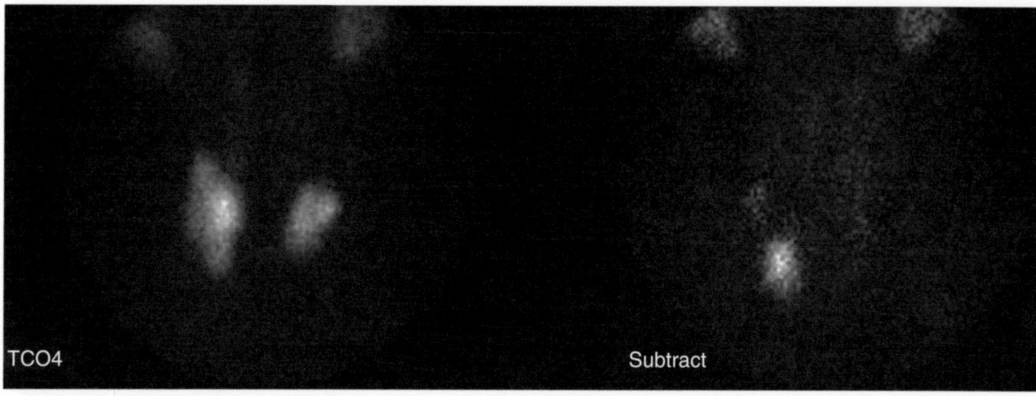

Fig. 14.3 In subtraction imaging, the image from the uptake of the thyroid-specific radionuclide (in this case, Tc-99m pertechnetate, *left*) is subtracted from the parathyroid/thyroid radionuclide (Tc-99m MIBI) image, resulting in an estimation of parathyroid tissue uptake (*right*)

Sestamibi Scan

Developed in the early 1990s, sestamibi parathyroid scanning is now widely available. This imaging modality, comprised of several different nuclear scintigraphic techniques, is the most popular procedure used for parathyroid localization and is collectively the most accurate, with a sensitivity and specificity of greater than 90 % for identifying parathyroid disease. Sestamibi scanning is particularly useful for identifying ectopic disease and has been shown to be more reliable for adenoma localization in patients with lower levels of vitamin D.

Often used in conjunction with ultrasound, this combination is highly reliable, as an ultrasound can anatomically identify a possible adenoma, while a nuclear medicine scan can differentiate it functionally from a lymph node or thyroid mass.

Tc-99m sestamibi is a lipid-soluble myocardial perfusion tracer that accumulates in the mitochondria of cells. Parathyroid adenomas are very vascular and have a high concentration of oxyphilic cells, which have increased mitochondrial content, increasing their sestamibi uptake. The sestamibi isotope, which emits gamma rays, is retained longer in the parathyroid adenoma cells than the adjacent thyroid due to this increased mitochondrial content. Thus, there is focal increased uptake on early and delayed images taken with a gamma camera in an adenoma, as compared to other surrounding tissue. The two most common techniques used are subtraction imaging and dual-phase imaging. Subtraction imaging can be especially helpful if a thyroid mass is present. Dual-phase imaging is less affected by motion artifact, making it a better option for SPECT imaging.

In subtraction imaging, both a thyroid-specific radionuclide and a thyroid- and parathyroid-specific radionuclide are administered. The most commonly used thyroid-specific radionuclides are either iodine-123 (^{123}I) or Tc-99 m sodium pertechnetate. The image from the uptake of the thyroid-specific radionuclide is subtracted from the parathyroid/thyroid radionuclide (Tc-99m sestamibi) image, resulting in an estimation of parathyroid tissue uptake (Fig. 14.3).

In the dual-phase technique, visualization of parathyroid adenomas is based on differential washout. In this process, initial images are taken 10 min after intravenous infusion, and subsequent images are taken at 2–3 h after sestamibi administration, based on the kinetics of the compound. Due to retention and delayed sestamibi washout, there should be persistent sestamibi visualization in the parathyroid adenomas in the delayed images, as compared to the initial set (Fig. 14.4). Hyperparathyroid patients with double adenomas and parathyroid hyperplasia have

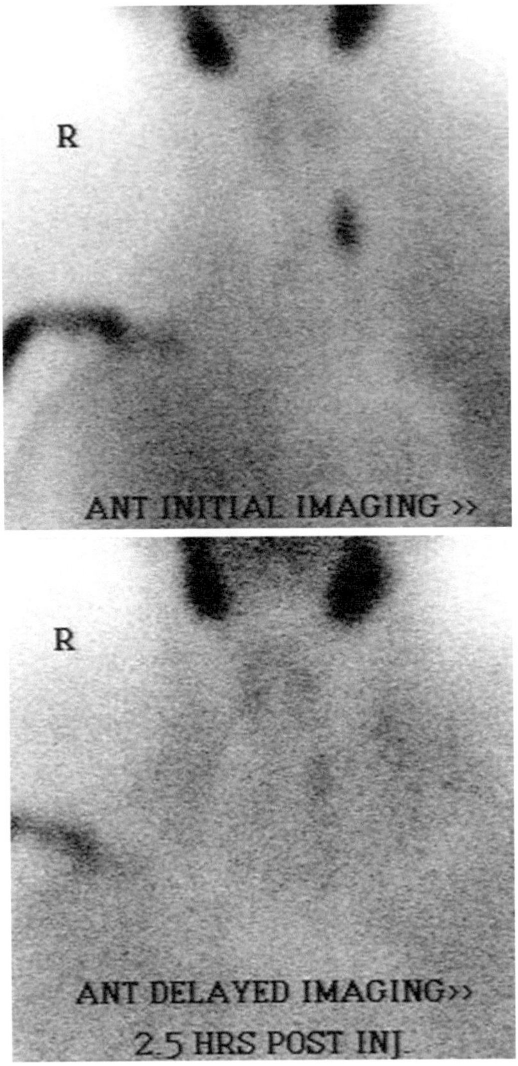

Fig. 14.4 Dual-phase technique. Early (10 min after intravenous infusion) and late (2–3 h after sestamibi infusion) show differential washout. There is typically persistent sestamibi visualization in parathyroid adenomas in the delayed images, although some adenomas, such as the one in this figure, show initial uptake and early washout

progressively less distinct or successful localization than those with single adenomas.

Sestamibi imaging was originally performed as two-dimensional (2D) planar scanning (Fig. 14.5). Such 2D scans have in some centers been replaced by SPECT (single proton emission computed tomography) scans, which provide three-dimensional (3D) reconstruction and

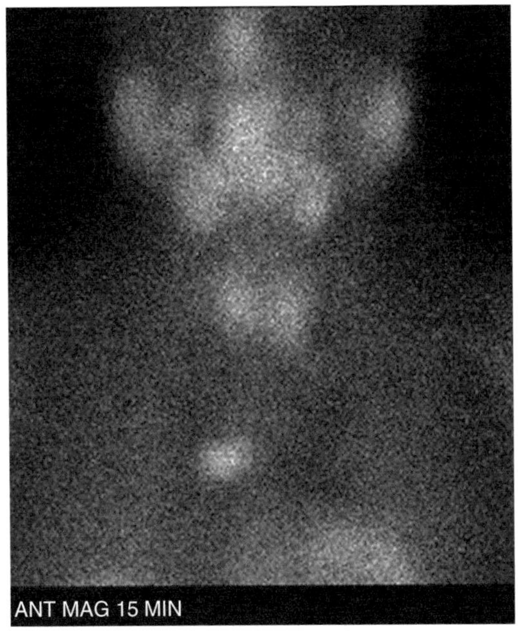

Fig. 14.5 Two-dimensional planar sestamibi scan, showing parathyroid uptake in a right inferior mediastinal adenoma

greater localizing information (Fig. 14.6). Furthermore, SPECT sestamibi scans have recently been fused with high-resolution, thin slice CT to localize disease even more precisely (Fig. 14.7). Several studies have found dual-phase SPECT/CT sestamibi imaging to be significantly superior to planar imaging in the detection of parathyroid lesions, especially when there is concomitant thyroid nodularity. However, other studies have found that SPECT/CT has no significant clinical value additional to that of conventional SPECT for parathyroid imaging except in locating ectopic parathyroid glands and that the additional time, radiation exposure, and expense do not justify the CT acquisition.

One of the main limitations of all variations of sestamibi scanning is the fact that, like ultrasound, it is highly operator dependent. It is most reliable for identifying large, solitary adenomas. False positives occur when there are other cell types that also have high mitochondrial content, such as Hurthle cell nodules in thyroid tissue.

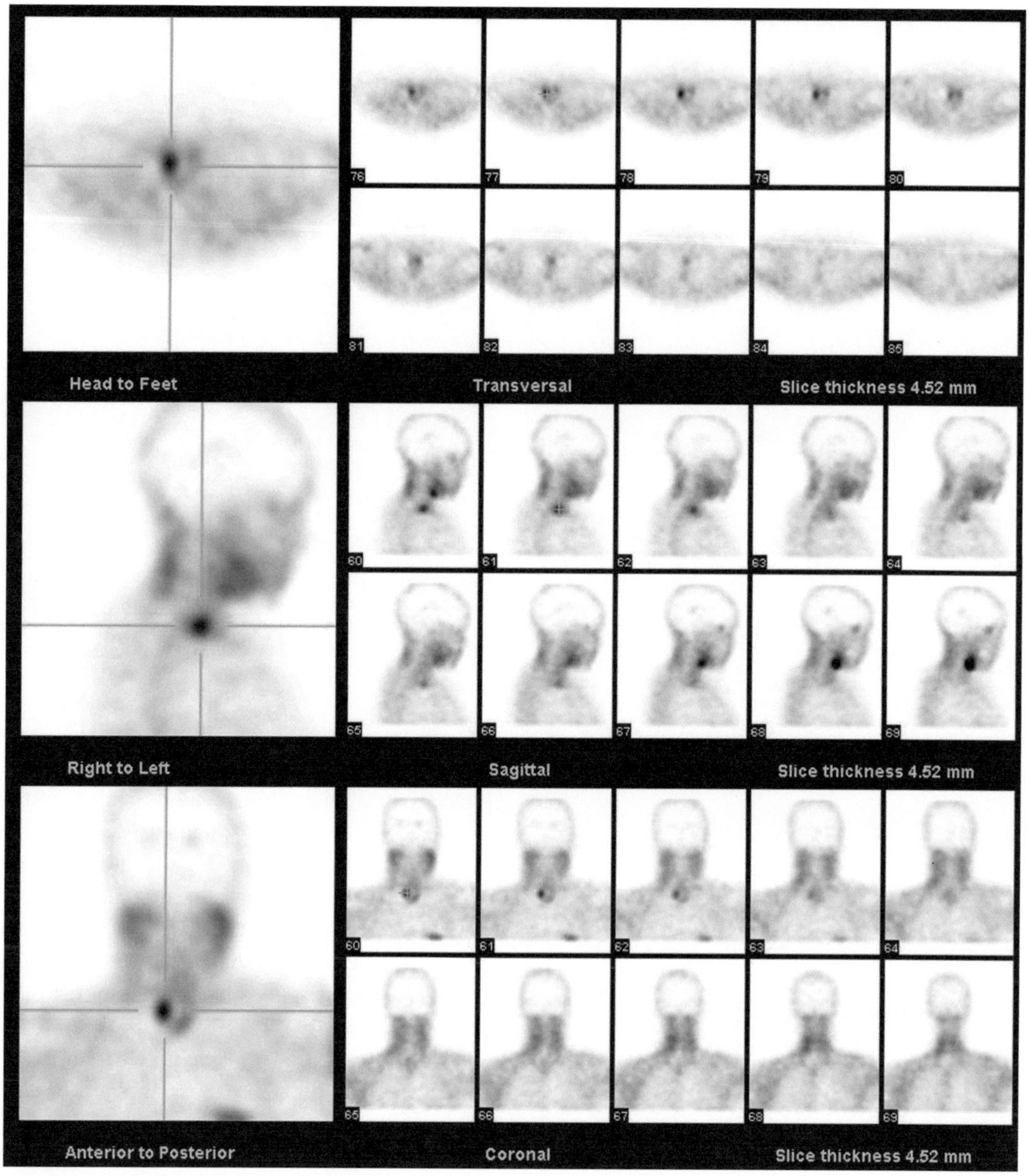

Fig. 14.6 SPECT sestamibi scan, showing axial, sagittal, and coronal 3D reconstructions and localization of a parathyroid adenoma to the right retrothyroid region

Also, brown fat, brown tumors, lymphoma, breast cancer, and thyroid carcinoma all have a propensity for increased uptake. False negatives often occur with adenomas with low oxyphilic count, which is seen in smaller adenomas and in multiglandular disease. False-negative sestamibi scanning has also been linked to patients with higher levels of vitamin D and lower levels of serum calcium, as well as patients with multigland disease (multiple adenomas or parathyroid hyperplasia.). Reviewing early, late, and subtraction pinhole images together with SPECT images maximizes parathyroid lesion detection accuracy. Also, the operating surgeon should review all sestamibi scans irrespective of what is reported, because there are often subtle findings that are pertinent but not reported on the formal interpretation.

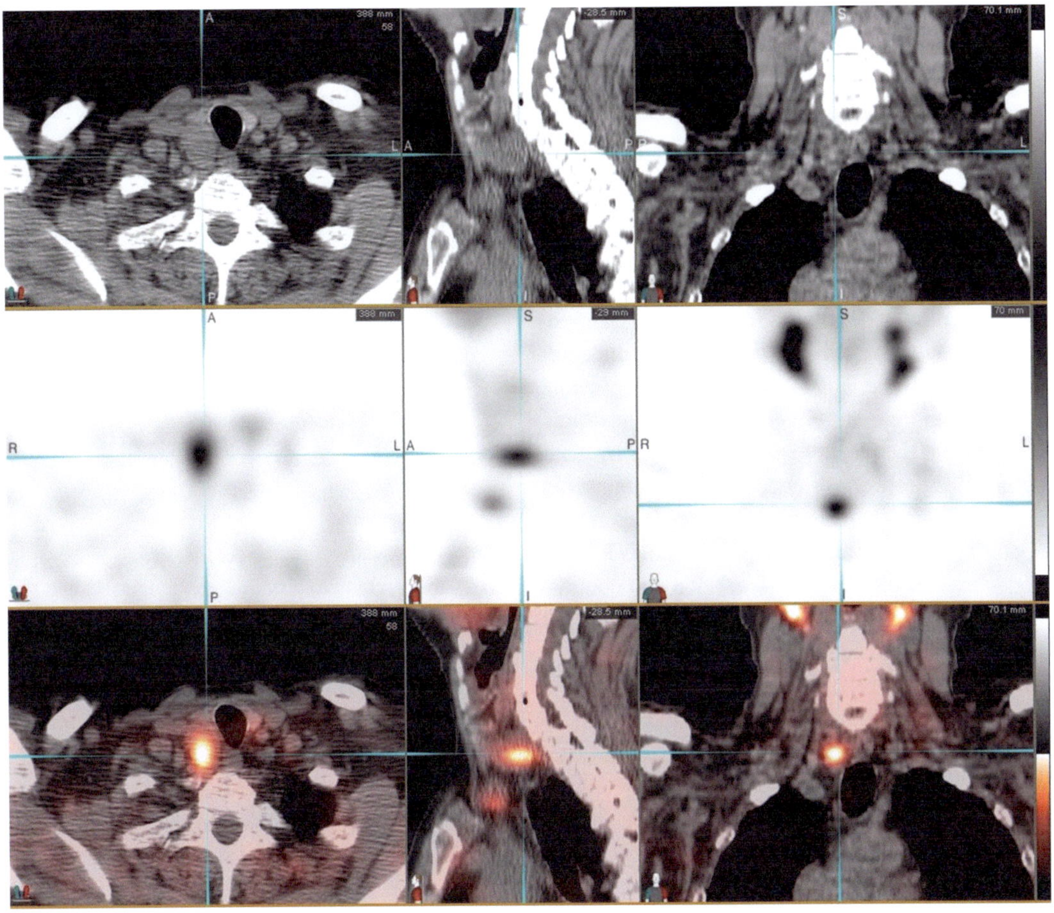

Fig. 14.7 SPECT/CT sestamibi fusion scans combine the advantages of cross-sectional imaging by CT with the functional imaging of sestamibi scintigraphy to yield a precise anatomic map such as seen for this right inferior parathyroid adenoma

Computed Tomography

Computed tomography (CT) is a second-line noninvasive imaging modality that is typically used to localize elusive parathyroid disease. Although not as sensitive as ultrasound or sestamibi scans, this imaging modality is useful for identifying ectopic disease (Fig. 14.8). It is available for use in most medical centers and can be used for guiding FNA biopsy of a lesion. In addition, it is less operator dependent than ultrasound or sestamibi imaging, and the images are easily stored in most databases.

The disadvantages of CT include its cost, exposure of the patient to radiation, and necessity for intravenous contrast. In addition, false positives

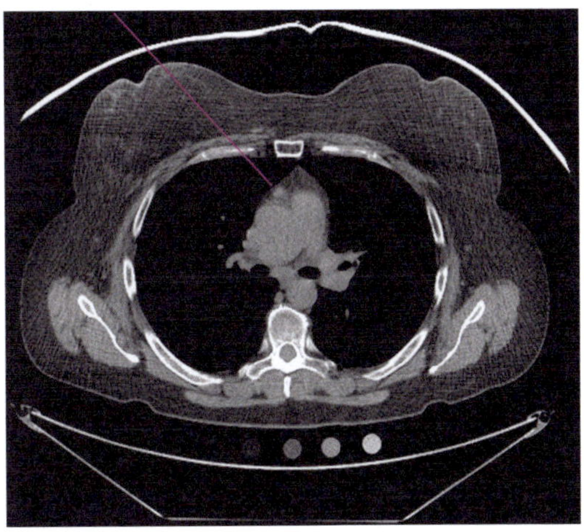

Fig. 14.8 CT can be useful for identifying ectopic disease, such as the mediastinal parathyroid adenoma located anterior to the ascending aorta in this patient (*line*)

are not uncommon, with lymph nodes most commonly mistaken for parathyroid adenomas. False negatives also result from parathyroid lesions being mistaken for lymph nodes.

The four-dimensional CT (4D-CT) imaging of the neck and upper mediastinum takes advantage of precise timing of contrast perfusion coordinated with acquisition of computed tomography data to identify the adenoma. It yields 3D multiphasic images, combined with the fourth or time dimension, to result in images at specified moments precontrast, during infusion, and 30 s after infusion. This imaging modality reveals both the anatomic location and the physiology of the lesion, by evaluating the perfusion characteristics. Parathyroid adenomas are characterized by rapid uptake of contrast with early washout of contrast. Lymph nodes are characterized by slow uptake of contrast with slow release. Thus, on the contrast-enhanced CT, a parathyroid adenoma will typically enhance earlier and more briefly than lymph nodes.

The 4D-CT has been shown in some centers to be more sensitive than ultrasound or sestamibi scan alone for precise localization of hyperfunctioning parathyroid glands, with a lateralization accuracy of 93 % and localization accuracy of 86 %. It has also been shown to be useful in localizing adenomas in the reoperative setting. The disadvantages of using this imaging modality are its cost, exposure of the patient to radiation, the necessity for contrast, and limited availability of this type of study, as compared to other imaging modalities.

MRI

The use of MRI for identification of parathyroid adenomas is mainly reserved for patients with nonlocalizing sestamibi and ultrasound studies and for previously operated patients with persistent hyperparathyroidism. MRI is also very useful for identifying ectopic disease, especially in the mediastinum (Fig. 14.9), and in cases when findings on nuclear medicine imaging and on ultrasound are discordant. Its use is limited due to its increased cost and need for expertise in interpreting the images.

On MRI, normal parathyroid glands are not seen. Adenomas are identified as soft tissue masses and are isointense to hyperintense as compared to thyroid tissue on T2-weighted images. They are isointense to hypointense on T1-weighted images as compared to thyroid tissue (Fig. 14.10). Parathyroid adenomas often enhance avidly with gadolinium on T1-weighted images. Dynamic or 4D-MRI can be performed in a manner similar to 4D-CT described above, where early uptake and subsequent washout of gadolinium from parathyroid adenomas can be detected if the scanning is timed carefully with the infusion of the contrast agent. Lymph nodes, which have similar signal intensities, can be mistaken for parathyroid adenomas on standard (nondynamic) MRI.

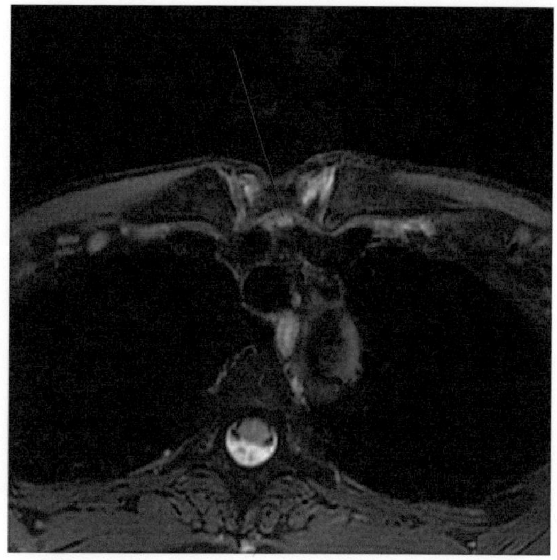

Fig. 14.9 MRI in a previously operated patient with persistent hyperparathyroidism, demonstrating ectopic disease in the retrosternal superior mediastinum (*line*)

PET/CT Scan

Like sestamibi scanning, PET/CT scanning is a functional imaging study that takes advantage of the hypermetabolic behavior of lesions, including parathyroid glands, and displays differential tracer retention and positron emission pictorially. Whereas there are case reports of the more commonly used fluorodeoxyglucose (FDG) revealing parathyroid lesions on PET scanning, more recent and larger series have described C-11 methionine (MET-PET) as highly accurate at localizing parathyroid lesions. There is limited experience to date with this type of scan, and it is significantly more costly than the alternative imaging studies.

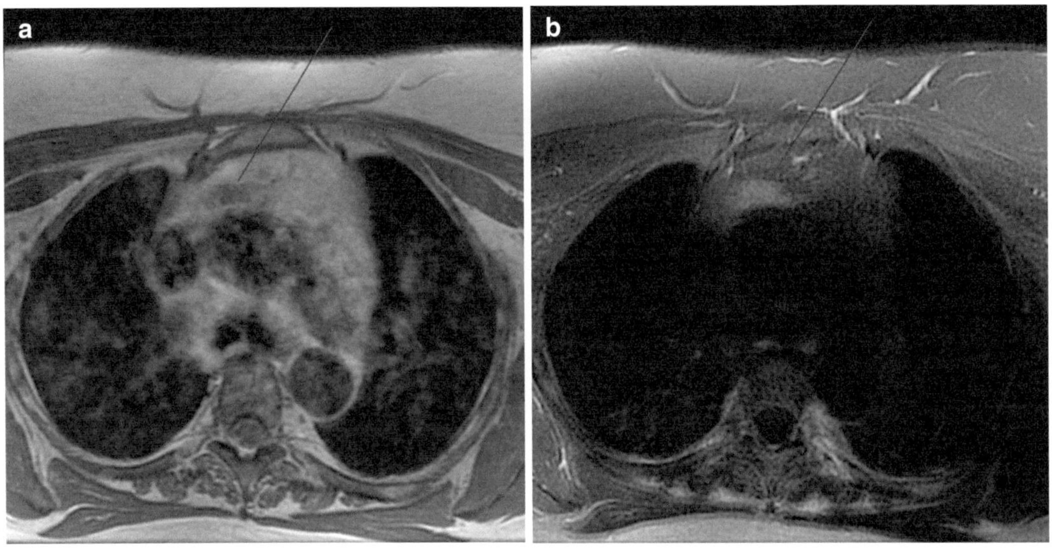

Fig. 14.10 On MRI, adenomas can be hypointense on T1-weighted images (**a**) and hyperintense on T2-weighted images (**b**), as seen in this example of a mediastinal parathyroid adenoma (*lines*)

Fine-Needle Aspiration

Fine-needle aspiration (FNA) can be guided by either ultrasound or CT (Fig. 14.11). It is very specific in distinguishing parathyroid tissue from nonparathyroid tissue, although distinction of parathyroid versus thyroid cytology can be challenging. When combined with testing for intact parathyroid hormone (PTH), FNA achieves a specificity of 95–100 %. The needle used for FNA is rinsed with saline and tested for intact PTH by the same chemical assay that is used for serum PTH. However, FNA is invasive and can lead to an inflammatory response at the biopsy site, which can have consequences for the surgical resection. There has been report of implantation of parathyroid tumor cells along the needle track, although separate literature attests to the safety of parathyroid FNA. Overall, FNA should only be considered in challenging cases.

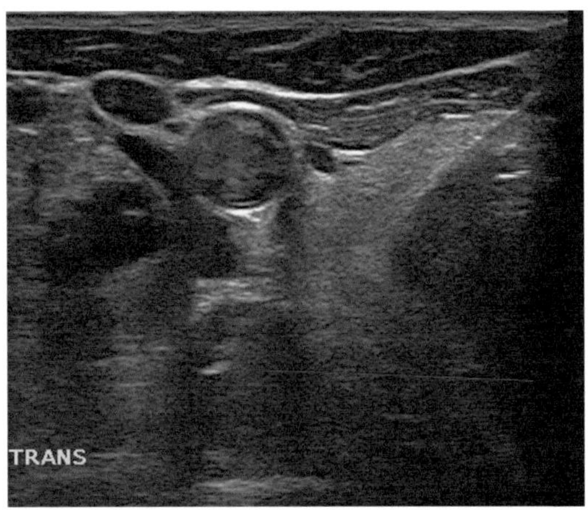

Fig. 14.11 Ultrasound-guided FNA of a deep parathyroid candidate lesion in a patient with prior unsuccessful exploration. The needle is rinsed with saline and analyzed for PTH (lines = needle tip and needle)

Selective Venous Sampling

Venous sampling for parathyroid hormone can also be used to determine the general location of a parathyroid adenoma. It is technically very challenging and success of the study is operator dependent. Blood samples are obtained from multiple bilateral sites within the venous circulation superior and inferior to the potential sites of a parathyroid tumor, and gradients in PTH are measured. It is mainly useful in complex revision operations when two or more preoperative imaging modalities have been inconclusive or unhelpful. Selective venous sampling has been shown to have a success rate of 86 % in identifying the location of a parathyroid adenoma in such patients. The use of the study is limited by its invasive nature, increased cost, need for interventional radiologist expertise, and exposure of the patient to radiation. However, recent reports of ultrasound-guided internal jugular vein sampling, even in the office setting, have renewed interest in the concept and use of PTH gradient testing for difficult cases, without the previously associated risks.

Parathyroid Arteriography

Although rarely used today due to its increased risks, this test is both specific and sensitive. Parathyroid adenomas are highly vascular, and thus angiographic imaging modalities may be utilized. Adenomas are identified as round- or oval-shaped lesions that display a vascular blush with angiographic injection. Success of the procedure is based on skill of the performing interventional radiologist. It is often utilized when other noninvasive imaging studies are equivocal. The risks of this procedure are devastating and include spinal cord injury and embolic infarction. More recently, noninvasive magnetic resonance angiography has been successfully used in the reoperative neck.

Conclusion

Accurate preoperative imaging methods have revolutionized the surgical approach to hyperparathyroidism and led to a trend toward minimally invasive, targeted procedures. While regional as well as individual surgeon preferences differ, the spectrum of choices available means that most parathyroid lesions can be localized prior to surgery. The nuclear medicine sestamibi scan, with or without SPECT/CT, is considered by most to be the optimal initial exam for localization of parathyroid adenomas. It is useful to compare this functional type of study to an anatomic study, such as an ultrasound, CT, or MRI, for precise three-dimensional targeting. Ultrasound, and increasingly surgeon-performed ultrasound, is cost effective, convenient, and highly reliable for localizing perithyroidal adenomas but has a limited role for adenomas in the mediastinum. The more expensive noninvasive imaging modalities, CT and MRI, are usually reserved for cases where nuclear medicine imaging and ultrasound are discordant or unrevealing or for revision cases. The use of invasive imaging modalities, namely, FNA, angiography, and venous sampling, is limited to cases where the noninvasive imaging modalities are nonlocalizing.

Recommended Reading

Abboud B, Sleilaty G, Rabaa L, Daher R, Abou Zeid H, Jabbour H, et al. Ultrasonography: highly accuracy technique for preoperative localization of parathyroid adenoma. Laryngoscope. 2008;118(9):1574–8.

Abraham D, Sharma PK, Bentz J, Gault PM, Neumayer L, McClain DA. Utility of ultrasound-guided fine-needle aspiration of parathyroid adenomas for localization before minimally invasive parathyroidectomy. Endocr Pract. 2007;13(4):333–7.

Adewole AD, Roman SA, Kraev AI, Kim AW. A fluorodeoxyglucose avid mediastinal parathyroid adenoma masquerading as metastatic bladder cancer. Interact Cardiovasc Thorac Surg. 2012;15(3):514–5.

Akerström G, Malmaeus J, Bergström R. Surgical anatomy of human parathyroid glands. Surgery. 1986;95(1):14–21.

Aschenbach R, Tuda S, Lamster E, Meyer A, Roediger H, Stier A, et al. Dynamic magnetic resonance angiography for localization of hyperfunctioning parathyroid glands in the reoperative neck. Eur J Radiol. 2012;81(11):3371–7.

Bancos I, Grant CS, Nadeem S. Risks and benefits of parathyroid fine-needle aspiration with parathyroid hormone washout. Endocr Pract. 2012;18(4):441–9.

Berber E, Parikh RT, Ballem N, Garner CN, Milas M, Siperstein AE. Factors contributing to negative parathyroid localization: an analysis of 1000 patients. Surgery. 2008;144(1):74–9.

Carneiro-Pla D. Effectiveness of "office"-based, ultrasound-guided differential jugular venous sampling (DJVS) of parathormone in patients with primary hyperparathyroidism. Surgery. 2009;146(6):1014–20.

Clayman GL. Targeted parathyroidectomy. In: Cohen JI, Clayman GL, editors. Atlas of head & neck surgery. Philadelphia: Elsevier; 2011. Print.

Elaraj DM, Sippel RS, Lindsay S, Sansano I, Duh QY, Clark OH, et al. Are additional localization studies and referral indicated for patients with primary hyperparathyroidism who have negative sestamibi scan results? Arch Surg. 2010;145(6):578–81.

Gayed IW, Kim EE, Broussard WF, Evans D, Lee J, Broemeling LD, et al. The value of 99mTc-sestamibi SPECT/CT over conventional SPECT in the evaluation of parathyroid adenomas or hyperplasia. J Nucl Med. 2005;46(2):248–52.

Gurney TA, Orloff LA. Otolaryngologist-head and neck surgeon-performed ultrasonography for parathyroid adenoma localization. Laryngoscope. 2008;118(2):243–6.

Haber RS, Kim CK, Inabnet WB. Ultrasonography for preoperative localization of enlarged parathyroid glands in primary hyperparathyroidism: comparison with (99m) technetium sestamibi scintigraphy. Clin Endocrinol. 2002;57(2):241–9.

Hunter GJ, Schellingerhout D, Vu TH, Perrier ND, Hamberg LM. Accuracy of four-dimensional CT for the localization of abnormal parathyroid glands in patients with primary hyperparathyroidism. Radiology. 2012;264(3):789–95.

Johnson NA, Tublin ME, Ogilvie JB. Parathyroid imaging: technique and role in the preoperative evaluation of primary hyperparathyroidism. Am J Roentgenol. 2007;188:1706–15.

Jones JJ, Brunaud L, Dowd C, Duh QY, Morita E, Clark OH. Accuracy of selective venous sampling for intact parathyroid hormone in difficult patients with recurrent or persistent hyperparathyroidism. Surgery. 2002;132(6):944–51.

Kandil E, Tufaro AP, Carson KA, Lin F, Somervell H, Farrag T, et al. Correlation of plasma 25-hydroxyvitamin D levels with severity of primary hyperparathyroidism and likelihood of parathyroid adenoma localization on sestamibi scan. Arch Otolaryngol Head Neck Surg. 2008;134:1071–5.

Kendrick ML, Charboneau JW, Curlee KJ, van Heerden JA, Farley DR. Risk of parathyromatosis after fine-needle aspiration. Am Surg. 2001;67(3):290–3.

Lau JH, Drake W, Matson M. The current role of venous sampling in the localization of endocrine disease. Cardiovasc Intervent Radiol. 2007;30(4):555–70.

Mahajan A, Starker LF, Ghita M, Udelsman R, Brink JA, Carling T. Parathyroid four-dimensional computed tomography: evaluation of radiation dose exposure during preoperative localization of parathyroid tumors in primary hyperparathyroidism. World J Surg. 2012;36(6):1335–9.

Mihai R, Gleeson F, Buley ID, Roskell DE, Sadler GP. Negative imaging studies for primary hyperparathyroidism are unavoidable: correlation of sestamibi and high-resolution ultrasound scanning with histological analysis in 150 patients. World J Surg. 2006;30(5):697–704.

Miller DL. Endocrine angiography and venous sampling. Radiol Clin North Am. 1993;31(5):1051–67.

Mitmaker J, Grogan RH, Duh QY. Guide to preoperative parathyroid localization testing. In: Randolph G, editor. Surgery of the thyroid and parathyroid glands. 2nd ed. Philadelphia: Elsevier; 2013.

Mortenson MM, Evans DB, Lee JE, Hunter GJ, Shellingerhout D, Vu T, et al. Parathyroid exploration in the reoperative neck: improved preoperative localization with 4D-computed tomography. J Am Coll Surg. 2008;206(5):888–95.

Nichols KJ, Tomas MB, Tronco GG, Rini JN, Kunjummen BD, Heller KS, et al. Preoperative parathyroid scintigraphic lesion localization: accuracy of various types of readings. Radiology. 2008;248(1):221–32.

Pata G, Casella C, Besuzio S, Mittempergher F, Salerni B. Clinical appraisal of 99m technetium-sestamibi SPECT/CT compared to conventional SPECT in patients with primary hyperparathyroidism and concomitant nodular goiter. Thyroid. 2010;20(10):1121–7.

Rodgers SE, Hunter GJ, Hamberg LM, Schellingerhout D, Doherty DB, Ayers GD, et al. Improved preoperative planning for directed parathyroidectomy with 4-dimensional computed tomography. Surgery. 2006;140(6):932–40.

Shafiei B, Hoseinzadeh S, Fotouhi F, Malek H, Azizi F, Jahed A, et al. Preoperative 99mTc-sestamibi scintigraphy in patients with primary hyperparathyroidism and concomitant nodular goiter: comparison of SPECT-CT, SPECT, and planar imaging. Nucl Med Commun. 2012;33(10):1070–6.

Shah S, Win Z, Al-Nahhas A. Multimodality imaging of the parathyroid glands in primary hyperparathyroidism. Minerva Endocrinol. 2008;33(3):193–202.

Siperstein A, Berber E, Barbosa GF, Tsinberg M, Greene AB, Mitchell J, et al. Predicting the success of limited exploration for primary hyperparathyroidism using ultrasound, sestamibi, and intraoperative parathyroid hormone: analysis of 1158 cases. Ann Surg. 2008;248(3):420–8.

Steward DL, Danielson GP, Afman CE. Parathyroid adenoma localization: surgeon-performed ultrasound versus sestamibi. Laryngoscope. 2009;116(8):1380–4.

Thomas DL, Bartel T, Menda Y, Howe J, Graham MM, Juweid ME. Single photon emission computed tomography (SPECT) should be routinely performed for the detection of parathyroid abnormalities utilizing technetium-99m sestamibi parathyroid scintigraphy. Clin Nucl Med. 2009;34(10):651–5.

Udelsman R, Pasieka JL, Sturgeon C, Young JE, Clark OH. Surgery for asymptomatic primary hyperparathyroidism: proceedings of the third international workshop. J Clin Endocrinol Metab. 2009;94(2):366–72.

Udelsman R, Lin Z, Donovan P. The superiority of minimally invasive parathyroidectomy based on 1650 consecutive patients with primary hyperparathyroidism. Ann Surg. 2011;253(3):585–91.

Untch BR, Adam MA, Scheri RP, Bennett KM, Dixit D, Webb C, et al. Surgeon-performed ultrasound is superior to 99Tc-sestamibi scanning to localize parathyroid adenomas in patients with primary hyperparathyroidism: results in 516 patients over 10 years. J Am Coll Surg. 2011;212(4):522–9.

Weber T, Maier-Funk C, Ohlhauser D, Hillenbrand A, Cammerer G, Barth TF, et al. Accurate preoperative localization of parathyroid adenomas with C-11 methionine PET/CT. Ann Surg. 2013;257:1124–8.

Yousem DM, Scheff AM. Thyroid and parathyroid gland pathology. Role of imaging. Otolaryngol Clin N Am. 1995;28(3):621–49.

15 Use of Intraoperative Parathyroid Hormone Assay

Keith S. Heller

Introduction

The availability of the rapid, intraoperative measurement of PTH (IOPTH) has changed the surgical approach to primary hyperparathyroidism (PHPT). Although bilateral cervical exploration with identification of all four parathyroid glands remains the standard to which all other surgical approaches are compared, the majority of patients undergoing surgery for PHPT in the United States undergo a less extensive exploration, limited to the removal of the single adenoma identified on preoperative imaging. This approach, frequently referred to as "minimally invasive parathyroidectomy" (MIP), is more accurately described as focused or single-gland exploration. MIP is not a surgical technique defined by the size of the incision or whether the procedure is performed endoscopically, robotically, or with video assistance. Rather it is a concept based on the fact that 80–85 % of patients with PHPT have a single adenoma and that while the location of this adenoma can be identified by preoperative imaging in most patients, preoperative imaging can only predict the presence of multiple hyperfunctioning parathyroid glands in 50 % of those patients in whom they occur. Based on these tenets, MIP is performed by removing the hyperfunctioning parathyroid gland identified on preoperative imaging and then measuring IOPTH. If IOPTH falls adequately, the procedure is terminated without identifying the remaining parathyroid glands. If all patients with PHPT had single adenomas or if preoperative imaging had a high sensitivity for the identification of those patients with multiple hyperfunctioning parathyroid glands, IOPTH would not be necessary. The crucial role of IOPTH is to predict the presence of additional hyperfunctioning parathyroid glands in those few patients, about 7 %, in whom imaging identifies one abnormal gland but who in fact have multiglandular disease. IOPTH does not necessarily confirm that parathyroid tissue that is removed is normal or abnormal. Rather it confirms that no residual hyperfunctioning parathyroid tissue remains in the neck.

K.S. Heller, MD, FACS
Department of Surgery, New York University Langone Medical Center, 530 First Avenue, HCC Suite 6H, New York, NY 10016, USA
e-mail: keith.heller@nyumc.org

History

The radioimmunoassay of PTH was first described by Berson, Yalow, and their associates in 1963. In 1988, Nussbaum et al. demonstrated that IOPTH fell to 40 % of baseline values within 15 min of the removal of a parathyroid adenoma and suggested that the "Intraoperative measurement of PTH by modification of this IRMA may complement surgical skill and histopathologic information and has the potential for providing guidance regarding the extent of neck exploration necessary for determining surgical care of

D.J. Terris, M.C. Singer (eds.), *Minimally Invasive and Robotic Thyroid and Parathyroid Surgery*,
DOI 10.1007/978-1-4614-9011-1_15, © Springer Science+Business Media New York 2014

hyperparathyroidism." Technical advances through the years have made the rapid intraoperative measurement of PTH by automated equipment either in the operating suite or in the central chemistry laboratory feasible. Dr. George Irvin, at the University of Miami, deserves recognition as the surgeon who was most responsible for demonstrating the clinical usefulness of IOPTH. Interestingly, in his initial report, IOPTH was used to decrease the failure rate in patients undergoing bilateral exploration, not to permit limited exploration. In multiple publications over the next two decades, his group has demonstrated that IOPTH could be used successfully to perform MIP with excellent immediate and long-term cure rates. Many other authors have confirmed his findings.

Technical Aspects

While it is convenient and expeditious to measure IOPTH in the OR suite, successful programs can function measuring IOPTH in the central chemistry lab if systems are developed to assure the rapid delivery of samples to the lab and the direct reporting of results to the OR. IOPTH values should be available within 30 min of being drawn and many systems can generate results in less than 20 min. Blood samples for IOPTH can be drawn from either an indwelling peripheral venous or intra-arterial cannula. We find the use of the jugular vein for routine sampling to be cumbersome, particularly through a small incision. In addition, the incision cannot be closed until the final sample is drawn. A baseline sample should be drawn as soon as the patient enters the operating room. In many patients, this intraoperative baseline is quite different from the most recent preoperative PTH. This sample should be obtained before the incision is made or the neck is palpated. Palpation of parathyroid adenomas can result in a sudden increase (spike) in IOPTH that can confound the interpretation of subsequent IOPTH values. Induction of general anesthesia may do this as well. The timing of subsequent IOPTH samples varies among institutions. Because the half-life of the intact PTH molecule is less than 2 min in most patients and almost never longer than 4 min, samples drawn 10 min after the hyperfunctioning gland is removed will usually demonstrate successful resolution of hyperparathyroidism. The decay curve is not simple first- or second-order kinetics, however, and IOPTH may take substantially longer to fall into the normal range when the baseline value is unusually high. It is important, and our practice, to obtain a sample at the time of excision of the enlarged parathyroid. Intraoperative manipulation of a hyperfunctioning parathyroid can result in a dramatic spike in IOPTH. Failure to recognize this may mislead the surgeon into thinking that IOPTH has not fallen adequately if samples are obtained only at 5 or 10 min after excision. In Fig. 15.1 it is demonstrated that if the "at excision" sample is not obtained, IOPTH levels at 5 and 10 min can suggest that additional hyperfunctioning parathyroid tissue is present and leads to unnecessary additional exploration. Another potential benefit of the "at excision" sample is that in some patients IOPTH has already decreased to an acceptable level, probably due to devascularization of the parathyroid, before it is actually removed, permitting early termination of the procedure. We usually draw samples at 15 and 20 min as well. While in many patients these prove unnecessary, in those patients in whom IOPTH decreases more slowly than normal or in whom there is an IOPTH spike at excision, substantial delay can result if additional samples are not drawn until the results of earlier samples are obtained.

There is no universal agreement on what constitutes an adequate decrease in IOPTH to assure cure. George Irvin and his associates rely on a 50 % decrease at 10 min from either the baseline or "at excision" IOPTH. Many surgeons feel uncomfortable terminating the procedure before the IOPTH has decreased more than 50 % from the baseline and into the normal range. Other permutations of this, all based on a percentage decrease at a set time interval, have been proposed. In most patients, IOPTH either falls dramatically after removal of the hyperfunctioning gland or falls hardly at all, making the decision to proceed with further exploration relatively simple. It should

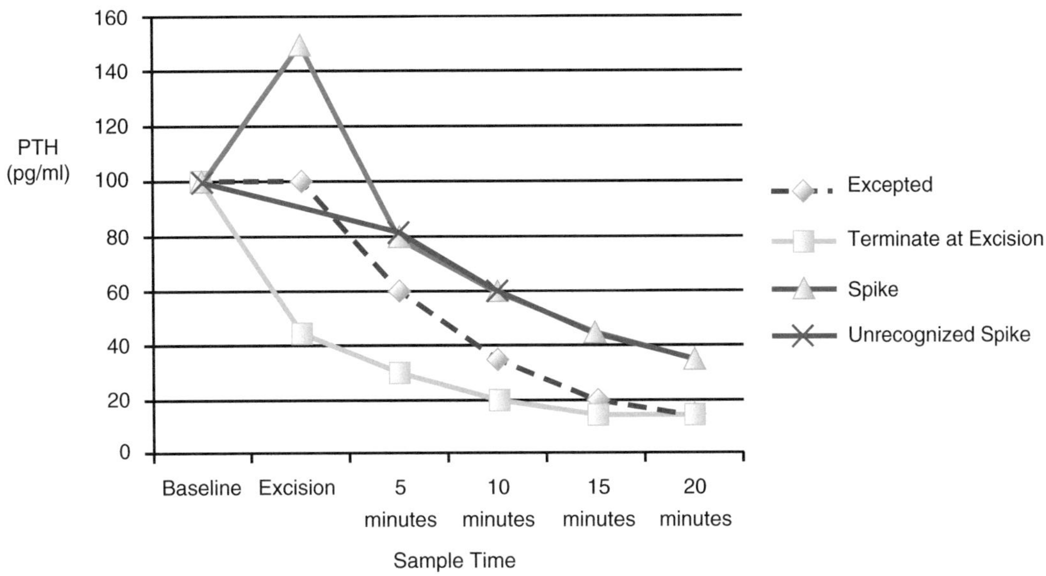

Fig. 15.1 Patterns of IOPTH decrease

also be noted that in some patients the baseline IOPTH is actually in the normal range. Even in these patients substantial decreases in IOPTH are usually observed following removal of the hyperfunctioning parathyroid(s).

Early in my experience, it became apparent that patients whose decrease in IOPTH level barely met the standard criteria had a higher incidence of persistent hyperparathyroidism postoperatively compared with those in whom the IOPTH decrease was dramatic. Requiring a greater decrease in IOPTH may result in fewer cases of persistent hyperparathyroidism after surgery but results in an increase in the number of unnecessary bilateral explorations. In a retrospective analysis of 194 patients, we found that persistent hyperparathyroidism after surgery almost always occurred in those patients whose final IOPTH was >40 pg/ml (although in all patients IOPTH decreased by at least 50 % and into the normal range) regardless of the percentage decrease from baseline. It would appear that the absolute final value of IOPTH is more predictive of success than the percentage decrease.

Some authors have suggested that MIP can be performed with a high success rate in many patients without the time and expense of IOPTH measurement. They argue that in a patient who only has a solitary adenoma that is localized by appropriate imaging, measurement of IOPTH is unnecessary. Kebebew et al. proposed a simple scoring system based on the results of preoperative sestamibi scans, ultrasonography, serum calcium level, and PTH that was 99 % accurate in predicting the presence of a single hyperfunctioning parathyroid. Others have suggested that the presence of concordant sestamibi and ultrasonography studies reliably predicts single-gland hyperparathyroidism and that measurement of IOPTH is not necessary in these patients. Our own experience differs from this. In patients with concordant sestamibi and ultrasonographic images demonstrating a solitary adenoma, 8 % of patients had additional enlarged hypercellular parathyroid glands found during further exploration performed because the decrease in IOPTH did not meet our criteria for successful surgery.

Other authors have criticized the entire concept of MIP based on IOPTH or radio guidance (see Chap. 5). Siperstein and his colleagues at the Cleveland Clinic have reported the results of their practice of measuring IOPTH while performing bilateral parathyroid exploration on all patients. In patients with preoperative imaging identifying a single adenoma and in whom IOPTH met the usual criteria for successful surgery following removal of the imaged parathyroid, 16 % were found to have additional enlarged hyperfunctioning parathyroid glands on bilateral exploration. This observation is difficult to reconcile with the results of many large series of focused, single-gland explorations in which the failure rate is only about 2 %. It would appear that either many patients will recur over time or that the enlarged, hypercellular parathyroid glands identified by Siperstein and his colleagues are of no clinical (and functional) significance.

There is another possible explanation for this observation. It has been well established that at least 15 % of patients whose calcium returns to normal after apparently successful parathyroidectomy have persistently elevated PTH postoperatively. In many patients, this is due to vitamin D deficiency or mild secondary hyperparathyroidism due to hypocalcemia. In some, however, the persistently elevated PTH is associated with normal vitamin D levels and calcium in the high normal range. These patients may indeed have mild persistent primary HPT and have been demonstrated to have a relatively high incidence of recurrent HPT with hypercalcemia. It is possible that those patients with additional enlarged, hypercellular parathyroid glands identified by Siperstein (which would not have been removed if exploration was terminated after an adequate decrease in IOPTH) may be responsible for this phenomenon.

Norman, in Tampa, was an early and enthusiastic advocate of MIP. Rather than assess the adequacy of parathyroidectomy by IOPTH, he used radio guidance to demonstrate that all hyperfunctioning parathyroid tissue had been removed. In a recent publication, he reported that long-term follow-up of his patients who had undergone limited exploration revealed a 6 % failure rate compared to a 99.4 % cure rate in those who had bilateral exploration. He concludes from this observation that limited exploration has an unacceptable high failure rate and should be abandoned. An alternative interpretation of his data, however, is that radio guidance is not an adequate substitute for IOPTH and that the difference in long-term outcome observed comparing limited with bilateral exploration would not have occurred had he determined the adequacy of surgery by IOPTH.

It will require many years of careful follow-up to confirm that MIP results in long-term cure rates of hyperparathyroidism comparable to bilateral exploration. Most studies published to date certainly support this. It is not adequate to follow serum calcium alone. At least 13 % of patients undergoing surgery for HPT are normocalcemic. In recent years in our practice, that figure has reached 19 %. These patients have significant clinical disease. Return of postoperative calcium levels to the normal range without knowledge of PTH levels is not a guarantee that the patient does not have mild persistent hyperparathyroidism. Serum calcium and PTH should be followed postoperatively, and in those patients with persistently elevated PTH, bone densitometry should be performed periodically. Lack of improvement or increase of bone loss would suggest that persistently elevated PTH, even in the presence of normocalcemia, is clinically significant. At the present time, there is insufficient data to suggest that MIP should be abandoned.

Other Uses of IOPTH

The measurement of IOPTH can help the surgeon in clinical situations other than MIP. There are many patients in whom bilateral exploration is necessary. Patients with inconclusive preoperative imaging or patients in whom imaging suggests multiple hyperfunctioning parathyroid glands are not candidates for MIP. Even the most experienced parathyroid surgeons can have difficulty differentiating normal from minimally enlarged, hyperfunctioning parathyroid glands, and persistent hyperparathyroidism can occur after bilateral exploration. Multiglandular parathyroid hyperplasia is not necessarily symmetrical. The presence of one obviously enlarged parathyroid does not mean that some of the smaller, relatively normal appearing glands are not hyperfunctioning. Frozen section biopsy of minimally enlarged parathyroid glands jeopardizes their viability. In addition, pathologists may not be able to differentiate normal from hypercellular parathyroid glands on frozen section when given a very small biopsy sample. When performing a bilateral exploration, persistence of IOPTH elevation following removal of an obviously enlarged parathyroid should prompt the removal or biopsy of additional parathyroid glands that appear relatively normal.

Conversely, while the goal in bilateral parathyroid exploration is to identify all four parathyroids, this is not always possible. If during the exploration an enlarged gland(s) is identified and one or more of the remaining glands cannot be identified, a decrease of IOPTH predictive of cure permits the surgeon to terminate the procedure rather than perform a difficult, time-consuming search for what is almost certainly a normal parathyroid. Before terminating an exploration of a patient suspected of having multiple hyperfunctioning parathyroid glands, the decrease of IOPTH should be well into the normal range, usually to less than 20 pg/ml, not simply more than 50 % of the baseline value.

This is especially true in reoperations on patients with recurrent or persistent hyperparathyroidism or in patients undergoing parathyroid exploration after previous thyroidectomy. Even when one has access to the previous operative and pathology reports, it is frequently difficult to be certain how many parathyroids were removed or damaged and how many remain in the neck. If during such a re-exploration an enlarged parathyroid is removed and IOPTH drops appropriately, further exploration to identify the remaining parathyroids, which may not even be present, can be avoided.

Carneiro-Pla has suggested the use of office-based ultrasound-guided bilateral jugular venous sampling to help localize parathyroid adenomas. This technique can also be used intraoperatively when a parathyroid adenoma cannot be found after thorough exploration. Blood samples are drawn directly from each jugular vein and IOPTH measured on each sample. A marked differential between the IOPTH in the two veins would prompt further exploration on the side with the higher value. This technique has proven useful in finding parathyroid adenomas cephalad to their usual locations.

IOPTH can also be used in conjunction with intraoperative FNA of thyroid nodules or other neck masses. If an intrathyroidal parathyroid is suspected during exploration, rather than perform a thyroid lobectomy, an intraoperative FNA can be performed and the needle rinsed with a small volume of saline which is sent for IOPTH. High PTH levels confirm the suspicion of a parathyroid gland. The same technique can be used to assess other neck masses rather than waiting for frozen section pathology.

Conclusion

IOPTH is an invaluable aid to the parathyroid surgeon. Access to this test permits the performance of MIP with a high likelihood of cure. Performance of MIP without IOPTH may result in a higher failure rate and should be discouraged. IOPTH is also valuable in difficult bilateral explorations and in reoperative surgery.

Recommended Reading

Alhefdhi A, Pinchot SN, Davis R, Sippel RS, Chen H. The necessity and reliability of intraoperative parathyroid hormone (PTH) testing in patients with mild hyperparathyroidism and PTH levels in the normal range. World J Surg. 2011;35(9):2006–9. Epub 2011/06/30.

Bergson EJ, Sznyter LA, Dubner S, Palestro CJ, Heller KS. Sestamibi scans and intraoperative parathyroid hormone measurement in the treatment of primary hyperparathyroidism. Arch Otolaryngol Head Neck Surg. 2004;130(1):87–91. Epub 2004/01/21.

Berson SA, Yalow RS, Aurbach GD, Potts JT. Immunoassay of bovine and human parathyroid hormone. Proc Natl Acad Sci USA. 1963;49(5):613–17. Epub 1963/05/01.

Carneiro DM, Solorzano CC, Nader MC, Ramirez M, Irvin 3rd GL. Comparison of intraoperative iPTH assay (QPTH) criteria in guiding parathyroidectomy: which criterion is the most accurate? Surgery. 2003;134(6):973–9; discussion 9–81. Epub 2003/12/12.

Carneiro-Pla D. Effectiveness of "office"-based, ultrasound-guided differential jugular venous sampling (DJVS) of parathormone in patients with primary hyperparathyroidism. Surgery. 2009;146(6):1014–20. Epub 2009/12/05.

Greene AB, Butler RS, McIntyre S, Barbosa GF, Mitchell J, Berber E, et al. National trends in parathyroid surgery from 1998 to 2008: a decade of change. J Am Coll Surg. 2009;209(3):332–43. Epub 2009/09/01.

Heller KS, Blumberg SN. Relation of final intraoperative parathyroid hormone level and outcome following parathyroidectomy. Arch Otolaryngol Head Neck Surg. 2009;135(11):1103–7. Epub 2009/11/18.

Hong JC, Morris LF, Park EJ, Ituarte PH, Lee CH, Yeh MW. Transient increases in intraoperative parathyroid levels related to anesthetic technique. Surgery. 2011;150(6):1069–75. Epub 2011/12/06.

Irvin 3rd GL, Dembrow VD, Prudhomme DL. Operative monitoring of parathyroid gland hyperfunction. Am J Surg. 1991;162(4):299–302. Epub 1991/10/01.

Kebebew E, Hwang J, Reiff E, Duh QY, Clark OH. Predictors of single-gland vs multigland parathyroid disease in primary hyperparathyroidism: a simple and accurate scoring model. Arch Surg. 2006;141(8):777–82; discussion 82. Epub 2006/08/23.

Libutti SK, Alexander HR, Bartlett DL, Sampson ML, Ruddel ME, Skarulis M, et al. Kinetic analysis of the rapid intraoperative parathyroid hormone assay in patients during operation for hyperparathyroidism. Surgery. 1999;126(6):1145–50; discussion 50–1. Epub 1999/12/22.

Mazzaglia PJ, Berber E, Kovach A, Milas M, Esselstyn C, Siperstein AE. The changing presentation of hyperparathyroidism over 3 decades. Arch Surg. 2008;143(3):260–6. Epub 2008/03/19.

Norman J, Lopez J, Politz D. Abandoning unilateral parathyroidectomy: why we reversed our position after 15,000 parathyroid operations. J Am Coll Surg. 2012;214(3):260–9. Epub 2012/01/24.

Nussbaum SR, Thompson AR, Hutcheson KA, Gaz RD, Wang CA. Intraoperative measurement of parathyroid hormone in the surgical management of hyperparathyroidism. Surgery. 1988;104(6):1121–7. Epub 1988/12/01.

Perrier ND, Ituarte P, Kikuchi S, Siperstein AE, Duh QY, Clark OH, et al. Intraoperative parathyroid aspiration and parathyroid hormone assay as an alternative to frozen section for tissue identification. World J Surg. 2000;24(11):1319–22. Epub 2000/10/19.

Richards ML, Thompson GB, Farley DR, Grant CS. An optimal algorithm for intraoperative parathyroid hormone monitoring. Arch Surg. 2011;146(3):280–5. Epub 2011/03/23.

Siperstein A, Berber E, Barbosa GF, Tsinberg M, Greene AB, Mitchell J, et al. Predicting the success of limited exploration for primary hyperparathyroidism using ultrasound, sestamibi, and intraoperative parathyroid hormone: analysis of 1158 cases. Ann Surg. 2008;248(3):420–8. Epub 2008/09/16.

Suliburk JW, Sywak MS, Sidhu SB, Delbridge LW. 1000 minimally invasive parathyroidectomies without intraoperative parathyroid hormone measurement: lessons learned. ANZ J Surg. 2011;81(5):362–5. Epub 2011/04/27.

Wang TS, Ostrower ST, Heller KS. Persistently elevated parathyroid hormone levels after parathyroid surgery. Surgery. 2005;138(6):1130–5; discussion 5–6. Epub 2005/12/20.

16 Minimally Invasive Non-endoscopic Parathyroidectomy

William S. Duke and David J. Terris

Introduction

Parathyroid surgery has changed significantly in the last 20 years, due largely to significant advances in early disease detection, improved preoperative localization modalities, and intraoperative adjuncts such as rapid parathyroid hormone (PTH) assays and handheld gamma probes. Prior to these advances, the surgical management of primary hyperparathyroidism (PHPT) mandated a large transverse cervical incision, bilateral neck exploration, identification of all four glands, and removal of any visibly abnormal glands. Though there are still clear indications for bilateral exploration, approximately 85 % of patients with PHPT have a single parathyroid adenoma. Given the largely focal nature of this disease process, as well as a global trend across surgical disciplines toward fewer open procedures, the development of minimally invasive surgery was a natural step in the treatment evolution of PHPT.

W.S. Duke, MD (✉)
Department of Otolaryngology,
Georgia Regents University, 1120 FifteenthStreet,
BP-4109, Augusta, GA 30912-4060, USA
e-mail: wduke@gru.edu

D.J. Terris, MD, FACS
Department of Otolaryngology–Head and Neck Surgery,
GRU Thyroid Center, Georgia Regents University,
1120 Fifteenth Street, BP-4109,
Augusta, GA 30912-4060, USA
e-mail: dterris@georgiahealth.edu

Minimally invasive surgery is in a broad sense a way of minimizing the tissue trauma required in traditional surgical exposures. However, there is currently no consensus as to what defines minimally invasive parathyroid surgery. This is due to the significant variations in surgical access options as well as differences in the potential extent of exploration performed in these procedures. Minimally invasive parathyroid surgery may refer to a bilateral exploration through an opening smaller than the Kocher incision used for the traditional procedure, a unilateral exploration only where two glands on the same side are identified, or focal surgery directed at only one gland. Though no strict definition exists, minimally invasive parathyroid surgery seeks to limit the length of the skin incision and minimize the extent of dissection to only that which is absolutely necessary to identify and remove the pathologic gland(s). This chapter primarily addresses the focused treatment of a single adenomatous gland through a minimally invasive open (non-endoscopic) approach. However, the concepts and techniques described are applicable to more extensive unilateral or bilateral, but still "minimally invasive," procedures.

Hyperparathyroidism Diagnosis

PHPT is characterized by hypercalcemia resulting from elevated PTH levels. PHPT is due to a single adenoma in 80–90 % of patients; multigland disease, such as double adenoma or diffuse

D.J. Terris, M.C. Singer (eds.), *Minimally Invasive and Robotic Thyroid and Parathyroid Surgery*, DOI 10.1007/978-1-4614-9011-1_16, © Springer Science+Business Media New York 2014

Table 16.1 Causes of hypercalcemia

Causes of hypercalcemia	
Parathyroid disease	*Drugs*
Adenoma	Lithium
Hyperplasia	Thiazide diuretics
MEN 1, MEN 2A	Vitamin D toxicity
Secondary hyperparathyroidism	Vitamin A toxicity
Tertiary hyperparathyroidism	Aminophylline
Carcinoma	*Miscellaneous*
Hyperparathyroidism-jaw tumor syndrome	Familial hypocalciuric hypercalcemia
Familial isolated hyperparathyroidism	Milk alkali syndrome
Malignancy	Granulomatous diseases
Ectopic PTH secretion	Immobilization
Parathyroid hormone-related protein	
Lytic bone lesions	
Ectopic vitamin D	
Endocrine	
Hyperthyroidism	
Adrenal insufficiency	
Pheochromocytoma	

hyperplasia, in 9–14 % of patients; and parathyroid carcinoma in fewer than 1 % of patients. Since demographic variations and assay differences preclude unified laboratory values to strictly define hyperparathyroidism, local reference ranges are adequate to establish the diagnosis.

Prior to calcium screening with routine blood chemistry tests, many patients with PHPT presented with a heterogeneous yet well-characterized spectrum of findings. The so-called traditional or symptomatic patients were frequently found to have renal disease such as nephrolithiasis, bone changes including osteopenia and pathologic fractures, gastrointestinal disturbances and gastric ulcers, fatigue, weakness, and mental status changes. Routine testing of blood calcium over the last five decades has led to a marked increase in the diagnosis of "asymptomatic" PHPT, which likely represents early detection in more than 80 % of patients with the disease. Though these patients lack the overt symptoms classically seen in advanced hyperparathyroidism, they may have subtle symptoms of malaise, fatigue, and neurocognitive deficits. These patients may undergo symptomatic disease progression if left untreated.

Calcium values are usually elevated or in the high normal range in patients with PHPT, though the levels may not be persistently elevated in those with mild or early disease. Patients with elevated calcium levels are further evaluated with PTH testing. The combination of hypercalcemia in the setting of an elevated or inadequately suppressed PTH level is strongly suggestive of PHPT. Other causes of hypercalcemia, particularly lithium use, should be evaluated as indicated and vitamin D levels should be obtained (Table 16.1). Patients should also be screened for conditions associated with multigland hyperplasia, including multiple endocrine neoplasia types 1 and 2A (MEN-1, MEN-2A), renal hyperparathyroidism, familial isolated hyperparathyroidism, and hyperparathyroidism-jaw tumor syndrome.

Familial hypocalciuric hypercalcemia (FHH), which is due to abnormalities in the calcium-sensing receptor (CaSR) in the parathyroid glands and kidneys, may cause both elevated calcium and PTH levels. This rare benign disorder does not require treatment and should be excluded prior to any surgical intervention. Patients may be screened with a calcium/creatinine clearance ratio (CCCR). Patients with FHH typically have a CCCR of less than 0.01, while those with PHPT have a ratio greater than 0.02. However, there is a great degree of overlap of these two diseases in patients with CCCRs between 0.01 and 0.02. Thus, those with a CCCR in this range may benefit from CaSR mutational analysis to clearly establish the diagnosis.

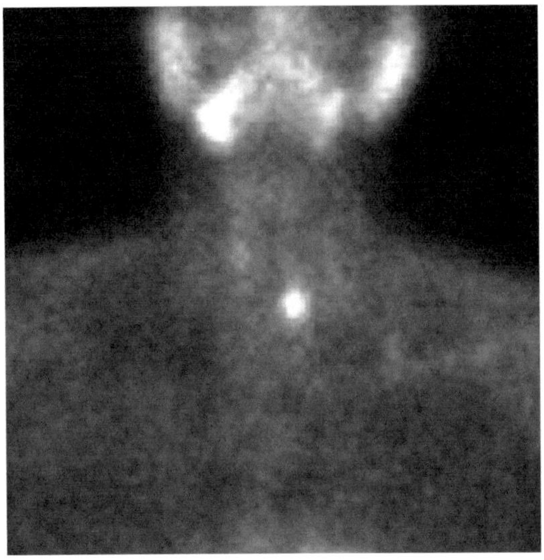

Fig. 16.1 Second phase of technetium-99m sestamibi scan obtained at 2 h showing uptake consistent with a left inferior parathyroid adenoma

Preoperative Imaging

Minimally invasive parathyroid surgery, in which fewer than four glands are sought, relies on identification of the likely abnormal gland location with preoperative imaging. This helps direct the surgeon to the side most likely to contain the abnormal gland and can offer information as to whether a superior or inferior gland is involved or if an ectopic adenoma is present. Studies suggest that performing at least two different imaging modalities can improve tumor localization and, when concordant, may result in successful surgery in 97 % of patients undergoing minimally invasive parathyroidectomy. It is important to recognize that these imaging modalities are not used to diagnose parathyroid disease but rather to help guide the surgeon in selecting the most appropriate procedure once the diagnosis is confirmed biochemically.

Technetium-99m sestamibi (sestamibi) is the most common imaging modality currently used (Fig. 16.1). The agent is concentrated in both the thyroid and parathyroid glands but takes longer to wash out of the parathyroid glands due to the relatively high mitochondrial content within parathyroid cells. The sensitivity of sestamibi varies between 50 and 90 % depending on the institution. The sensitivity may drop in the presence of thyroid nodules, which are found in more than a third of all patients that are imaged. A negative sestamibi does not necessarily preclude treatment with a minimally invasive procedure. This modality may be of limited use in detecting small adenomas, and the accuracy may vary based on calcium and PTH levels, patient body mass index, or in patients taking calcium channel blockers. Ultrasound or another imaging modality may identify the single adenoma and therefore render the patient a candidate for a minimally invasive procedure. However, a negative sestamibi may impart a higher risk of multigland disease, up to 47 % in some series, so the surgeon should be prepared to perform a bilateral exploration in these patients if necessary.

Sestamibi is useful in detecting ectopic parathyroid glands, identifying up to 75 % of cases in one series. The test is often combined with single photon emission computed tomography (SPECT) to improve anatomic localization of a sestamibi-positive lesion. Sestamibi-SPECT has also been shown to improve single adenoma detection compared with standard planar sestamibi techniques and has an overall sensitivity of 78.9 %. Sestamibi-SPECT is now routinely performed as the initial imaging modality in many institutions and is recommended in all cases of previously failed surgery.

Ultrasound using a high-frequency linear array transducer is also frequently used to evaluate the parathyroid glands preoperatively and has an overall sensitivity of 76 % for single-gland disease. It is often combined with a sestamibi scan, which increases detection sensitivity to 89–98 %. There are many advantages of ultrasound, including the speed and accessibility of the procedure, a relatively low cost, and the lack of radiation exposure. Perhaps the most important advantages are the ability of the surgeon to personally perform the study and visualize the anatomic location of the adenoma and the opportunity to evaluate for the presence of any concurrent thyroid disease, such as nodules or thyroiditis, which may significantly affect surgical planning.

Normal parathyroid glands are typically not appreciated on cervical ultrasound. Parathyroid adenomas usually present as round or ovoid solid hypoechoic masses. They are generally separated from the thyroid gland by an echogenic band. The presence of a polar vascular pedicle on Doppler mode rather than a central hilar vascular pattern can help distinguish adenomas from lymph nodes. Ultrasound will typically detect eutopic glands larger than 1 cm, but its sensitivity decreases in the presence of multigland disease, when the glands are usually not as large as in the case of single-gland adenomas. Ultrasound may visualize the location of some ectopic gland locations in the neck, such as an intrathyroidal adenoma, but its utility is limited in cases of mediastinal or retropharyngeal lesions.

Computed tomography (CT) and magnetic resonance imaging (MRI) have been used to provide cross-sectional anatomic imaging of abnormal parathyroid glands. The utilization of these modalities has traditionally been limited because of their use of contrast, decreased sensitivity, and significant radiation exposure (with CT). Therefore, these studies have primarily been reserved for cases with unsuccessful localization with ultrasound and sestamibi, ectopic glands, and reoperative procedures. The development of advanced imaging techniques such as 4D-CT, in which contrast uptake and washout are combined with CT imaging to identify parathyroid lesions, may contribute to improved imaging accuracy and help identify cases of multigland disease.

Medical Treatment

Though surgery is the only cure for PHPT, there are patients who may not be candidates for the procedure. These may be asymptomatic individuals who do not yet meet the established guidelines for surgical intervention or who may have other medical comorbidities that place them at high risk of a perioperative adverse event. Nonsurgical options include surveillance with regular evaluation by a primary care physician or endocrinologist, correction of any underlying vitamin D deficiency, a normocalcemic diet, and medical intervention. Agents potentially useful in the treatment of PHPT include bisphosphonates, hormone replacement therapy in postmenopausal women, or the use of calcimimetics. Bisphosphonates and hormone replacement therapy may help decrease bone turnover and improve bone mineral density, but have not been shown to durably reduce PTH or calcium levels. Calcimimetics, such as cinacalcet, modulate the CaSR, increasing the receptor's sensitivity to circulating calcium and thereby decreasing PTH release. Cinacalcet may decrease calcium and PTH levels, but does not significantly improve bone density. It is important that patients be counselled that medical treatment may help mediate some of the metabolic effects of their condition, but does not cure them of their disease.

Surgical Intervention

Indications

Surgery is the only curative treatment for PHPT and is more cost effective than prolonged medical therapy. Parathyroid surgery is indicated in patients with symptomatic hyperparathyroidism or in asymptomatic patients who meet the guidelines established by the 2002 and 2009 NIH consensus panels (Table 16.2). Patients with non-localizing imaging studies or those with disorders known to involve multiple glands generally undergo a bilateral neck exploration.

Candidates for successful minimally invasive non-endoscopic parathyroid surgery are patients with presumed single-gland disease, who have localizing preoperative imaging studies. However, it is critical for surgeons to be aware that even in cases with concordant preoperative imaging studies, multiglandular disease can be present. The surgeon should therefore always be prepared to convert to a bilateral exploration if indicated.

Surgery

Traditional parathyroid surgery requires a long transverse neck incision (typically 7–10 cm), elevation of subplatysmal flaps, and bilateral

Table 16.2 Indications for parathyroidectomy

Indications for parathyroidectomy in asymptomatic patients	
1. Serum calcium elevated more than 1 mg/dL above upper limits of normal	4. Age <50 years old
2. Glomerular filtration rate <60 mL/min	5. Patient requests surgery or is poor candidate for long-term observation
3. Bone mineral density T-score <–2.5 at any site or prior fragility fracture	

Adapted from Bilezikian J, Potts J, Fuleihan G, et al. Summary statement from a workshop on asymptomatic primary hyperparathyroidism: a perspective for the 21st century. J Endocrinol Metab. 2002;87(12):5353–61 and Bilezikian J, Khan A, Potts J. Guidelines for the management of asymptomatic primary hyperparathyroidism: summary statement from the third international workshop. J Clin Endocrinol Metab. 2009;94(2):335–9

neck exploration to expose all four parathyroid glands. Glands that appear abnormal are removed. Some surgeons confirm the presence of hypercellular tissue in the suspicious gland by comparing it to frozen section biopsy specimens from the normal-appearing glands. Drains are often placed and patients are typically admitted to the hospital for postoperative monitoring. This approach, with a success rate of 95 %, was considered the standard of care prior to widespread use of preoperative localization studies. It remains the standard by which the effectiveness of all minimally invasive approaches is judged. Bilateral exploration is still indicated in patients with disease entities associated with diffuse hyperplasia, such as renal hyperparathyroidism, MEN-1, and MEN-2A.

Though diverse in execution and the use of ancillary aids, minimally invasive parathyroid surgery is defined by a reduction either in the size of the incision or in the overall extent of dissection and resultant tissue trauma. Minimally invasive non-endoscopic parathyroidectomy utilizes a small incision, with initial dissection focused solely in the quadrant of the presumed abnormal gland (as seen on preoperative imaging). The procedure is subsequently directed by intraoperative findings and the results of the rapid intraoperative PTH (IOPTH) assay.

The planned cervical incision is marked while the patient is awake and upright in the holding area. This helps ensure the incision will be concealed within a naturally occurring skin crease (Fig. 16.2). The patient is placed supine on the operating table and general anesthesia is induced. Intubation is generally performed with a standard endotracheal tube, though in selected or revision cases a laryngeal EMG endotracheal tube (Medtronic ENT, Jacksonville, FL) may be used. Generally no shoulder roll is required, but the headrest of the bed is lowered slightly to provide gentle neck extension. The operating table is then rotated 180° so the patient's lower extremities are facing the anesthesia team. This allows placement of an intravenous line in one of the patient's feet for IOPTH assessment and obviates the need for an arterial line. An ultrasound repeated at this time by the surgeon can confirm the findings of the preoperative studies and provide precise

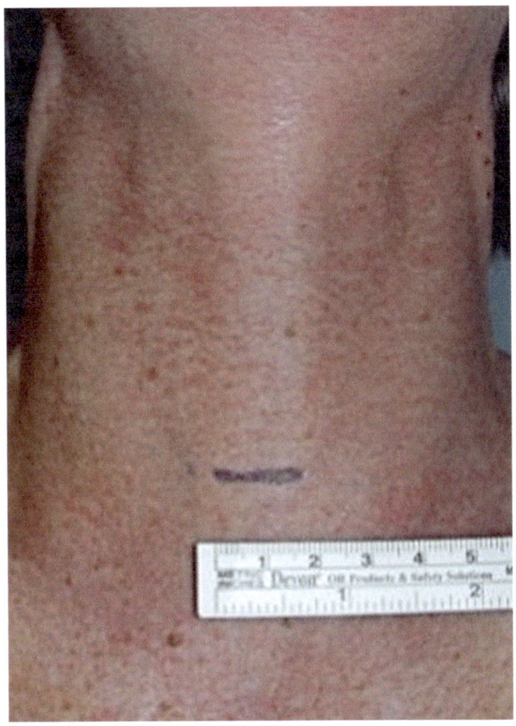

Fig. 16.2 Planned 1.5-cm midline incision in a naturally occurring skin crease

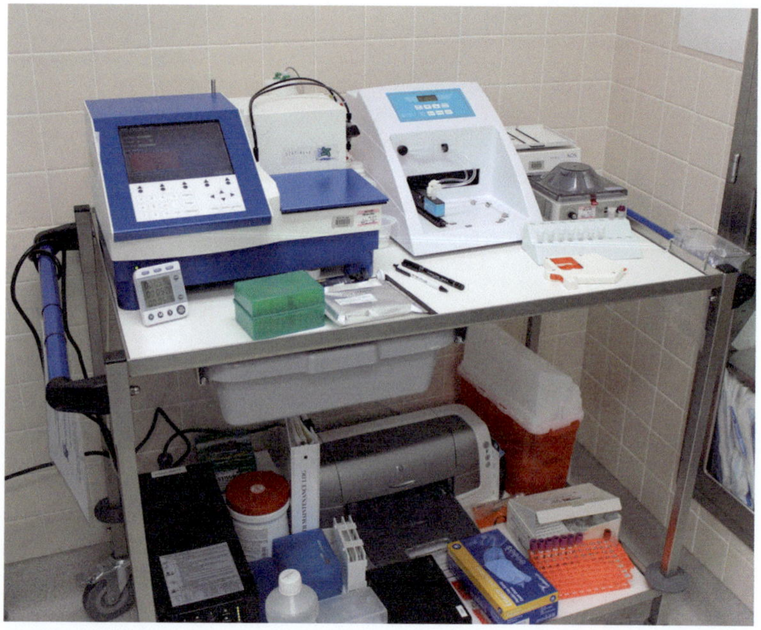

Fig. 16.3 Mobile intraoperative PTH assay equipment in operating room

guidance for the upcoming dissection. The planned incision site is infiltrated with 0.25 % bupivacaine with 1:200,000 epinephrine (Hospira, Lake Forest, IL), and a sterile prep is applied to the neck. A baseline IOPTH level is drawn prior to incision. The IOPTH assay is preferably performed by a technician with mobile equipment in the operating room, eliminating the transport time required to send the sample to the main laboratory (Fig. 16.3).

A knife is used to make a 2- to 2.5-cm skin incision, and the dissection is carried through the subcutaneous tissue. Careful attention is given to absolute hemostasis, as any bleeding from superficial tissue layers can obscure critical visualization of deeper structural details. The medial aspects of the platysma, if encountered, are divided to the lateral extent of the incision. No subplatysmal flaps are elevated. The strap muscles are separated vertically in the midline and the thyroid isthmus is identified. The strap muscles on the side of the suspected adenoma are bluntly elevated off the anterior and lateral aspect of the thyroid lobe and secured under Terris thyroid retractors (Medtronic ENT, Jacksonville, FL).

Attention is then directed toward the most likely location of the pathologic gland, as predicted by localization studies. The majority of parathyroid adenomas lie in predictable locations within the central neck compartment, but up to 13 % of patients have supernumerary glands, which may be pathologic, and as many as 11 % of patients have more than 1 adenoma. The superior glands are usually located within a 2-cm area whose center is 1 cm cranial to the intersection of the recurrent laryngeal nerve and the inferior thyroid artery. The location of the inferior parathyroid glands is more variable. They are typically located within 1 cm of the inferior aspect of the thyroid gland, anterior to a coronal plane drawn through the recurrent laryngeal nerve, but may be intimately associated with the thymus or thyrothymic tract in up to 26 % of patients.

To explore the superior gland, the thyroid lobe is retracted ventrally and medially with the Terris retractors, exposing the posterior aspect of the thyroid lobe and the paratracheal region. This exposure can usually be accomplished without division of the middle thyroid vein. The inferior parathyroid gland may be found by gently dissecting the soft tissue ventral to inferior pole of the thyroid gland or may be identified dorsal to the gland by gentle retraction of the thyroid lobe.

The ability to visually distinguish a normal from abnormal gland is crucial to minimally invasive parathyroid surgery, as there are often no

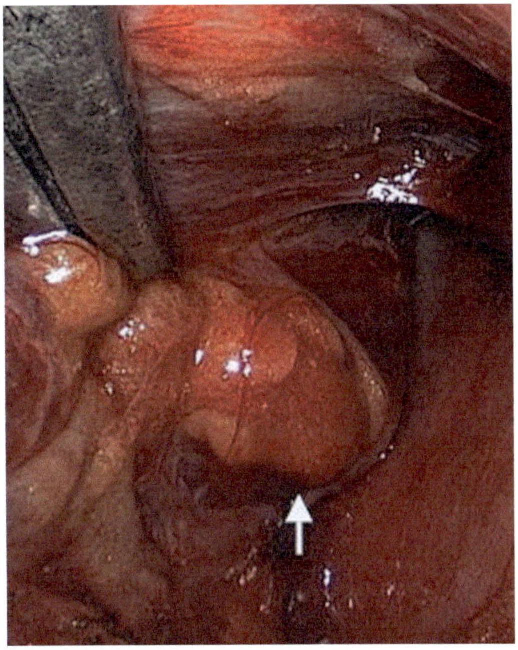

Fig. 16.4 Normal parathyroid gland (*arrow*) demonstrating the caramel color and surrounding fat

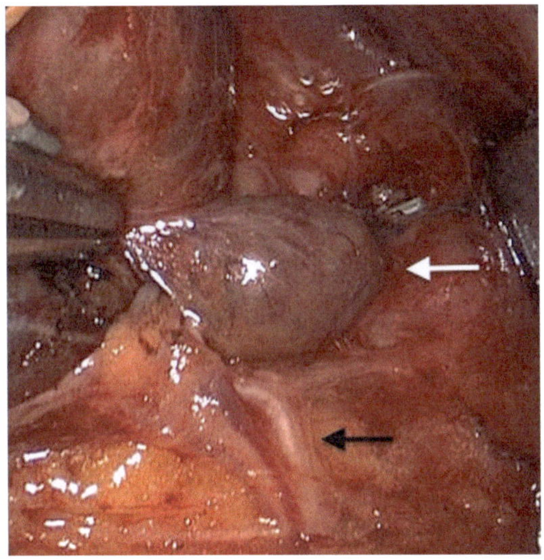

Fig. 16.5 Parathyroid adenoma (*white arrow*) and recurrent laryngeal nerve (*black arrow*)

normal glands exposed for reference. Normal parathyroid glands are typically flat, are light brown to tobacco in color, and are 3–8 mm long with an average weight of 40 mg. They are usually surrounded by or capped with fat (Fig. 16.4). Parathyroid adenomas are typically larger, more rounded, rubbery, and a darker red brown in color (Fig. 16.5). Gentle spreading of overlying fat may help reveal the enlarged glands. Once identified, blunt dissection with spatulas is used to gently liberate the gland from the surrounding soft tissue, until only the vascular pedicle remains attached to the gland. Soft tissue adherent to the capsule of the gland may be gently grasped to facilitate retraction and dissection, but care should be taken to avoid grabbing or excessive manipulation of the gland itself, as this may stimulate release of stored parathyroid hormone and alter subsequent IOPTH levels.

The recurrent laryngeal nerve may be identified and is preserved during this dissection. Once free from the surrounding tissue, the vascular pedicle of the adenoma may be transected with electrocautery or ligated with vessel clips and sharply divided if it is near the recurrent laryngeal nerve. Frozen sections are not generally used. Once the suspicious gland has been removed, the surgical field is irrigated, hemostasis is assured, and half a sheet of Surgicel (Ethicon, Inc., Somerville, NJ) is placed into the wound bed. The strap muscles are reapproximated in the midline with a single 3–0 Vicryl (Ethicon, Inc., Somerville, NJ) figure-of-eight suture. The subcutaneous tissue is closed with buried interrupted 4–0 Vicryl (Ethicon, Inc., Somerville, NJ) sutures, and the skin edges are closed with DermaFlex adhesive (Chemence Medical Products, Inc., Alpharetta, GA) and a single transverse Steri-Strip (3M Corporation, St. Paul, MN). No drains or external sutures are used (Fig. 16.6).

Post-excisional IOPTH levels are drawn 5 and 10 min after removal of the abnormal gland. This may be extended to a 15-min interval if necessary. Obtaining levels at these time points allows the surgeon to assess the PTH decline and make a decision about the likelihood of a successful operation. The 5-min level is particularly useful because the operation can often be terminated after this value is ascertained. The procedure is considered successful and terminated if the post-extirpation IOPTH level has fallen at least 50 % below the baseline value and is within the normal

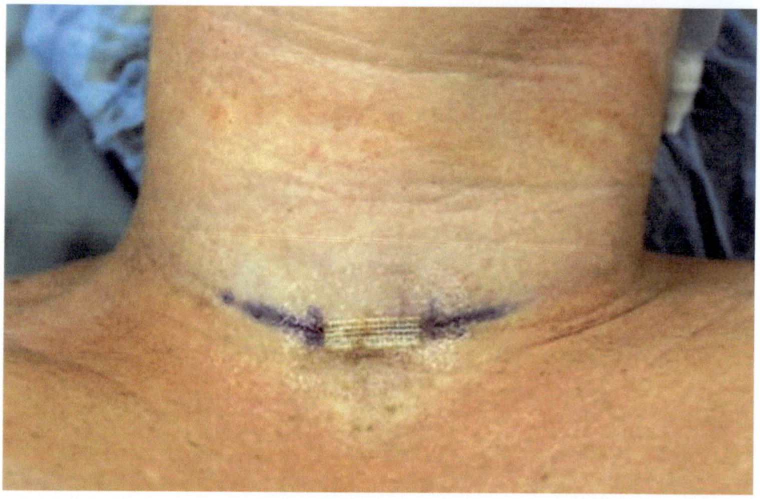

Fig. 16.6 Final appearance of the closed incision with ¼-in. Steri-Strip embedded in skin glue to facilitate removal of the adhesive at 3 weeks postoperatively

range. Patients are discharged home on the day of surgery with a short-term prescription for an oral calcium supplement.

When the IOPTH fails to decrease as anticipated, the surgeon should be suspicious of the presence of multigland disease. If there is any doubt about the ability to adequately identify the glands or if an ectopic gland is suspected, the procedure should be converted to a standard bilateral exploration and all potential gland locations explored as indicated.

Modifications

There are numerous modifications of the previously described minimally invasive non-endoscopic parathyroidectomy technique, which may be tailored to the individual preferences of the surgeon and needs of the patient. While these modifications are reviewed in detail in other chapters of this text, they are briefly introduced here to demonstrate the versatility of the minimally invasive approach.

The procedure can be performed under local anesthesia using a cervical block and monitored anesthesia care. This may allow patients with medical comorbidities that preclude the safe use of general anesthesia to undergo the procedure.

As mentioned earlier, the focused approach can be expanded to either a unilateral or bilateral exploration if necessary, often through the same small incision. This may be useful for identifying and obtaining a biopsy of a second, normal-appearing gland in institutions that rely on frozen section analysis rather than IOPTH assays or in cases where the previously suspected abnormal gland on preoperative imaging appears to be normal on intraoperative inspection. Proceeding with a bilateral exploration through the same minimally invasive incision is generally easier in patients without large thyroid nodules or a history of thyroiditis, though these conditions are not necessarily contraindications to a minimally invasive procedure.

Though typically described with a midline incision, the minimally invasive procedure may be performed through a lateral approach in carefully selected patients with posteriorly located adenomas. Rather than dividing the strap muscles in the midline, dissection is directed between the lateral aspect of the strap muscles and the sternocleidomastoid muscle to access the region posterior to the thyroid gland. This approach may offer fast, more direct access to deep adenomas and may be more comfortable for patients undergoing local anesthesia for their procedure.

Endoscopic modifications of minimally invasive parathyroid surgery are also possible, though more stringent patient selection criteria apply than for other procedures. Patients generally should have well-localized adenomas in the absence of a large goiter, diffuse hyperplasia, or a history of previous neck surgery. The operation may be performed through a midline or lateral approach with the assistance of a 30° endoscope, and bilateral exploration is possible if a midline incision is used.

The minimally invasive radioguided modification takes advantage of the preferential retention of technetium-99m sestamibi by the parathyroid glands compared to the thyroid gland and surrounding soft tissue. After injection of sestamibi on the day of surgery, a standard minimally invasive non-endoscopic parathyroidectomy is performed. Once the suspicious gland has been removed, a handheld gamma probe is used to measure the radioactivity in both the excised gland and over the patient's right shoulder. A radioactivity reading in the excised gland that exceeds 20 % of the background level suggests successful removal of the pathologic gland.

Success Rates

To become a reasonable alternative, any new surgical technique must yield outcomes that are at least equivalent to the conventional approach. Multiple studies have now confirmed that minimally invasive parathyroidectomy procedures performed by experienced providers in properly selected patients produce results that are comparable to traditional open four-gland exploration. Durable biochemical cures are reliably obtained in 95–99 % of patients undergoing a minimally invasive parathyroid procedure, identical to the 97 % success rate reported for the classic approach. Overall complication rates of 1–3 % in minimally invasive procedures also compare favorably to a 3.1 % complication rate in conventional explorations. Operating times are significantly reduced with the minimally invasive approach, although the IOPTH assay adds to the overall procedure time. The ability to perform the PTH assay in the OR decreases specimen transport time, and the incision may be closed while the assay is being performed. The hospital length of stay is reduced in patients undergoing minimally invasive parathyroidectomy, with most patients discharged on the day of surgery. Minimally invasive parathyroidectomy has been shown to be more cost effective than long-term medical therapy or traditional parathyroidectomy, but the actual cost differences will vary by choices in preoperative imaging, the use of intraoperative adjuncts, and the type of anesthesia administered.

Complications

There are no specific complications unique to a minimally invasive non-endoscopic parathyroidectomy. In addition to the standard risks inherent in any surgical procedure, patients undergoing any parathyroid surgery are at risk for hypocalcemia, recurrent laryngeal nerve (RLN) injury, and persistence or recurrence of their disease. The risk of permanent RLN injury is less than 1 % when the procedure is performed by experienced surgeons. Transient hypocalcemia may occur in up to 35 % of patients undergoing parathyroid surgery and may be persistent in up to 4 % of cases. The effects of any transient hypocalcemia in the immediate postoperative period may be mitigated by the use of prophylactic calcium and vitamin D supplementation.

Persistence and recurrence rates are both low, as evidenced by the high success rates in minimally invasive procedures. Persistent disease, defined as hypercalcemia and elevated PTH levels within 6 months of the initial procedure, typically occurs when residual hyperfunctioning parathyroid tissue remains after the initial operation. Recurrence refers to biochemical evidence of PHPT that occurs after at least 6 months of normal postoperative laboratory results. The most common cause for persistence or recurrence is a single eutopic adenoma that was not located on the initial exploration. Other causes include a missed double adenoma, inadequate treatment of multigland hyperplasia, an ectopic adenoma, conversion of normal glands to hyperfunctional glands in patients with familial syndromes, and parathyromatosis or residual parathyroid carcinoma. Re-exploration via a non-endoscopic minimally invasive approach may still be feasible in appropriately selected patients.

There are instances when conversion from a minimally invasive approach to a conventional, open bilateral neck exploration may be warranted. Common causes for conversion include failed localization of the pathologic gland, concern for an ectopic gland, failure of the IOPTH levels to decline after adenoma removal, multigland disease, concern for parathyroid carcinoma, concomitant thyroid disease, and suspicion of failed localization. Published rates of conversion vary from 3 to 17 %.

Conclusion

The last several decades have resulted in a significant change in the dogma of parathyroid surgery. Though there are still clear indications for bilateral open exploration, the majority of patients that now present with PHPT are candidates for a minimally invasive non-endoscopic approach to cure their disease. This transformation has been driven by improved preoperative localization strategies and innovative intraoperative adjuncts, which, along with increased surgeon experience, has made the minimally invasive parathyroidectomy a well-established, safe, and efficacious treatment of PHPT.

Recommended Reading

Berber E, Parikh R, Ballem N, et al. Factors contributing to negative parathyroid localization: an analysis of 1000 patients. Surgery. 2008;144(1):74–9.

Bilezikian J, Potts J, Fuleihan G, et al. Summary statement from a workshop on asymptomatic primary hyperparathyroidism: a perspective for the 21st century. J Clin Endocrinol Metab. 2002;87(12):5353–61.

Bilezikian J, Khan A, Potts J. Guidelines for the management of asymptomatic primary hyperparathyroidism: summary statement from the third international workshop. J Clin Endocrinol Metab. 2009;94(2):335–9.

Chazen J, Gupta A, Dunning A, Phillips C. Diagnostic accuracy of 4D-CT for parathyroid adenomas and hyperplasia. Am J Neuroradiol. 2012;33:429–33.

Cheung K, Wang T, Farrokhyar F, et al. A meta-analysis of preoperative localization techniques for patients with primary hyperparathyroidism. Ann Surg Oncol. 2012;19:577–83.

Cho N, Gawande A, Sheu E, et al. Critical role of identification of the second gland during unilateral parathyroid surgery: a prospective review of 119 patients with concordant localization. Arch Surg. 2011;146(5):512516.

Christensen S, Nissen P, et al. Discriminative power of three indices of renal calcium excretion for the distinction between familial hypocalciuric hypercalcemia and primary hyperparathyroidism: a follow-up study on methods. Clin Endocrinol. 2008;69:713–20.

Crea N, Pata G, Casella C, et al. Predictive factors for postoperative severe hypocalcaemia after parathyroidectomy for primary hyperparathyroidism. Am Surg. 2012;78(3):352–8.

Denham D, Norman J. Cost-effectiveness of preoperative sestamibi scan for primary hyperparathyroidism is dependent solely upon the surgeon's choice of operative procedure. J Am Coll Surg. 1998;186(3):293–304; discussion 304–5.

Eastell R, Arnold A, Brandi M, et al. Diagnosis of asymptomatic primary hyperparathyroidism: proceedings of the third international workshop. J Clin Endocrinol Metab. 2009;94(2):340–50.

Erbil Y, Barbaros U, Tukenmez M, et al. Impact of adenoma weight and ectopic location of parathyroid adenoma on localization study results. World J Surg. 2008;32:566–71.

Fancy T, Gallagher D, Hornig J. Surgical anatomy of the thyroid and parathyroid glands. Otolaryngol Clin N Am. 2010;43:221–7.

Gracie D, Hussain S. Use of minimally invasive parathyroidectomy techniques in sporadic primary hyperparathyroidism: systematic review. J Laryngol Otol. 2012;126:221–7.

Grayev A, Gentry L, Hartman M, et al. Presurgical localization of parathyroid adenomas with magnetic resonance imaging at 3.0 T: an adjunct method to supplement traditional imaging. Ann Surg Oncol. 2012;19:981–9.

Heizmann O, Viehl C, Schmid R, et al. Impact of concomitant thyroid pathology on preoperative workup for primary hyperparathyroidism. Eur J Med Res. 2009;14:37–41.

Heller K, Blumberg S. Relation of final intraoperative parathyroid hormone level and outcome following parathyroidectomy. Arch Otolaryngol Head Neck Surg. 2009;135(11):1103–7.

Hunter J. Minimally invasive surgery: the next frontier. World J Surg. 1999;23:422–4.

Kamaya A, Quon A, Jeffrey R. Sonography of the abnormal parathyroid gland. Ultrasound Q. 2006;22(4):253–62.

Kandil E, Malazai A, Alrasheedi S, Tufano R. Minimally invasive/focused parathyroidectomy in patients with negative sestamibi scan results. Arch Otolaryngol Head Neck Surg. 2012;138(3):223–5.

Kebebew E, Hwang J, Reiff E, et al. Predictors of single-gland vs multigland parathyroid disease in primary hyperparathyroidism: a simple and accurate scoring model. Arch Surg. 2006;141:777–82; discussion 782.

Keutgen X, Buitrago D, Filicori F, et al. Calcimimetics versus parathyroidectomy for treatment of primary hyperparathyroidism: retrospective chart analysis of a prospective database. Ann Surg. 2012;255(5):981–5.

Khan A, Grey A, Shobak D. Medical management of asymptomatic primary hyperparathyroidism: proceedings of the third international workshop. J Clin Endocrinol Metab. 2009;94(2):373–81.

Miccoli P, Materazzi G, Bonari G, et al. Minimally invasive video-assisted parathyroidectomy. Oper Tech Otolaryngol. 2008;19:22–5.

Moore F. Oral calcium supplements to enhance early hospital discharge after bilateral surgical treatment of the thyroid gland or exploration of the parathyroid glands. J Am Coll Surg. 1994;178:11–6.

Moreno M, Callender G, Woodburn K, et al. Common locations of parathyroid adenomas. Ann Surg Oncol. 2011;18:1047–51.

Nagar S, Reid D, Czako P, et al. Outcomes analysis of intraoperative adjuncts during minimally invasive parathyroidectomy for primary hyperparathyroidism. Am J Surg. 2012;203(2):177–81.

Norman J, Chheda H, Farrell C. Minimally invasive parathyroidectomy for primary hyperparathyroidism: decreasing operative time and potential complications while improving cosmetic results. Am Surg. 1998; 64(5):391–5.

Pellitteri P. Intraoperative assessment of parathyroid hormone. Oper Tech Otolaryngol. 2009;20:60–5.

Phillips C, Shatzkes D. Imaging of the parathyroid glands. Semin Ultrasound CT MR. 2012;33:123–9.

Prager G, Czerny C, Kurtaran A. Minimally invasive open parathyroidectomy in an endemic goiter area. Arch Surg. 2001;136:810–6.

Prager G, Czerny C, Ofluoglu S, et al. Impact of localization studies on feasibility of minimally invasive parathyroidectomy in an endemic goiter region. J Am Coll Surg. 2003;196(4):541–8.

Richards M, Thompson G, Farley D, Grant C. An optimal algorithm for intraoperative parathyroid hormone monitoring. Arch Surg. 2011;146(3):280–5.

Ritter H, Milas M. Bilateral parathyroid exploration for hyperparathyroidism. Oper Tech Otolaryngol. 2009;20:44–53.

Ruda J, Hollenbeak C, Stack B. A systematic review of the diagnosis and treatment of primary hyperparathyroidism from 1995 to 2003. Otolaryngol Head Neck Surg. 2005;132:359–72.

Sharma J, Mazzaglia P, Milas M, et al. Radionuclide imaging for hyperparathyroidism (HPT): which is best technetium-99m sestamibi modality. Surgery. 2006;140(6):856–63; discussion 863–5.

Shindo M, Rosenthal J. Minimal access parathyroidectomy using the focused lateral approach: technique, indication and results. Arch Otolaryngol Head Neck Surg. 2007;133(12):1227–34.

Silverberg S, Lewiecki M, Mosekilde L, et al. Presentation of asymptomatic primary hyperparathyroidism: proceedings of the third international workshop. J Clin Endocrinol Metab. 2009;94(2):351–65.

Siperstein A, Berber E, Mackey R, et al. Prospective evaluation of sestamibi scan, ultrasonography, and rapid PTH to predict the success of limited exploration for sporadic primary hyperparathyroidism. Surgery. 2004;136(4):872–8; discussion 878–80.

Smith N, Magnuson J, Vidrine D, et al. Minimally invasive parathyroidectomy: use of intraoperative parathyroid hormone assays after 2 preoperative localization studies. Arch Otolaryngol Head Neck Surg. 2009;135(11):1108–11.

Stack B. Minimally invasive radioguided parathyroidectomy. Oper Tech Otolaryngol. 2009;20:54–9.

Starker L, Fonseca A, Carling T, Udelsman R. Minimally invasive parathyroidectomy. Int J Endocrinol. 2001;206502:1–8. Published Online 2011 May 23.

Suliburk J, Perrier N. Primary hyperparathyroidism. Oncologist. 2007;12:644–53.

Udelsman R. Six hundred fifty-six consecutive explorations for primary hyperparathyroidism. Ann Surg. 2002;235(5):665–72.

Udelsman R. Approach to the patient with persistent or recurrent primary hyperparathyroidism. J Clin Endocrinol Metab. 2011;96(10):2950–8.

Udelsman R, Carling C. Focused approach to parathyroidectomy. World J Surg. 2008;32:1512–7.

Udelsman R, Pasieka J, Sturgeon C, Clark O. Surgery for asymptomatic primary hyperparathyroidism: proceedings of the third international workshop. J Clin Endocrinol Metab. 2009;94(2):366–72.

Udelsman R, Lin Z, Donovan P. The superiority of minimally invasive parathyroidectomy based on 1650 consecutive patients with primary hyperparathyroidism. Ann Surg. 2011;253(3):585–91.

Van Husen R, Kim L. Accuracy of surgeon-performed ultrasound in parathyroid localization. World J Surg. 2004;28:1122–6.

Vasher M, Goodman A, Politz D, Norman J. Postoperative calcium requirements in 6,000 patients undergoing outpatient parathyroidectomy: easily avoiding symptomatic hypocalcemia. J Am Coll Surg. 2012;211(1):49–54.

Westerdahl J, Bergenfelz A. Unilateral versus bilateral neck exploration for primary hyperparathyroidism: five year follow-up of a randomized controlled trial. Ann Surg. 2007;246(6):976–80; discussion 980–1.

Zanocco K, Angelos P, Sturgeon C. Cost-effectiveness analysis of parathyroidectomy for asymptomatic primary hyperparathyroidism. Surgery. 2006;140(6):874–81; discussion 881–2.

Minimally Invasive Video-Assisted Parathyroidectomy

17

Marco Raffaelli and Celestino P. Lombardi

Introduction

Bilateral neck exploration (BNE) with identification of four parathyroid glands and the removal of macroscopically pathologic parathyroid tissue has long been the standard surgical procedure for patients with primary hyperparathyroidism (pHPT). This approach can achieve a cure rate of more than 95 % in experienced hands. However, most patients (>85 %) with pHPT have a single parathyroid adenoma. Given this, less invasive parathyroidectomy procedures (i.e., unilateral neck exploration) have been developed with the goal of reducing surgical trauma and postoperative pain, shortening recovery times, and limiting complications. Since the early 1980s, these techniques have become widely adopted. Studies have demonstrated that these focused techniques are safe and at least as effective as standard BNE while providing numerous advantages, including decreased incidence of postoperative hypocalcemia, shorter operative times, reduced postoperative pain, faster recovery periods, and improved cosmetic results. In an effort to further reduce the invasiveness of these procedures, surgeons incorporated the use of endoscopes.

M. Raffaelli, MD (✉) • C.P. Lombardi, MD
Division of Endocrine and Metabolic Surgery,
Department of Surgery, Istituto di Semeiotica Chirurgica,
Università Cattolica del Sacro Cuore,
Policlinico A. Gemelli, L.go A. Gemelli 8,
Rome 00168, Italy
e-mail: marcoraffaelli@rm.unicatt.it

Background

The first endoscopic parathyroidectomy was performed by Gagner in 1996. This technique employed ports and gas insufflation to maintain the operative space. Purely endoscopic procedures were met with only limited enthusiasm because they were technically demanding and often required long operative times with extended periods of CO_2 insufflation. The introduction of video-assisted procedures obviated the need for gas insufflation. Several video-assisted techniques have been described, including the lateral approach reported by Henry. The lateral approach appears to be effective and safe but is significantly limited by the inability to perform a bilateral exploration if necessary.

Minimally invasive video-assisted parathyroidectomy (MIVAP), first described by Miccoli, is the most widely adopted of the video-assisted parathyroidectomy techniques. This technique is relatively easy to learn and implement, as it reproduces the steps of conventional parathyroidectomy. The endoscope is used only as a tool to allow the same operation to be performed but through a smaller skin incision. The endoscope in these cases provides tremendous magnification and resolution of the operative bed.

The limited dissection, small incision, and midline approach characteristic of MIVAP result in numerous benefits for patients. Avoiding neck hyperextension and extensive dissection results in less postoperative pain. The minimal incision, as small as 1.5 cm, guarantees a better cosmetic

D.J. Terris, M.C. Singer (eds.), *Minimally Invasive and Robotic Thyroid and Parathyroid Surgery*, DOI 10.1007/978-1-4614-9011-1_17, © Springer Science+Business Media New York 2014

result. Several comparative studies have indeed demonstrated the advantages of MIVAP in terms of reduced postoperative pain, improved cosmetic outcomes, and higher patient satisfaction over both conventional and open, non-endoscopic minimally invasive parathyroidectomies. Another merit of this technique, in contrast to any of the procedures utilizing a lateral approach, is the possibility of performing a bilateral neck exploration when necessary through the same central incision. In line with national standards, our department does not perform parathyroid surgery on an outpatient basis. However, in settings where ambulatory surgery is practiced, MIVAP, which can be completed under locoregional anesthesia, is an ideal technique. Importantly, several studies have shown that these benefits of MIVAP can be realized without longer operative times compared to other minimally invasive approaches.

Selection Criteria

Indications for MIVAP

With increasing experience, the indications for MIVAP have significantly widened. All patients with pHPT are now potential candidates for MIVAP. However, patients with sporadic pHPT, in whom a single adenoma is suspected based on preoperative localizing studies, are ideal candidates for MIVAP. These focused procedures result in the most benefit for patients.

As the endoscope can be rotated and placed in every direction, all levels of the neck and the upper mediastinum can be visualized. Consequently, patients with caudally located pathologic glands (i.e., retrosternal, intrathymic) can undergo MIVAP. In cases of suspected multiglandular disease (including patients with multiple endocrine neoplasia), a video-assisted bilateral exploration can be planned. This same bilateral approach can be used in patients with limited or uncertain preoperative localization information.

In terms of contraindications, greater comfort with MIVAP has allowed an increasing number of patients to benefit from this approach. Early in the experience, a history of neck surgery, persistent or recurrent hyperparathyroidism, the presence of a substernal adenoma, or a concurrent goiter all were considered contraindications for MIVAP. However, based on the experience of the surgeon and the particular details of a case, MIVAP can sometimes be utilized in these settings. Another technical limitation concerns large parathyroid adenomas (>30 mm). Indeed, dissection and extraction of large adenomas through a small incision can result in capsule rupture with the theoretical risk of parathyromatosis. No case of this complication has been reported to date.

In order to achieve the best results, surgeons should be well trained in both endocrine and endoscopic surgeries. Moreover, as with all new surgical procedures, a learning curve exists with MIVAP and should be taken into account. Finally, to optimize the results, efficiency, and safety of MIVAP, a dedicated team of surgeons, assistants, and nurses should be assembled to perform these procedures.

Procedural Details

Anesthesia

When this procedure was first implemented, it was performed under general anesthesia with orotracheal intubation. With increasing experience, MIVAP can be routinely performed under locoregional anesthesia, with superficial modified or deep cervical block.

Patients and Surgical Team Position

The patient is placed in the supine position with the neck slightly extended. The surgical team consists of a primary surgeon and two assistants, one to handle the endoscope and the second to hold the retractors (Fig. 17.1). Efforts have been made to eliminate the need for a second assistant, with the use of a scope holder, for example. However, at this time, MIVAP remains a procedure requiring two assistants. This represents one of the main limitations of MIVAP.

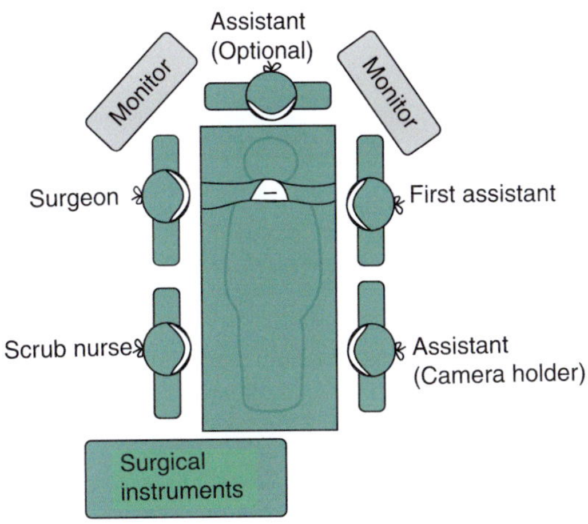

Fig. 17.1 Minimally invasive video-assisted parathyroidectomy (MIVAP): setup of the operative room and surgical team

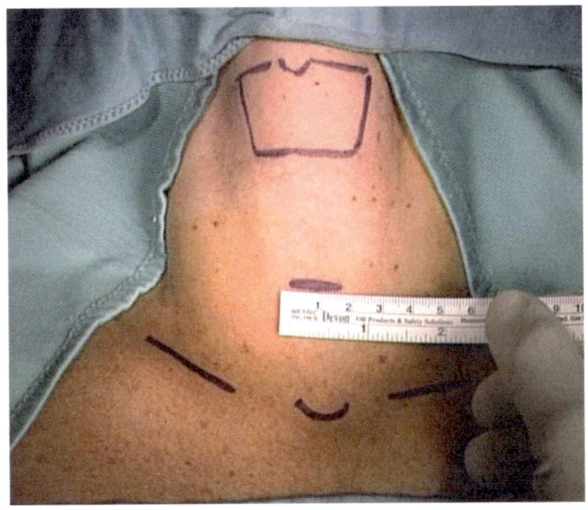

Fig. 17.2 In MIVAP, a 1.5–2-cm incision is routinely used

The monitor is placed at the head of the patient, across from the surgeon, who is positioned on the right side of the patient. A second monitor is usually positioned across from the scope-holding assistant, who stands on the left side of the patient (Fig. 17.1). This setup allows for easy viewing of the monitors, eliminating the need for any awkward positioning. The second assistant stands at the head of the bed, between the two monitors.

Surgical Technique

A small (1.5–2 cm), midline skin incision is made between the cricoid cartilage and the sternal notch (Fig. 17.2). The skin incision in MIVAP is often placed higher than in conventional parathyroidectomy. Precise placement of the incision may also be impacted by the location of the apparent adenoma on preoperative imaging.

After the skin incision is carried through the subcutaneous tissues and platysma muscle, the *linea alba*, between the strap muscles, is opened as widely as possible. When initially developed, MIVAP utilized a short period of CO_2 insufflation to facilitate dissection of the thyroid lobe from the strap muscles. The use of gas insufflation has now been completely abandoned. The thyroid lobe is separated from the overlying strap muscles by means of small conventional retractors (Farabeuf retractors), which are also used to maintain the operative space. Following this, the thyroid lobe is medially retracted, while the strap muscles are retracted laterally. At this point, the endoscope (5 mm – 30°) and the dedicated small surgical instruments (2 mm in diameter) are introduced through the incision (Fig. 17.3). The endoscope is maintained in position with two hands by the assistant. The absence of a trocar allows the position of the endoscope to be precisely changed, thus constantly providing optimal visualization of the operative site. This represents an important advantage of the video-assisted procedure over purely endoscopic techniques. In MIVAP, the endoscope is usually angled upwards, oriented toward the head of the patient. The angle of the endoscope can be changed to expose and explore the upper mediastinum when required.

Critical to obtaining exposure is the complete release of the thyroid gland from the strap muscles. This allows the view necessary to fully explore the likely sites of the parathyroid glands. Inadequate dissection and rotation of the thyroid gland medially can lead to difficulty identifying an adenoma.

After unfurling the thyroid gland from the tracheoesophageal groove, the recurrent laryngeal

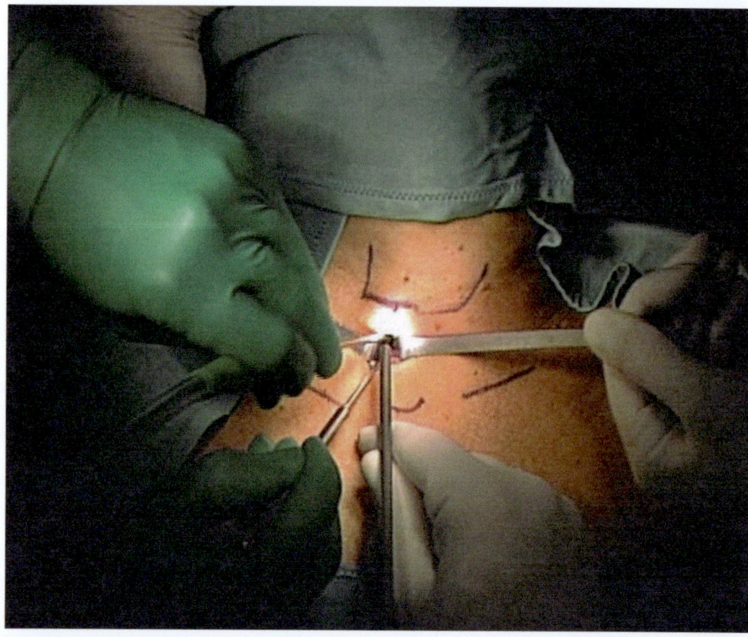

Fig. 17.3 After creating the operative space, the endoscope and surgical instruments are introduced through the skin incision without any trocar utilization

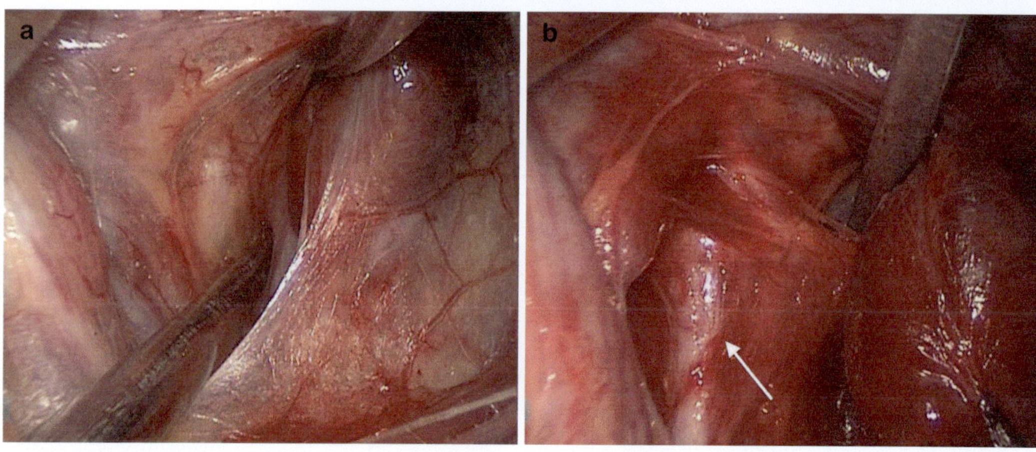

Fig. 17.4 (**a**), A large left superior parathyroid adenoma identified with the aid of the endoscope. The left thyroid lobe is retracted medially to the left of the image. (**b**), The left superior adenoma has been progressively dissected and its pedicle prepared. The recurrent laryngeal nerve is indicated by the *arrow*

nerve can be identified, usually in close proximity to the inferior thyroid artery. Following this, a targeted exploration is carried out, almost exclusively with blunt dissection, to identify the abnormal gland. The magnification of the endoscope permits, in most cases, the nerve and the parathyroid glands to be easily recognized. This is particularly true if the principles of blunt and bloodless dissection are respected.

After being identified (Fig. 17.4a), the pathologic parathyroid gland is bluntly dissected under endoscopic vision, using dedicated spatulas and spatula-shaped aspirator (Karl STORZ, Tuttlingen, Germany) (Fig. 17.4b). The pedicle of the adenoma is usually clipped with titanium clips or ligated with conventional ligature. After dividing the pedicle, the adenoma is extracted through the skin incision (Figs. 17.5 and 17.6). IO-PTH assay

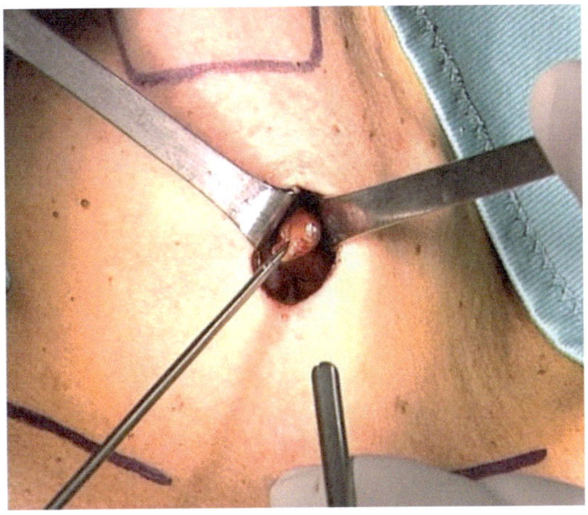

Fig. 17.5 After clipping and cutting the vascular pedicle, the adenoma is extracted through the skin incision

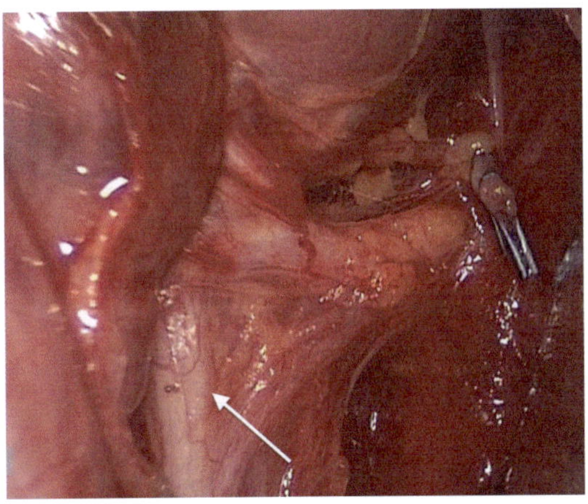

Fig. 17.6 Final check of the recurrent nerve (*arrow*) and the clipped pedicle after completing the parathyroidectomy

should confirm the removal of all pathologic tissue. After assuring adequate hemostasis, the strap muscles are sutured along the midline. The skin is closed by means of a subcuticular running suture or with a skin sealant. No drain is placed.

In case of suspicion of multiglandular disease (whether because of inadequate IO-PTH decrease, 2-gland enlargement recognized during unilateral exploration, or if no localization is provided by preoperative imaging studies), bilateral parathyroid exploration can be accomplished using the same video-assisted technique through the single, central skin incision.

Outcomes

A number of retrospective series have reported on the outcome and the medium-term results of MIVAP. The largest of these series, from the Miccoli group, assessed 350 cases of MIVAP after a 6-year experience. They reported a cure rate of 98.3 %. After an average follow-up of 35.1 months, persistent disease was evident in four cases. In regard to complications, the authors reported a 2.7 % rate of transient hypocalcemia, 0.8 % rate of definitive nerve palsy, and a 0.3 % rate of postoperative bleeding. Other studies have uniformly shown similar excellent cure and complication rates.

With appropriate patient selection and adequate surgeon experience, the need to convert to conventional BNE is usually infrequent, even in an endemic goiter region. The need to convert to an open approach or BNE is usually related to difficulty identifying the diseased gland(s), challenging dissection because of a large goiter or adenoma, thyroiditis or previous surgery, suspicion of thyroid malignancy, suspicion of multiglandular disease, or an ectopically located adenoma.

Studies have shown favorable benefits of MIVAP compared to BNE and open minimally invasive parathyroidectomy. One prospective, randomized trial compared MIVAP with BNE, in terms of operative time, postoperative pain, complications, cosmetic result, and costs. The results showed a significant decrease in operative time, postoperative pain, and postoperative inactivity period with MIVAP. Patient satisfaction with the cosmetic outcome was significantly superior in the group of patients who underwent MIVAP. Despite the need for two assistants (a frequently cited concern with MIVAP), no significant differences in terms of overall costs were found between the two procedures. Several studies comparing open minimal invasive parathyroidectomy with MIVAP have shown that the two approaches have similar results with regard to cure and morbidity rates and operative time. MIVAP appears to offer improved cosmesis, significantly better postoperative physical functioning, and perhaps shorter postoperative hospital stays.

Conclusions

MIVAP represents the apex of minimally invasive parathyroidectomy techniques. While requiring two assistants and limited specialized equipment, it is a relatively easy-to-learn procedure, which can be performed in most surgical centers. The widespread adoption of MIVAP attests to the multiple benefits it provides to patients.

Recommended Reading

Agarwal G, Barraclough BH, Reeve TS, Delbridge LW. Minimally invasive parathyroidectomy using the "focused" lateral approach. II. Surgical technique. Aust N Z J Surg. 2002;72:147–51.

Alesina PF, Hinrichs J, Kribben A, Walz MK. Minimally invasive video-assisted parathyroidectomy (MIVAP) for secondary hyperparathyroidism: report of initial experience. Am J Surg. 2010;199:851–5.

Alesina PF, Hinrichs J, Heuer M, Hofmeister S, Meier B, Walz MK. Feasibility of video-assisted bilateral neck exploration for patients with primary hyperparathyroidism and failed or discordant localization studies. Langenbecks Arch Surg. 2013;398:107–11.

Barbaros U, Erbil Y, Yildirim A, Saricam G, Yazici H, Ozarmağan S. Minimally invasive video-assisted subtotal parathyroidectomy with thymectomy for secondary hyperparathyroidism. Langenbecks Arch Surg. 2009;394:451–5.

Barczyński M, Cichoń S, Konturek A, Cichoń W. Minimally invasive video-assisted parathyroidectomy versus open minimally invasive parathyroidectomy for a solitary parathyroid adenoma: a prospective, randomized, blinded trial. World J Surg. 2006;30:721–31.

Bergenfelz A, Lindblom P, Tibblin S, Westerdahl J. Unilateral versus bilateral neck exploration for primary hyperparathyroidism: a prospective randomized trial. Ann Surg. 2002;236:543–51.

Bergenfelz A, Kanngiesser V, Zielke A, Nies C, Rothmund M. Conventional bilateral cervical exploration versus open minimally invasive parathyroidectomy under local anaesthesia for primary hyperparathyroidism. Br J Surg. 2005;92:190–7.

Bergenfelz A, Jansson S, Mårtensson H, Reihnér E, Wallin G, Kristoffersson A, Lausen I. Scandinavian quality register for thyroid and parathyroid surgery: audit of surgery for primary hyperparathyroidism. Langenbecks Arch Surg. 2007;392:445–51.

Bergenfelz AOJ, Hellman P, Harrison B, Sitges-Serra A, Dralle H, European Society of Endocrine Surgeons. Positional statement of the European Society of Endocrine Surgeons (ESES) on modern techniques in pHPT surgery. Langenbecks Arch Surg. 2009;394:761–4.

Berti P, Materazzi G, Picone A, Miccoli P. Limits and drawbacks of video-assisted parathyroidectomy. Br J Surg. 2003;90:743–7.

De Pasquale L, Bianchi P, Barabino M, Bestetti A, Bastagli A. Radio-guided video-assisted parathyroidectomy. A preliminary report. Surg Endosc. 2001;15:1456–8.

Dralle H, Lorenz K, Nguyen-Thanh P. Minimally invasive video-assisted parathyroidectomy – selective approach to localize single gland adenoma. Langenbecks Arch Surg. 1999;384:556–62.

Duh QY. Surgical approach to primary hyperparathyroidism (bilateral approach). In: Clark OH, Duh Q, editors. Textbook of endocrine surgery. Philadelphia: WB Saunders; 1997.

Gagner M. Endoscopic subtotal parathyroidectomy in patients with primary hyperparathyroidism. Br J Surg. 1996;83:875.

Goldstein RE, Blevins L, Delbeke D, Martin WH. Effect of minimally invasive radioguided parathyroidectomy on efficacy, length of stay, and costs in the management of primary hyperparathyroidism. Ann Surg. 2000;231:732–42.

Hallfeldt KK, Trupka A, Gallwas J, Horn K. Minimally invasive video-assisted parathyroidectomy. Surg Endosc. 2001;15:409–12.

Henry JF, Defechereux T, Gramatica L, de Boissezon C. Minimally invasive videoscopic parathyroidectomy by lateral approach. Langenbecks Arch Surg. 1999;384:298–301.

Henry JF, Raffaelli M, Iacobone M, Volot F. Video-assisted parathyroidectomy via the lateral approach vs conventional surgery in the treatment of sporadic primary hyperparathyroidism: results of a case–control study. Surg Endosc. 2001a;15:1116–9.

Henry JF, Iacobone M, Mirallie E, Deveze A, Pili S. Indications and results of video-assisted parathyroidectomy by a lateral approach in patients with primary hyperparathyroidism. Surgery. 2001b;130:999–1004.

Hessman O, Westerdahl J, Al-Suliman N, Christiansen P, Hellman P, Bergenfelz A. Randomized clinical trial comparing open with video-assisted minimally invasive parathyroid surgery for primary hyperparathyroidism. Br J Surg. 2010;97:177–84.

Irvin GL, Carneiro DM. Rapid parathyroid hormone assay guided exploration. Oper Tech Gen Surg. 1999;1:18–27.

Kitagawa W, Shimizu K, Kumita S, Akasu H, Kumazaki T, Tanaka S. Radioguided parathyroidectomy for primary hyperparathyroidism combined with video-assisted surgery using the solid-state multi-crystal gamma camera. J Surg Oncol. 2002;80:173–5.

Kitano H, Fujimura M, Hirano M, Kataoka H, Kinoshita T, Seno S, Kitajima K. Endoscopic surgery for a parathyroid functioning adenoma resection with the neck region-lifting method. Otolaryngol Head Neck Surg. 2000;123:465–6.

Lombardi CP, Raffaelli M, Traini E, De Crea C, Corsello SM, Sollazzi L, Pontecorvi A, Bellantone R.

Advantages of a video-assisted approach to parathyroidectomy. ORL J Otorhinolaryngol Relat Spec. 2008;70:313–8.

Lombardi CP, Raffaelli M, Traini E, De Crea C, Corsello SM, Bellantone R. Video-assisted minimally invasive parathyroidectomy: benefits and long-term results. World J Surg. 2009;33:2266–81.

Lorenz K, Miccoli P, Monchik JM, Düren M, Dralle H. Minimally invasive video-assisted parathyroidectomy: multiinstitutional study. World J Surg. 2001; 25:704–7.

Maweja S, Sebag F, Hubbard J, Giorgi R, Henry JF. Immediate and medium-term results of intraoperative parathyroid hormone monitoring during video-assisted parathyroidectomy. Arch Surg. 2004;139:1301–3.

Melck AL, Armstrong MJ, Yip L, Carty SE. Case-controlled comparison of video-assisted and conventional minimally invasive parathyroidectomy. Am Surg. 2012;78:125–32.

Miccoli P, Pinchera A, Cecchini G, Conte M, Bendinelli C, Vignali E, Picone A, Marcocci C. Minimally invasive, video-assisted parathyroid surgery for primary hyperparathyroidism. J Endocrinol Invest. 1997; 20:429–30.

Miccoli P, Bendinelli C, Berti P, Vignali E, Pinchera A, Marcocci C. Video-assisted versus conventional parathyroidectomy in primary hyperparathyroidism: a prospective randomized study. Surgery. 1999;126:1117–22.

Miccoli P, Berti P, Conte M, Raffaelli M, Materazzi G. Minimally invasive video-assisted parathyroidectomy: lesson learned from 137 cases. J Am Coll Surg. 2000;191:613–8.

Miccoli P, Berti P, Materazzi G, Massi M, Picone A, Minuto MN. Results of video-assisted parathyroidectomy: single institution's six-year experience. World J Surg. 2004;28:1216–8.

Miccoli P, Minuto M, Cetani F, Ambrosini CE, Berti P. Familial parathyroid hyperplasia: is there a place for minimally invasive surgery? Description of the first treated case. J Endocrinol Invest. 2005a;28:942–3.

Miccoli P, Barellini L, Monchik JM, Rago R, Berti P. Randomized clinical trial comparing regional and general anaesthesia in minimally invasive video-assisted parathyroidectomy. Br J Surg. 2005b;92:814–8.

Miccoli P, Berti P, Materazzi G, Ambrosini CE, Fregoli L, Donatini G. Endoscopic bilateral neck exploration versus quick intraoperative parathormone assay (qPTHa) during endoscopic parathyroidectomy: a prospective randomized trial. Surg Endosc. 2008; 22:398–400.

Mourad M, Ngongang C, Saab N, Coche E, Jamar F, Michel JM, Maiter D, Malaise J, Squifflet JP. Video-assisted neck exploration for primary and secondary hyperparathyroidism. Surg Endosc. 2001;15:1112–5.

Naitoh T, Gagner M, Garcia-Ruiz A, Heniford BT. Endoscopic endocrine surgery in the neck. An initial report of endoscopic subtotal parathyroidectomy. Surg Endosc. 1998;12:202–6.

Norman J, Chheda H. Minimally invasive parathyroidectomy facilitated by intraoperative nuclear mapping. Surgery. 1997;122:998–1003.

Ohshima A, Simizu S, Okido M, Shimada K, Kuroki S, Tanaka M. Endoscopic neck surgery: current status for thyroid and parathyroid diseases. Biomed Pharmacother. 2002;56:48s–52s.

Okido M, Shimizu S, Kuroki S, Yokohata K, Uchiyama A, Tanaka M. Video-assisted parathyroidectomy for primary hyperparathyroidism: a new approach involving a skin-lifting method. Surg Endosc. 2001;15:1120–3.

Palazzo FF, Delbridge LW. Minimal-access/minimally invasive parathyroidectomy for primary hyperparathyroidism. Surg Clin North Am. 2004;84:717–34.

Russel CF, Dolan SJ, Laird JD. Randomized clinical trial comparing scan-directed unilateral versus bilateral exploration for parathyroidectomy due to solitary adenoma. Br J Surg. 2006;93:418–21.

Russell C. Unilateral neck exploration for primary hyperparathyroidism. Surg Clin North Am. 2004;84:705–16.

Santini J. Chirurgie des glandes parathyroïdes. In: Encyclopedie Médico-Chirurgicale. Traité de Techniques Chirurgicales – Tête et cou. Paris: Elsevier; 1997. p. 46–465.

Tibblin S, Bondeson AG, Ljungberg O. Unilateral parathyroidectomy in hyperparathyroidism due to a single adenoma. Ann Surg. 1982;195:245–52.

Westerdahl J, Bergenfelz A. Unilateral versus bilateral neck exploration for primary hyperparathyroidism: 5-year follow up of a randomized controlled trial. Ann Surg. 2007;249:976–80.

Yeung GH, Ng JW. The technique of endoscopic exploration for parathyroid adenoma of the neck. Aust N Z J Surg. 1998;68:147–50.

18 Radioguided Parathyroidectomy

Sarah C. Oltmann and Herbert Chen

Introduction

Radioguidance has broad applications in parathyroid surgery and should be considered a crucial tool in parathyroid surgeons' armamentariums. Technetium 99m sestamibi, injected the day of surgery, is preferentially retained by parathyroid tissue. This characteristic of parathyroid tissue can be harnessed to facilitate multiple facets of these surgeries, including gland localization, tissue identification, and metabolic assessment. We find that radioguidance is helpful in all parathyroid cases, from minimally invasive to reoperations to bilateral neck explorations.

Selection Criteria and Preoperative Planning

Once the clinical diagnosis of hyperparathyroidism has been made, and the patient is felt to be a surgical candidate, operative planning can commence.

S.C. Oltmann, MD
Department of Surgery,
University of Wisconsin, Madison, WI, USA

H. Chen, MD (✉)
Division of General Surgery,
Department of Surgery, University of Wisconsin,
600 Highland Avenue, Clinical Science
Center K3/705, Madison, WI 53792-7375, USA
e-mail: chen@surgery.wisc.edu

Those patients with a diagnosis of primary hyperparathyroidism should undergo preoperative imaging in efforts to identify or localize the abnormal gland and allow for a more directed surgical approach when possible. This can be done via ultrasound, technetium 99m sestamibi scanning, or CT, based on institutional resources and imaging quality. It is important to stress that the diagnosis of hyperparathyroidism is a clinical one, and imaging only serves to assist in operative planning. Negative imaging studies do not refute the clinical diagnosis, and surgical intervention should not be delayed. Negative imaging does not prohibit the patient from being a candidate from a radioguided approach.

For those patients with secondary or tertiary hyperparathyroidism, or hyperparathyroidism secondary to MEN, preoperative localization studies are not needed as these generally represent multi-gland disease and hyperplasia.

In patients with persistent or recurrent disease, attempts at re-localization with imaging should be made. This ideally would include cross-sectional imaging (MIBI with SPECT, or CT) to further delineate the area of radioactivity in a three-dimensional setting, especially if initial images were two-dimensional only.

In summary, all patients can potentially benefit from the use of radioguidance during parathyroidectomy, and the only exclusion criteria should be pregnancy and radiation-dose limitations. The use of the low-dose (10 mCi) technetium 99m sestamibi has been shown to be safe for both patients and the operative team.

D.J. Terris, M.C. Singer (eds.), *Minimally Invasive and Robotic Thyroid and Parathyroid Surgery*, DOI 10.1007/978-1-4614-9011-1_18, © Springer Science+Business Media New York 2014

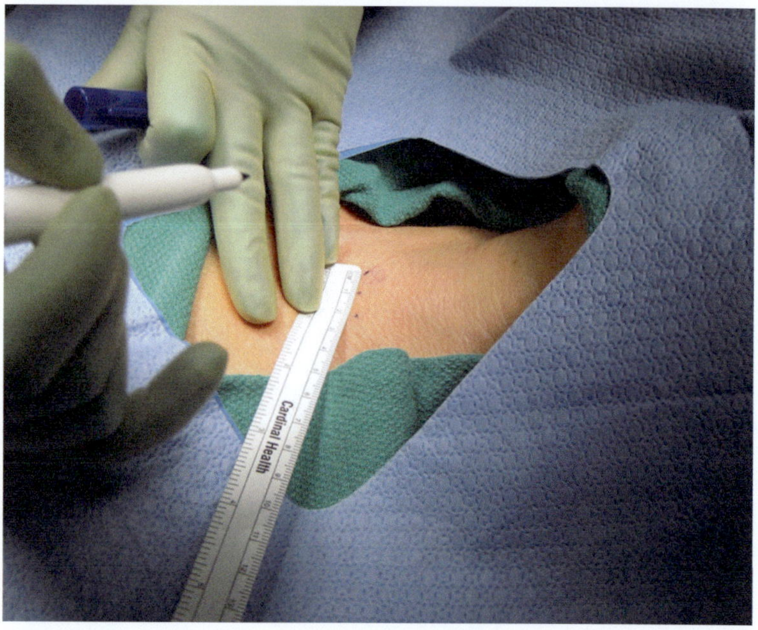

Fig. 18.1 The incision is marked and measured

Procedural Details

Patients undergo an intravenous injection of 10 mCi technetium 99m sestamibi 30 min to 3 h prior to surgery. We generally do not obtain any images on the day of surgery. The day of surgery injection serves to provide signal for intraoperative gamma detection. For those patients who are traveling a great distance to have surgery performed, or who present emergently in hypercalcemic crisis and need intervention done during that admission, a higher dose of 20 mCi technetium 99m sestamibi can be given, with images obtained at 15 and 90 min, and surgery planned within 2–2.5 h of the injection.

Once in the operating room, the patient is positioned. At our institution, we routinely use general anesthesia with either an endotracheal tube or a laryngeal mask. However, the minimally invasive approach can easily be performed under local anesthesia with monitored anesthesia care as well.

After induction of anesthesia, a baseline parathyroid hormone level is drawn from a peripheral vein, generally from the foot. Internal jugular draws are reserved only for those patients with significant peripheral vascular disease and limited access points. They can also be used to help with localization by obtaining samples from the bilateral internal jugular veins.

Surgeon-performed ultrasound can be conducted at this time to verify gland localization and further assist with incision placement.

The patient is then prepped and draped in usual sterile fashion.

We mark out our 2-cm incision mid neck, in a preexisting skin crease (Fig. 18.1). Alternatively, it can be placed directly over the diseased parathyroid if a lateral approach is planned.

Prior to making the incision, a baseline assessment of background radioactivity is measured by placing the gamma probe over the thyroid isthmus (Fig. 18.2). For this procedure, we use an 11-mm collimated gamma probe (Neoprobe 2000, Ethicon Endo-Surgery Breast Care, Cincinnati, OH). A second background count can be obtained by placing the probe over the left shoulder, if preferred.

Once the background number has been obtained, the incision is made. Dissection is carried down through the platysma, and the straps are divided in the midline if using an anterior approach. For the lateral approach the sternocleidomastoid muscle is separated from the strap and omohyoid muscles.

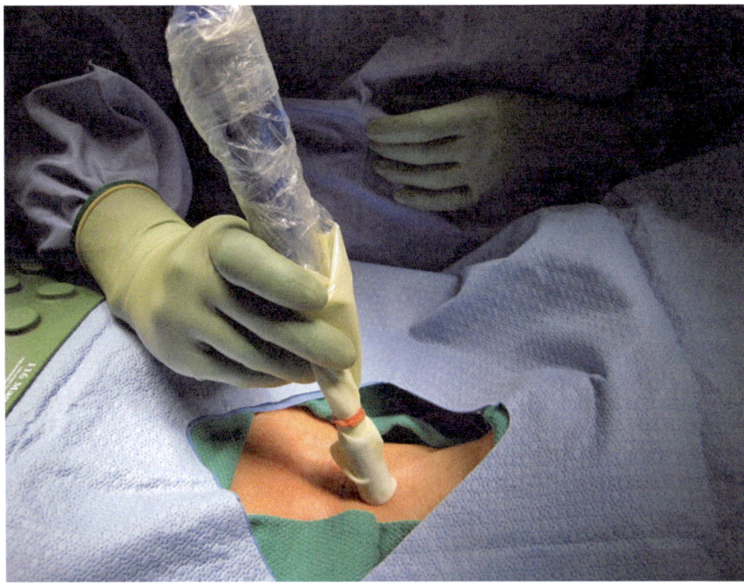

Fig. 18.2 Prior to the incision, the background radioaction count is established with the gamma probe

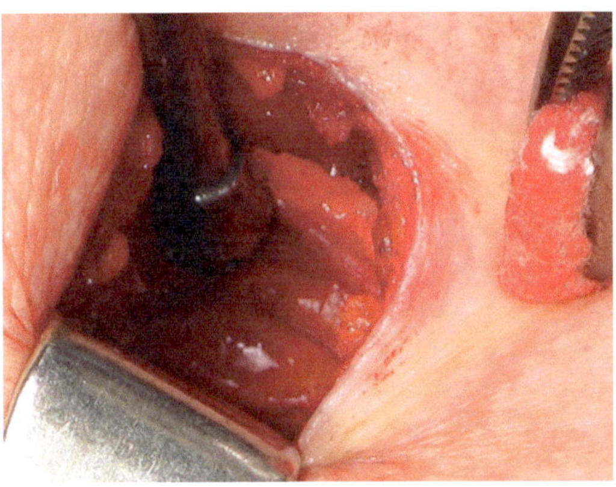

Fig. 18.3 The pathologic gland is identified

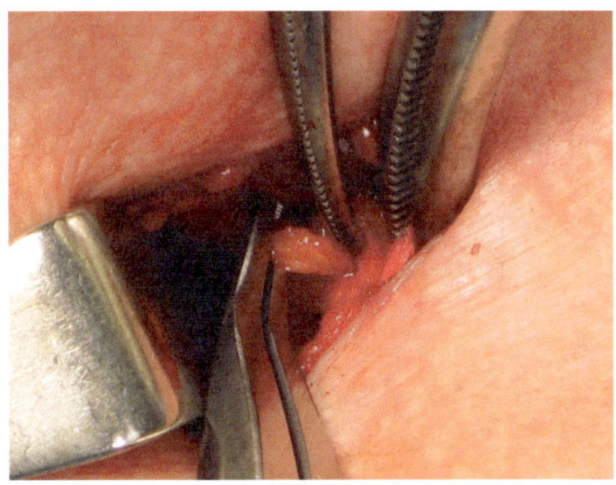

Fig. 18.4 The vascular pedicle of the pathologic gland is isolated and divided

For those patients who do not have any localization on preoperative imaging, radioactivity counts can be taken on both sides of the neck, or more specifically, the four quadrants of the neck. The area of highest activity gives the surgeon an idea as to where to start dissection.

If the gland is not quickly identified during dissection, the gamma probe can be inserted into the wound to provide the surgeon with a trajectory and area of highest activity to further localize ectopic glands.

Glands identified by the surgeon can then be assessed in vivo for radioactivity over that of baseline (Fig. 18.3). If appearing to be consistent with a diseased gland, the vascular pedicle is isolated and controlled (Fig. 18.4). The specimen is then excised, with the timer starting for intraoperative parathyroid hormone monitoring. Ex vivo counts of the excised gland are taken with the tissue balanced on the tip of the probe to ensure no background is picked up from the patient (Fig. 18.5). Counts greater than 20 % of background are thought to represent pathologic parathyroid tissue and confirm the presence of parathyroid tissue within the specimen. Lymph nodes, fat, and normal parathyroid tissue will not have counts this high.

As the gamma probe only helps localize and then confirm the excision of pathologic tissue, we recommend the concomitant use of intraoperative parathyroid hormone monitoring to confirm that all hyperfunctioning parathyroid tissue has been removed.

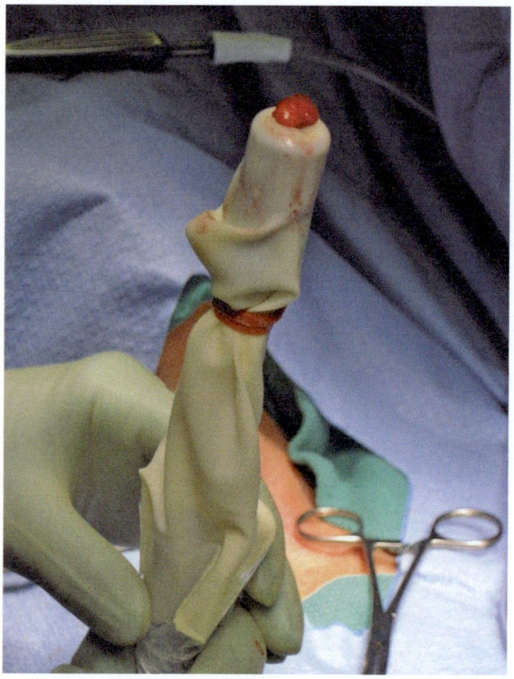

Fig. 18.5 After the gland is excised, ex vivo radiation counts are taken. This is done with the gland balanced on the tip of the probe to ensure no background activity is picked up from the patient

Once satisfied that all hyperfunctioning tissue has been excised, hemostasis is meticulously obtained. The wound is then injected with local anesthetic (Fig. 18.6). The strap muscles are then reapproximated, as is the platysma. We use a running, knotless subcuticular closure for the skin (Fig. 18.7a, b). Steri-Strips are then applied.

The majority of patients are able to go home the same day as surgery. Ice packs are routinely used at our institution to minimize tissue swelling and aid in pain control. Oral analgesics are generally all that is needed to achieve adequate pain control. We routinely discharge our patients with oral calcium supplementation. Patients are instructed to take additional doses for any symptoms of hypocalcemia (numbness, tingling, cramping).

Serum calcium and parathyroid hormone levels are checked at the time of the postoperative follow-up visit, occurring 1 week after surgery.

Pearls and Pitfalls

Consistent use of the radioguided technique allows the surgeon to become facile with interpreting the count data. For this reason, we routinely use this approach for all our parathyroid surgeries, and not just the cases with the potential to be more complex.

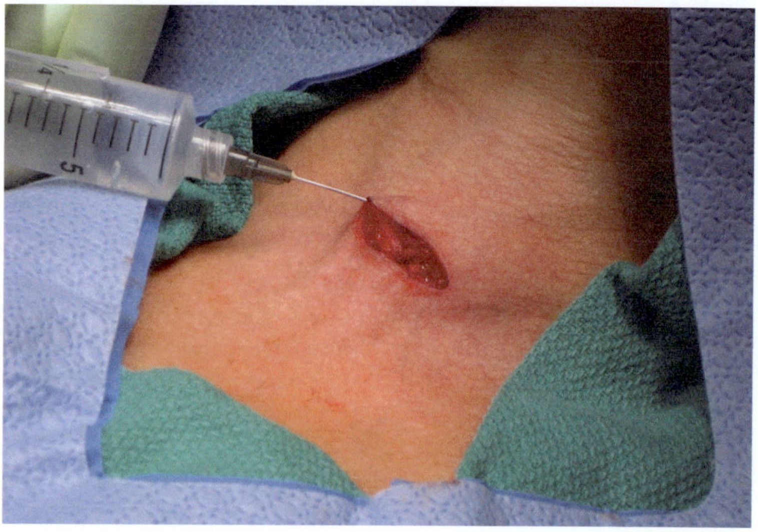

Fig. 18.6 To minimize postoperative pain the wound is injected with a local anesthetic at the end of the case

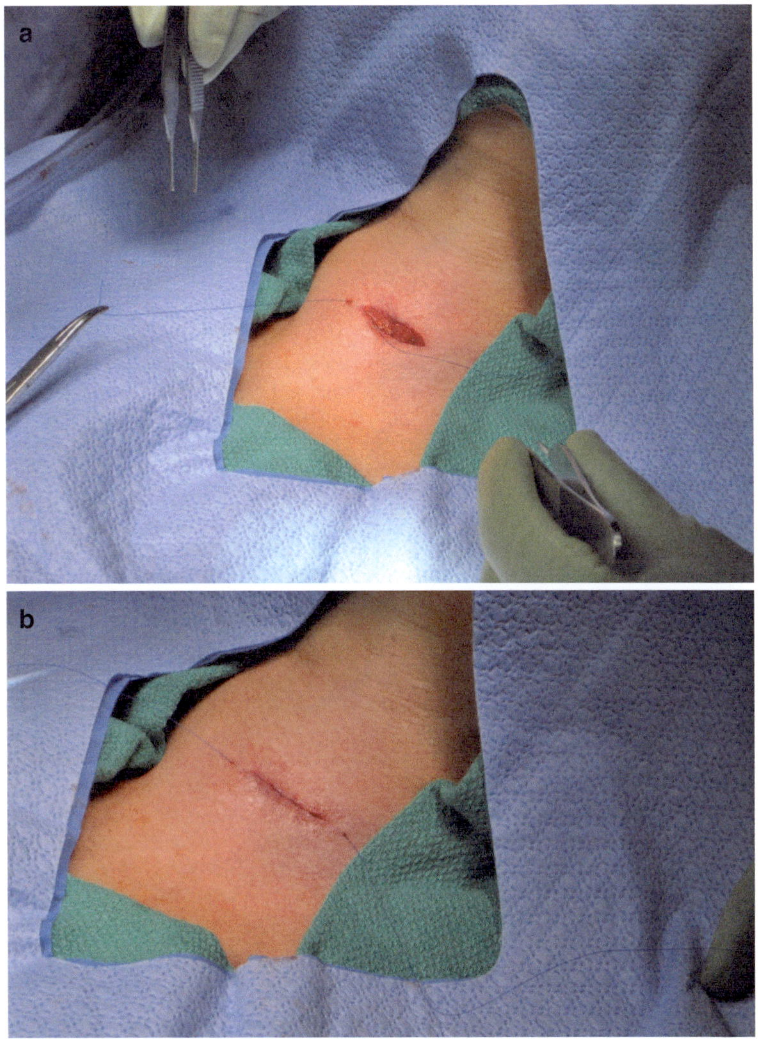

Fig. 18.7 (**a**) The wound is closed with a subcuticular closure. (**b**) Completed wound closure

Improper angling of the probe can pick up increased background levels from the heart, carotid arteries, or salivary glands. Thyroid uptake is not always uniform, and can be particularly confounding in patients with nodular thyroid disease. To ensure that the area of increased counts truly represents pathologic parathyroid tissue, the count elevation should exist when holding the probe at multiple angles to the tissue in question.

Glands located in the mediastinum can also be identified with the use of radioguidance and provide the means for a less invasive resection. Those glands localized in the mediastinum on preoperative sestamibi scan can still be accessed via a left video-assessed thoracoscopic approach with the laparoscopic gamma probe assisting with localization. For these patients, this approach offers a less morbid option compared with the traditional median sternotomy.

To ensure best uptake of the tissues, surgery should ideally occur roughly 1 h after injection. The longer after injection, the less sensitive the gamma probe becomes. After 6 h, the gamma probe is less useful. For these reasons, coordination within your medical system is crucial to ensure the patients receive their injections on time and are able to return to the preoperative area without delay. As the gamma probe used for parathyroid surgery is the same machine and setup used for sentinel lymph node procedures in breast and melanoma surgery, most institutions already have the needed equipment.

Recommended Reading

Ardito G, Revelli L, Giustozzi E, Giordano A. Radioguided parathyroidectomy in forearm graft for recurrent hyperparathyroidism. Br J Radiol. 2012;85:e1–3.

Bekis R, Celik P, Uysal B, Kocdor MA, Atila K, Saydam S, et al. Exposure of surgical staff in surgical probe applications in radioguided parathyroidectomy. Eur Arch Otorhinolaryngol. 2008;265:1545–8.

Cayo A, Chen H. Radioguided reoperative parathyroidectomy for persistent primary hyperparathyroidism. Clin Nucl Med. 2008;33:668–70.

Chen H, Mack E, Starling JR. Radioguided parathyroidectomy is equally effective for both adenomatous and hyperplastic glands. Ann Surg. 2003;238:332–8.

Chen H, Pruhs Z, Starling J, Mack E. Intraoperative parathyroid hormone testing improves cure rates in patients undergoing minimally invasive parathyroidectomy. Surgery. 2005;138:583–90.

Chen H, Sippel BS, Schaefer S. The effectiveness of radioguided parathyroidectomy in patients with negative technetium Tc 99m-sestamibi scans. Arch Surg. 2009;144:643–8.

Cutress RI, Manwaring-White C, Dixon K, Dhir A, Skene AI. Gamma probe radioguided parathyroid forearm surgery in recurrent hyperparathyroidism. Ann R Coll Surg Engl. 2009;91:1–3. On-line Case Report.

Garcia-Talavera P, Gonzalez C, Garcia-Talavera JR, Martin E, Martin M, Gomez A. Radioguided surgery of primary hyperparathyroidism in a population with a high prevalence of thyroid pathology. Eur J Nucl Med Mol Imaging. 2010;37:2060–7.

Lal A, Bianco J, Chen H. Radioguided parathyroidectomy in patients with familial hyperparathyroidism. Ann Surg Oncol. 2006;14:739–43.

Martinez DA, King DR, Romshe C, Lozano RA, Morris JD, O'Dorisio MS, et al. Intraoperative identification of parathyroid gland pathology: a new approach. J Pediatr Surg. 1995;9:1306–9.

Murphy C, Norman J. The 20% rule: a simple, instantaneous radioactivity measurement defines cure and allows elimination of frozen sections and hormone assays during parathyroidectomy. Surgery. 1999;126:1023–9.

Nichol PF, Mack E, Bianco J, Hayman A, Starling JR, Chen H. Radioguided parathyroidectomy in patients with secondary and tertiary hyperparathyroidism. Surgery. 2003;134:713–9.

Norman J, Chheda H. Minimally invasive parathyroidectomy facilitated by intraoperative nuclear mapping. Surgery. 1997;122:998–1004.

O'Herrin JK, Weigel T, Wilson M, Chen H. Radioguided parathyroidectomy via VATS combined with intraoperative parathyroid hormone testing: the surgical approach of choice for patients with mediastinal parathyroid adenomas? J Bone Miner Res. 2002;17:1368–71.

Olson J, Repplinger D, Bianco J, Chen H. Ex vivo radioactive counts and decay rates of tissue resected during radioguided parathyroidectomy. J Surg Res. 2006;136:187–91.

Pitt SC, Panneerselvan R, Sippel RS, Chen H. Influence of morbid obesity on parathyroidectomy outcomes in primary hyperparathyroidism. Am J Surg. 2010;199:410–5.

Sippel RS, Bianco J, Chen H. Radioguided parathyroidectomy for recurrent hyperparathyroidism caused by forearm graft hyperplasia. J Bone Miner Res. 2003;18:939–42.

Thyroid Surgery 2020

19

Peter Angelos and Raymon H. Grogan

Prediction is very difficult, especially about the future.
Niels Bohr, Winner of Nobel Prize in Physics, 1922

Introduction

An invitation to write a chapter predicting future developments in any field is a double-edged sword. At the time that the predictions are made, they can never be wrong since the future is unknown. At the point that they can be proven wrong, they are rarely reviewed since few in the future care what was predicted in the past. Writing a chapter about the future also has the benefit of being inherently subjective since, by definition, predictions can never be evidence based. Given the restrictions noted above, we will, in the upcoming paragraphs, consider some of the innovations that have characterized thyroid surgery in the last few decades and suggest possible directions for future development.

Innovation in surgery has largely been characterized by surgeons creatively attempting to solve intraoperative problems for their patients. As such, the drive to innovate (i.e., to make changes for the good) is grounded in the belief that something should be able to be done better. Although determining whether a new approach is actually beneficial for patients requires a scientific approach and the accumulation of data, the actual drive to try a new approach, is often based on the serendipity of adapting a technique or technology to solve a specific clinical problem. For this reason, innovation generally requires the belief that a problem exists.

P. Angelos, MD, PhD, FACS (✉)
Department of Surgery, The University of Chicago Medicine, 5841 S. Maryland Avenue, MC 4052, Chicago, IL 60637, USA
e-mail: pangelos@surgery.bsd.uchicago.edu

R.H. Grogan, MD
Endocrine Surgery Research Program, Department of Surgery, The University of Chicago Medicine, Chicago, IL USA

A Look Back

In order to thoughtfully consider the potential changes in thyroidectomy in the future, it is helpful to look at the recent past. In the last few decades, thyroid surgery has become increasingly common as rates of papillary thyroid cancer have risen worldwide. A number of changes have occurred with the operation over that time: (1) performing thyroid surgery as an outpatient procedure; (2) neuromonitoring of the recurrent laryngeal nerve during thyroid surgery; and (3) making the scar smaller or moving it to a location away from the neck. We will consider these changes and what has driven their development as a tool to help predict future changes.

Although a small number of surgeons have performed outpatient thyroidectomies for many years, in the last decade, the numbers of patients treated this way have significantly increased. The move to outpatient surgery has been an innovation that is primarily driven by surgeons rather than by patients. Although many patients are happy not to spend a night in the hospital, the economic incentives for discharge are primarily for the insurance company or the hospital. Thus,

D.J. Terris, M.C. Singer (eds.), *Minimally Invasive and Robotic Thyroid and Parathyroid Surgery*, DOI 10.1007/978-1-4614-9011-1_19, © Springer Science+Business Media New York 2014

the push for outpatient surgery has largely been reflective of the more general shift to outpatient surgery in order to save money.

In recent years, neuromonitoring technologies have been increasingly used as a way to try to reduce the risks of recurrent laryngeal nerve (RLN) injury during thyroidectomy. Many studies have looked at how neuromonitoring affects the actual risks of nerve injury, yet only one has shown a statistically significant improvement in RLN injury rates with use of neuromonitoring. Barczynski and colleagues showed a statistically significant reduction in rates of transient RLN injury (but not in permanent RLN injury) with use of neuromonitoring. When looking to determine what has driven the move toward increasing use of neuromonitoring technology in recent years, a number of important factors can be identified. RLN injuries, although not common after thyroidectomy, remain a problem in a small number of patients and an ongoing source of worry for patients and surgeons. The morbidity of a RLN injury can be significant and a complication that all surgeons try to avoid for their patients' benefit. In addition, RLN injuries are a common cause of malpractice claims against surgeons and, as such, a clear source of added concern to thyroid surgeons.

A third major change in thyroid surgery in the last 10–15 years has been the push to make the incisions smaller and/or move them to a less noticeable location than the anterior base of the neck. Numerous chapters in the present volume have addressed various approaches to minimally invasive or remote access thyroid surgery. To some extent, the widespread interest in these approaches can be traced to the public's fascination with almost anything that is described as "minimally invasive." In addition, the technology that has allowed these approaches to be successful is appealing to surgeons who have widely accepted that surgery that can be performed in a minimally invasive manner is desirable.

These many different approaches to remove a thyroid gland without a large incision in the front of the neck can be seen as a response to "the problem of the scar on the neck." How much of a problem this really is for patients is certainly quite variable and something that does not lend itself to objective measurement. However, as is commonly the case, innovation in surgery occurs when there is some dissatisfaction with the status quo. When the issue is a visible scar on the neck, even if it is not particularly bothersome for many patients, the fact that some patients see it as a clear problem has driven much of the creative attempts to shorten or hide the scars.

Possible Future Directions

In the upcoming years, we anticipate that thyroid surgery will continue to change in response to the desires of surgeons and their patients. As the economic pressures on all surgical care increase, there will likely be a continued movement to reducing costs for thyroid surgery and as a result, many more patients will likely be treated as outpatients. Whether one considers this an advance or not depends on one's perspective, but if outpatient thyroid surgery can be safely performed for increasing numbers of patients, it will certainly save money for any healthcare system.

The future likely also holds significant promise for increasing use of new technology to make thyroid surgery, even via remote incisions, less invasive. If, for example, robotic technology were to allow for smaller devices, then the potential to significantly shrink the incisions used would be quite high. We anticipate that in the years to come, the various remote access and small incision approaches to thyroidectomy will become faster and more closely approximate the operative times for conventional open operations. This will do much to reduce the economic disincentives to some of the newest techniques. However, because of the difficulty of showing changes in the risks of thyroid surgery since they occur at such a low rate, we anticipate that there will always be a large number of thyroidectomies performed through low transverse collar incisions.

What additional changes in thyroid surgery are less likely, but would be wonderful if they occurred? We are hopeful that future approaches will help to reduce the rates of morbidity associated with thyroid surgery. Any techniques or technologies that would allow for lower rates of

RLN injury and hypoparathyroidism would be welcome additions to the arsenal of options for thyroid surgeons. Although as noted above, current RLN monitors do not reduce the risk of permanent RLN injuries, perhaps such future neuromonitoring devices would successfully reduce the rates of this complication. The options for continuous vagal stimulation during thyroidectomy may prove the basis for the next generation of neuromonitoring devices or some innovative approach, not currently described, may be effective. We do not anticipate that any technology will ever replace the necessity for meticulous technique on the part of the surgeon, but we are hopeful that the future will see options that will make the likelihood of injuring the RLN or superior laryngeal nerve increasingly rare.

With respect to preserving parathyroid glands during thyroidectomy, little in the way of new approaches has been offered in decades. Without doubt, increasing visualization with magnification has the potential to improve parathyroid preservation, but other approaches may also be more helpful in the future. If it were possible to more accurately identify the parathyroid glands intraoperatively, surgeons would be better able to preserve them. This could be accomplished by administering an agent to the patient so that the parathyroid glands become more appreciably different from the adjacent thyroid and other soft tissue. Alternatively, if parathyroid hormone levels could be followed in real time throughout a thyroidectomy, it would be possible to look for parathyroid glands for autotransplantation perhaps before it was too late.

Another avenue for future progress in thyroid surgery could potentially surround the diagnosis of thyroid cancer in thyroid nodules. If fewer patients needed surgery for indeterminate nodules, healthcare costs could be reduced. In addition, if it were possible to reliably identify thyroid cancer in indeterminate thyroid nodules intraoperatively, fewer patients would face a second operation to treat thyroid cancer.

Among those patients with known thyroid cancer, any technique that would allow the surgeon to more readily assess the adequacy of the total/near-total thyroidectomy intraoperatively would be beneficial to patients. If it were possible to assess the residual thyroid tissue either hormonally or via some specific altering of thyroid tissue so that it is more distinctly different from the surrounding tissue, then some patients would be saved from the increased morbidity associated with the need to perform completion thyroidectomies.

In a similar manner, patients with known thyroid cancer would benefit from techniques or technologies that would allow a surgeon to better assess lymph nodes intraoperatively. If surgeons could determine which patients had positive lymph nodes more accurately, then only those patients who have positive nodes would get node dissections. In this fashion, the risks to those patients who would not benefit from node dissection would be reduced. Among those patients with positive nodes from thyroid cancer, any technique that could allow for the intraoperative assessment of the adequacy of lymph node clearance would be a significant benefit for patients. Such information would allow surgeons to more closely tailor the patient's operation to the patient's specific condition.

Conclusions

Thyroid surgery has dramatically changed over the last century and a half. In 1866, Dr. Samuel Gross wrote:

> But no sensible man will, on slight considerations, attempt to extirpate a goitrous thyroid gland. If a surgeon should be so adventurous, or fool-hardy, as to undertake the enterprise, I shall not envy him his feelings, while engaged in the performance of it, or after he has completed it, should he be so fortunate as to do this. Every step he takes will be environed by with difficulty, every stroke of his knife will be followed by a torrent of blood, and lucky will it be for him if his victim live long enough to enable him to finish his horrid butchery.

Certainly, things have changed since Dr. Gross' time. Thyroid surgery has become a very safe procedure from which the vast majority of patients rapidly recover. However, if we remain sensitive to the complications that continue to occur in our patients, we will continue to strive in the future to improve the operation. Although none of the items suggested above may occur in the next 10 years, it remains valuable to contemplate what could make thyroid surgery a better operation for our patients. Although not all new ideas are good ideas, unless we remain dissatisfied with the current state of affairs, we will not seek new options for how to make operations better. In future years, we hope that surgeons will continue to strive to improve surgery for our patients while maintaining a level of skepticism of new techniques and technologies that will allow us to seek the data to ensure that what we may believe is better for patients actually results in improved outcomes.

Recommended Reading

Abadin S, Kaplan EL, Angelos P. Malpractice litigation following thyroidectomy: the role of recurrent laryngeal nerve injuries, 1989 to 2009. Surgery. 2010;148:718–22; discussion 722–3.

Barczynksi M, Konturek A, Chichon S. Randomized clinical trial of visualization versus neuromonitoring of recurrent laryngeal nerves during thyroidectomy. Br J Surg. 2009;96:240–6.

Dralle H, Sekulla C, Lorenz K, Brauckhoff M, Machens A, et al. Intraoperative monitoring of the recurrent laryngeal nerve in thyroid surgery. World J Surg. 2008;32:1358–66.

Gross SD. A system of surgery; pathological, diagnostic, therapeutic and operative. Philadelphia: Henry C. Lea; 1866. p. 394.

Hermann M, Hellebart C, Freissmuth M. Neuromonitoring in thyroid surgery: prospective evaluation of electrophysiological responses for the prediction of recurrent laryngeal nerve injury. Ann Surg. 2004;240:9–17.

Lo Gerfo P. Local/regional anesthesia for thyroidectomy: evaluation as an outpatient procedure. Surgery. 1998; 124:975–9.

Sun GH, DeMonner S, Davis MM. Epidemiological and economic trends in inpatient and outpatient thyroidectomy in the United States, 1996–2006. Thyroid. 2013;23:727–33.

Parathyroid Surgery 2020

20

Janice L. Pasieka

Confucius said *study the past if you would define the future*. To envision what parathyroid surgery will look like in 2020, one needs to understand just how far we have evolved since the parathyroid gland was first identified in an Indian Rhinoceros by Richard Owen in 1850. Ivor Sandstrom, a Swedish medical student, went on to describe the *glandulae parathyroideae* in humans in 1880. A decade later Eugene Gley began to elucidate the importance of the parathyroid glands in calcium homeostasis when he recognized the loss of parathyroid gland caused tetany in dogs. In 1903, Max Askanazy noted the association of enlarged parathyroid glands with von Recklinghausen bone disease (osteitis fibrosa cystica). Many thought the parathyroid enlargement was compensatory, and initially, patients with osteitis fibrosa cystica were treated with parathyroid extract and/or grafts. In 1915, Friedrich Schlagenhaufer suggested that the enlarged parathyroid tumors were the primary cause of the bone disease and recommended surgical excision. It was 10 years later, in 1925, that Felix Mandl performed the first parathyroidectomy in Vienna, excising an enlarged parathyroid gland in a patient suffering from bone disease. The patient's calcium dropped significantly postoperatively and the bone disease, overtime, improved. Unfortunately the disease reoccurred 6 years later. Around the same time in North America, surgeons also embarked on neck explorations for what was later termed "hyperparathyroidism" (HPT). In their 1929 article Barr et al described the condition of osteitis fibrosa cystica associated with muscle weakness, renal stones, high serum calcium, and elevated urinary calcium caused by a solitary parathyroid adenoma. As experience mounted, surgeons soon learned that not all patients had solitary adenomas and recognized the need to explore all four parathyroid glands to rule out the 19 % of patients with multi-gland disease. A bilateral neck exploration (BNE) became the standard surgical approach for this disease. The strategy of a unilateral exploration (ULE) was first suggested by Roth et al. in 1975 and subsequently championed by Tibblin et al. in the early 1980s. The principle of a ULE was the removal of one abnormal gland and identification of a normal gland on the ipsilateral side. Developed long before accurate preoperative imaging, the choice of which side to start the operation was arbitrary. It was not until the development of preoperative imaging did this more limited approach gain acceptance. Minimally invasive surgical techniques in general surgery lead many surgical pioneers to experiment within the realm of endocrine surgery. More directed approaches for parathyroid pathology were explored with the development of various surgical adjuncts.

J.L. Pasieka, MD, FRCSC, FACS (✉)
Department of Surgery,
North Tower,
1403 29th Street NW, T2N 2T9
Calgary, Alberta, Canada
e-mail: janice.pasieka@albertahealthservices.ca

D.J. Terris, M.C. Singer (eds.), *Minimally Invasive and Robotic Thyroid and Parathyroid Surgery*,
DOI 10.1007/978-1-4614-9011-1_20, © Springer Science+Business Media New York 2014

This chapter describes the evolution of the diagnosis of HPT and the developments in preoperative imaging and surgical adjuncts that have expanded the surgical armamentarium that surgeons utilize today. By reflecting on the past, I hope to be able to speculate on what surgery for HPT will look like in 2020.

Diagnosis

Historically, patients presented with the clinical manifestations of long-standing HPT and end-organ damage such as osteitis fibrosa cystica, nephrolithiasis, and muscle atrophy. Other symptoms such as pancreatitis, peptic ulcer disease, and metal disturbances were added to the growing list of symptoms associated with HPT. Fuller Albright can be credited for studying and documenting the clinical manifestation of HPT in the initial decades of this disease. The ability to measure PTH was not developed until the late 1960s. Widespread use of serum channel autoanalyzers in the 1970s allowed for earlier detection of this disease. Approximately 70–80 % of patients diagnosed with HPT today have none of the classical manifestations of the disease. Compared to the initial presentation of this disease, only 20–30 % of patients today have nephrolithiasis, overt skeletal disease is rare, but osteoporosis is increasing and acute pancreatitis and hypercalcemic crisis are uncommon. However, many studies have demonstrated that HPT patients suffer from vague nonspecific symptoms that are difficult to quantify yet appear to improve following parathyroidectomy. Thus over time, HPT has evolved from a clinical diagnosis with end-organ damage to a biochemical one with vague symptomatology. So much so that HPT can be detected before calcium levels are elevated, so call normocalcemic HPT. With earlier detection, it has been demonstrated the patients operated on between after 1995 had a smaller gland weights and lower preoperative serum calcium levels compared to those operated on between before 1995. This trend of earlier detection could potentially lead to a decreased sensitivity in preoperative imaging and increased rate of failed explorations.

Imaging

In 1983, Ferlin et al. described for the first time a novel method of localizing parathyroid adenomas utilizing two different radioisotopes, technetium-99 and thalium-201. This was based on the concept that technetium was taken up by the thyroid alone, and thallium by both thyroid and parathyroid glands. Double-isotope subtraction scans were labor intense and had a much lower sensitivity of localizing the diseased parathyroid gland compared to an experienced endocrine surgeon. The development of technetium-99m sestamibi (Tc-99m MIBI) in 1989 increased both the use and the sensitivity of nuclear imaging. Tc-99m MIBI is taken up by both thyroid and parathyroid tissue but washes out faster from the thyroid gland. Anatomical detail is enhanced with the addition of single-photon emission computed tomography/computed tomography (SPECT/CT). Although this technique can localize single-gland disease 80 % of the time, unfortunately the sensitivity of Tc-99m MIBI remains poor in multi-gland disease with a sensitivity of only 63 %.

High-resolution ultrasound (US) has become more commonly utilized for preoperative imaging. It provides excellent anatomical detail, is noninvasive, and is inexpensive. It also has the ability to detect concomitant thyroid nodules that must be addressed prior to surgical exploration. Although operative dependent, US has been shown to have an accuracy of 70–80 % for solitary disease, much less for multi-gland disease (35 %). As a result many centers use the combination of US and Tc-99m MIBI, increasing the accuracy in solitary disease to >94 %.

Other techniques such as axial imaging with CT and MRI have been shown to be useful in the re-operative setting. Four-dimensional CT imaging (4DCT), with the additional dimension being time, has improved on the other imaging modalities. In a study of 75 patients, 4DCT had a greater sensitivity for localization of the parathyroid adenoma (88 %) compared to MIBI (65 %) and US (57 %). However, the same group has recently analyzed this technique and found it did not appear to shorten operative time or failure rates.

As such the clinical benefit of 4DCT in first-time HPT patients must be weighed against the increased cost and increased radiation exposure to the patient.

Despite the increased technological advances in preoperative imaging, multi-gland disease remains a challenge. Surgical exploration still is the best localizing modality when done by an experienced endocrine surgeon. What is important to remember is that none of the imaging modalities are diagnostic. The indication for any preoperative imaging modality is for surgical planning only. Patients in whom imaging failed to localize disease are still surgical candidates and the majority will be cure with a BNE.

Surgical Technique

Given that the definition of minimally invasive parathyroidectomy (MIP) is "any surgical access to a selected single gland," it can be said that the first parathyroidectomy was a focused, "MIP" operation. When it became apparent early in the surgical experience that up to 20 % of patients had multi-gland disease, BNE became the standard operation for HPT. With the majority of patients having solitary adenomas, in 1975, Roth et al. first proposed that a unilateral approach would be adequate for the majority of patients as long as the surgeon recognized one abnormal and one normal parathyroid gland on the same side. Unilateral exploration met with early resistance given that 50 % of the time, the surgeon had to convert to a BNE because selection of the operative side was arbitrary. Once preoperative imaging became more reliable, surgeons started to see the benefit of a more focused approach to this disease. In a randomized control trial, Bergenfelz et al. demonstrated that ULE patients had lower incidence of postoperative hypocalcemia and shorter operative time with the same cure rate (97 %) compared to a BNE.

With the development of intraoperative PTH (iPTH) came the move from purely morphologically based operations (BNE, ULE) to utilizing this adjunct to indicate when all abnormally functioning parathyroid tissue was removed. Others experimented with another adjunct borrowed from the sentinel node experience in breast and melanoma. Utilizing a gamma probe to find and measure the radioactivity of excised tissue, several surgeons found that this technique allowed for a focused approach without the need for iPTH or frozen section to confirm parathyroid tissue.

With the development of better preoperative imaging and surgical adjuncts that demonstrated when all autonomously functioning parathyroid tissue was removed, the era of MIP was born. The focused open approach to a single gland demonstrated several advantages over a BNE. An anterior cervical approach allowed for regional anesthesia in selected patients, shorter incisions, and decreased morbidity while maintaining an excellent cure rate of 95–97 %. Advances in surgical endoscopic techniques allowed for the development of a variety of MIP surgical approaches. Miccoli introduced the video-assisted technique, Henry introduced the endoscopic approach, and various "scarless" approaches from the axilla or anterior chest with the use of gasless techniques or robotic surgery have been described. In a review of the literature, currently robotic techniques for parathyroid surgery appear to be reasonable for mediastinal tumors, but there is lack of data to support an advantage over an open cervical approach for the majority of patients. Natural orifice surgery has been applied to thyroid surgery, so it is conceivable that parathyroidectomy maybe be next. The wisdom of development of such a procedure has been questioned.

What Will Parathyroid Surgery Look Like in 2020?

Parathyroid surgery in 2020 will likely have geographic diversity. Not all health-care systems will be able to afford the emerging technology presently driving the changes in the surgical approach to HPT. The utilization of preoperative imaging must remain cost-effective, safe for the patient, and easily accessible. Ultrasound and/or Tc-99m MIBI scan will likely continue to play a key role in the preoperative planning of patients that are suitable for MIP. Three-dimensional virtual imaging will likely become more mainstream in the surgical world in developed nations by 2020. It is only a matter of time before Tc-99m MIBI scans can be superimposed on a 3D virtual model. This will allow the surgeon to plan the ideal operative approach and conceivably allow for simulator training preoperatively.

With the growing number of patients undergoing MIP, utilization of iPTH has increased. Recent advances in the development of a fast iPTH point-of-care assay will allow for faster and simpler means of measuring PTH in the operating room. However, the cost-effectiveness of iPTH has been questioned by some. Intraoperative PTH was found to be advantageous in only 3 % of patients, making BNE, or one could argue a traditional ULE, still the most cost-effective surgical strategy for centers unable to afford this adjunct.

The open focused MIP techniques are more cost-effective than any of the endoscopic or robotic techniques, especially when performed under regional block. Expertise in these more costly endoscopic techniques will likely remain focused in a few centers throughout the world, yet for most, a cervical approach will remain the most commonly performed operation. It is said however, that *history has way of repeating itself.* If true, does that mean we are moving from the era of MIP back to a BNE? Although several authors have reported excellent results with MIP, recently some surgeons have started question whether this technology-driven phenomenon has gone too far. The Achilles' heel for the parathyroid surgeon will always be multi-gland disease. Both iPTH and concordant preoperative imaging have been shown to be inaccurate in multi-gland disease. Siperstein et al in their large prospective study of over 900 patients undergoing BNE found that the combination of localizing studies and iPTH failed to identify multi-gland disease in 16 % of patients. They questioned whether long-term follow-up of these patients will demonstrate a greater recurrence than reported to date. Large prospective databases, with long-term follow-up, are starting to notice a greater recurrence rate in patients undergoing MIP versus a BNE. Schneider et al. analyzed more than 1,000 cases and found overall that there was no difference in the recurrence rate between MIP and BNE (2.5 vs. 1.9 %). Yet when considering the period beyond 8 years alone, there was an 8 % recurrence rate in MIP-treated patients compared to zero in the BNE. This has led one of the MIP staunchest advocate to abandon MIP and return to BNE. Furthermore, there is an ongoing body of literature reporting an increased rate of elevated PTH levels postoperatively in patients considered cured. Elevated PTH with concomitant normal serum calcium has been found to occur between 11 and 44 % of postoperative patients. Although this can occur following a bilateral exploration (36 %), focused approaches have demonstrated a higher incidence of this phenomenon (64 %). A recent 10-year follow-up of MIP patients with persistently elevated PTH demonstrated a 5 % recurrence rate. It is therefore conceivable that many of the 16 % of patients that Siperstein et al. found with multi-gland disease on further exploration will ultimately recur if followed long enough. The clinical relevance of this anomaly is unclear. Let us not forget, however, that the first parathyroidectomy patient recurred 6 years later. Hopefully by 2020 we will have elucidated the clinical significance of this finding with more long-term prospective follow-up studies.

Finally, nonsurgical techniques for HPT are under investigation. Surgery for other slow-growing tumors such as hepatocelluar carcinoma and neuroendocrine tumors has changed over the past decade with the development of ablative techniques such as radiofrequency ablation (RFA) and ethanol injections. Although most of these techniques have been for unresectable disease, the technology does exist and can be adapted to the neck region. Both ethanol and RFA have been utilized for locoregional control in thyroid cancer patients. Injury to the RLN was seen in those treated with RFA in the central compartment, yet it is likely just a matter of time before smaller probes are developed allowing for more precise application. Ethanol injection for HPT was initially reported by the Mayo Clinic group in 1998. In this study, 12/36 patient treated were eucalcemic on follow-up, demonstrating the feasibility of this technique. Little has been written since that report until recently. In 2011 Chen et al. reported their results of percutaneous ethanol injection in persistent or recurrent secondary HPT. Forty-five of the 49 patients have a clinically significant decrease in their PTH. Kovatcheva et al. reported a pilot study utilizing high-intensity focused ultrasound on four patients with HPT. Three patients normalized their calcium and two had normalization of their PTH at follow-up. It is therefore conceivable that nonoperative, percutaneous techniques for ablation of parathyroid adenoma will be part of the surgical strategies offered to patients in the future. It is therefore important that endocrine surgeons be part of this developing technology.

The history of parathyroid surgery illustrates how surgical pioneers, along with technical advances, have changed the surgical paradigm for this disease. We started with removal on one gland, only to find a BNE was needed to ensure long-term cure. More recently, with the development of better imaging and iPTH, we have moved towards a more focused approach to this disease. George Santayana said, *those who do not learn from history are doomed to repeat it.* I would therefore like to dedicate this chapter to my surgical mentors, Norman W Thompson and Bertil Hamberger, two endocrine surgical leaders who taught me the sound principles of parathyroid surgery in the era of BNE. It is those principles that have allowed me to recognize that these technological advances and adjuncts are only tools, and not substitutes, for diligent surgical exploration. Surgery for parathyroid disease will continue to evolve well beyond 2020. However, it is paramount that the next generation of endocrine surgeons has within their armamentarium an ability to safely and effectively perform a BNE and to properly select patients for a less invasive approach.

Recommended Reading

Abbott DE, Cantor SB, Grubbs EG, et al. Outcomes and economic analysis of routine preoperative 4-dimensional CT for surgical intervention in de novo primary hyperparathyroidism: does clinical benefit justify the cost? J Am Coll Surg. 2012;214:629–37; discussion 637–9.

Albright F. A page out of history of hyperparathyroidism. J Clin Endocrinol Metab. 1948;8:637–57.

Almquist M, Bergenfelz A, Martensson H, Thier M, Nordenstrom E. Changing biochemical presentation of primary hyperparathyroidism. Langenbecks Arch Surg. 2010;395:925–8.

Askanazy M. Ueber ostitis deformans ohne osteides. Arb Pathol Inst Tubingen. 1904;4:398–422.

Barr DP, Bulger HA, Dixon HH. Hyperparathyroidism. JAMA. 1929;92:951–2.

Bergenfelz A, Lindblom P, Tibblin S, Westerdahl J. Unilateral versus bilateral neck exploration for primary hyperparathyroidism: a prospective randomized controlled trial. Ann Surg. 2002;236:543–51.

Bergenfelz A, Kanngiesser V, Zielke A, Nies C, Rothmund M. Conventional bilateral cervical exploration versus open minimally invasive parathyroidectomy under local anaesthesia for primary hyperparathyroidism. Br J Surg. 2005;92:190–7.

Bergenfelz AO, Jansson SK, Wallin GK, et al. Impact of modern techniques on short-term outcome after surgery for primary hyperparathyroidism: a multicenter study comprising 2,708 patients. Langenbecks Arch Surg. 2009;394:851–60.

Bilezikian JP, Silverberg SJ. Normocalcemic primary hyperparathyroidism. Arq Bras Endocrinol Metabol. 2010;54:106–9.

Caron NR, Pasieka JL. What symptom improvement can be expected after operation for primary hyperparathyroidism? World J Surg. 2009;33:2244–55.

Carsello CB, Yen TW, Wang TS. Persistent elevation in serum parathyroid hormone levels in normocalcemic patients after parathyroidectomy: does it matter? Surgery. 2012;152:575–83.

Carty SE, Roberts MM, Virji MA, Haywood L, Yim JH. Elevated serum parathormone level after "concise parathyroidectomy" for primary sporadic hyperparathyroidism. Surgery. 2002;132:1086–92; discussion 1092–3.

Chen H, Mack E, Starling JR. Radioguided parathyroidectomy is equally effective for both adenomatous and hyperplastic glands. Ann Surg. 2003;238:332–7; discussion 337–8.

Chen H, Mack E, Starling JR. A comprehensive evaluation of perioperative adjuncts during minimally invasive parathyroidectomy: which is most reliable? Ann Surg. 2005;242:375–80; discussion 380–3.

Chen HH, Lin CJ, Wu CJ, et al. Chemical ablation of recurrent and persistent secondary hyperparathyroidism after subtotal parathyroidectomy. Ann Surg. 2011;253:786–90.

Cirocchi R, Trastulli S, Boselli C, et al. Radiofrequency ablation in the treatment of liver metastases from colorectal cancer. Cochrane Database Syst Rev. 2012;6, CD006317.

Cope O. The story of hyperparathyroidism at the Massachusetts General Hospital. N Engl J Med. 1966;274:1174–82.

D'Agostino J, Diana M, Vix M, Soler L, Marescaux J. Three-dimensional virtual neck exploration before parathyroidectomy. N Engl J Med. 2012;367(11): 1072–3.

Donatini G, Materazzi G, Miccoli P. The endoscopic approach to the neck: a review of the literature and an overview of the various techniques. Surg Endosc. 2012;26:287.

Doppman JL. Reoperative parathyroid surgery; localization procedures. Prog Surg. 1986;18:117–32.

Eastell R, Arnold A, Brandi ML, et al. Diagnosis of asymptomatic primary hyperparathyroidism: proceedings of the third international workshop. J Clin Endocrinol Metab. 2009;94:340–50.

Felger EA, Kandil E. Primary hyperparathyroidism. Otolaryngol Clin North Am. 2010;43:417–32, x.

Ferlin G, Borsato N, Camerani M, Conte N, Zotti D. New perspectives in localizing enlarged parathyroids by technetium-thallium subtraction scan. J Nucl Med. 1983;24:438–41.

Foley CS, Agcaoglu O, Siperstein AE, Berber E. Robotic transaxillary endocrine surgery: a comparison with conventional open technique. Surg Endosc. 2012;26: 2259–66.

Fraker DL, Harsono H, Lewis R. Minimally invasive parathyroidectomy: benefits and requirements of localization, diagnosis, and intraoperative PTH monitoring. long-term results. World J Surg. 2009;33: 2256–65.

Fraser WD. Hyperparathyroidism. Lancet. 2009;374: 145–58.

Genc V, Agcaoglu O, Berber E. Robotic endocrine surgery: technical details and review of the literature. J Robot Surg. 2012;6:85–97.

Goldfarb M, Gondek S, Irvin 3rd GL, Lew JI. Normocalcemic parathormone elevation after successful parathyroidectomy: long-term analysis of parathormone variations over 10 years. Surgery. 2011;150: 1076–84.

Harman CR, Grant CS, Hay ID, et al. Indications, technique, and efficacy of alcohol injection of enlarged parathyroid glands in patients with primary hyperparathyroidism. Surgery. 1998;124:1011–9; discussion 1019–20.

Harness JK. Invited commentary on "Scan-directed unilateral cervical exploration for parathyroid adenoma: a legitimate approach?". World J Surg. 1990;14:409.

Harris R, Ryu H, Vu T, et al. Modern approach to surgical intervention of the thyroid and parathyroid glands. Semin Ultrasound CT MR. 2012;33:115–22.

Henry JF, Defechereux T, Gramatica L, de Boissezon C. Minimally invasive videoscopic parathyroidectomy by lateral approach. Langenbecks Arch Surg. 1999;384:298–301.

Hessman O, Westerdahl J, Al-Suliman N, Christiansen P, Hellman P, Bergenfelz A. Randomized clinical trial comparing open with video-assisted minimally invasive parathyroid surgery for primary hyperparathyroidism. Br J Surg. 2010;97:177–84.

Ikeda Y, Takami H. Endoscopic parathyroidectomy. Biomed Pharmacother. 2000;54 Suppl 1:52s–656.

Irvin 3rd GL, Prudhomme DL, Deriso GT, Sfakianakis G, Chandarlapaty SK. A new approach to parathyroidectomy. Ann Surg. 1994;219:574–9; discussion 579–81.

Irvin 3rd GL, Sfakianakis G, Yeung L, et al. Ambulatory parathyroidectomy for primary hyperparathyroidism. Arch Surg. 1996;131:1074–8.

Irvin 3rd GL, Carneiro DM, Solorzano CC. Progress in the operative management of sporadic primary hyperparathyroidism over 34 years. Ann Surg. 2004;239:704–8; discussion 708–11.

Jarrige V, Nieuwenhuis JH, van Son JP, Martens MF, Vissers JL. A fast intraoperative PTH point-of-care assay on the Philips handheld magnotech system. Langenbecks Arch Surg. 2011;396:337–43.

Kovatcheva RD, Vlahov JD, Shinkov AD, et al. High-intensity focused ultrasound to treat primary hyperparathyroidism: a feasibility study in four patients. AJR Am J Roentgenol. 2010;195:830–5.

Kunstman JW, Udelsman R. Superiority of minimally invasive parathyroidectomy. Adv Surg. 2012;46: 171–89.

Lew JI, Solorzano CC. Surgical management of primary hyperparathyroidism: state of the art. Surg Clin North Am. 2009;89:1205–25.

Miccoli P, Bendinelli C, Conte M, Pinchera A, Marcocci C. Endoscopic parathyroidectomy by a gasless approach. J Laparoendosc Adv Surg Tech A. 1998;8:189–94.

Miccoli P, Materazzi G, Berti P. Natural orifice surgery on the thyroid gland using totally transoral video-assisted thyroidectomy: report of the first experimental results for a new surgical method: are we going in the right direction? Surg Endosc. 2010;24:957–8; author reply 959–60.

Mihai R, Palazzo FF, Gleeson FV, Sadler GP. Minimally invasive parathyroidectomy without intraoperative parathyroid hormone monitoring in patients with primary hyperparathyroidism. Br J Surg. 2007;94:42–7.

Mihai R, Barczynski M, Iacobone M, Sitges-Serra A. Surgical strategy for sporadic primary hyperparathyroidism an evidence-based approach to surgical strategy, patient selection, surgical access, and reoperations. Langenbecks Arch Surg. 2009;394:785–98.

Naitoh T, Gagner M, Garcia-Ruiz A, Heniford BT. Endoscopic endocrine surgery in the neck. An initial report of endoscopic subtotal parathyroidectomy. Surg Endosc. 1998;12:202–5; discussion 206.

Norman J, Politz D. 5,000 parathyroid operations without frozen section or PTH assays: measuring individual parathyroid gland hormone production in real time. Ann Surg Oncol. 2009;16:656–66.

Norman J, Lopez J, Politz D. Abandoning unilateral parathyroidectomy: why we reversed our position after 15,000 parathyroid operations. J Am Coll Surg. 2012;214:260–9.

Owen R. On the anatomy of the Indian Rhinoceros. Tran Zool Soc Lon. 1862;4:31–58.

Rahbar K, Colombo-Benkmann M, Haane C, et al. Intraoperative 3-D mapping of parathyroid adenoma using freehand SPECT. EJNMMI Res. 2012;2:51.

Riss P, Scheuba C, Asari R, Bieglmayer C, Niederle B. Is minimally invasive parathyroidectomy without QPTH monitoring justified? Langenbecks Arch Surg. 2009;394:875–80.

Rodgers SE, Hunter GJ, Hamberg LM, et al. Improved preoperative planning for directed parathyroidectomy with 4-dimensional computed tomography. Surgery. 2006;140:932–40; discussion 940–1.

Roth SL, Wang C-A, Potts JT. The team approach to primary hyperparathyroidism. Hum Pathol. 1975;6:645–8.

Russell C. Unilateral neck exploration for primary hyperparathyroidism. Surg Clin North Am. 2004;84:705–16.

Schlagenhaufer F. Zwei falle von parathyroideatumoren. Wien Kiln Wochenschr Zentral. 1915;28:1362.

Schneider DF, Mazeh H, Sippel RS, Chen H. Is minimally invasive parathyroidectomy associated with greater recurrence compared to bilateral exploration? Analysis of more than 1,000 cases. Surgery. 2012;152: 1008–15.

Shiina S, Tateishi R, Imamura M, et al. Percutaneous ethanol injection for hepatocellular carcinoma: 20-year outcome and prognostic factors. Liver Int. 2012;32: 1434–42.

Shin JE, Baek JH, Lee JH. Radiofrequency and ethanol ablation for the treatment of recurrent thyroid cancers: current status and challenges. Curr Opin Oncol. 2013;25:14–9.

Sidhu S, Neill AK, Russell CF. Long-term outcome of unilateral parathyroid exploration for primary hyperparathyroidism due to presumed solitary adenoma. World J Surg. 2003;27:339–42.

Silverberg SJ, Lewiecki EM, Mosekilde L, Peacock M, Rubin MR. Presentation of asymptomatic primary hyperparathyroidism: proceedings of the third international workshop. J Clin Endocrinol Metab. 2009;94: 351–65.

Siperstein A, Berber E, Barbosa GF, et al. Predicting the success of limited exploration for primary hyperparathyroidism using ultrasound, sestamibi, and intraoperative parathyroid hormone: analysis of 1158 cases. Ann Surg. 2008;248:420–8.

Stalberg P, Sidhu S, Sywak M, Robinson B, Wilkinson M, Delbridge L. Intraoperative parathyroid hormone measurement during minimally invasive parathyroidectomy: does it "value-add" to decision-making? J Am Coll Surg. 2006;203:1–6.

Terris DJ, Stack BCJ, Gourin CG. Contemporary parathyroidectomy: exploiting technology. Am J Otolaryngol. 2007;28:408–14.

Terris DJ, Weinberger PM, Farrag T, Seybt M, Oliver JE. Restoring point-of-care testing during parathyroidectomy with a newer parathyroid hormone assay. Otolaryngol Head Neck Surg. 2011;145:557–60.

Thompson NW. The history of hyperparathyroidism. Acta Chir Scand. 1990;156:5–21.

Tibblin S, Bondeson A-G, Ljungberg O. Unilateral parathyroidectomy in hyperparathyroidism due to single adenoma. Ann Surg. 1982;195:245–52.

Twigt BA, van Dalen T, Vollebregt AM, Kortlandt W, Vriens MR, Borel Rinkes IH. The additional value of intraoperative parathyroid hormone assessment is marginal in patients with nonfamilial primary hyperparathyroidism: a prospective cohort study. Am J Surg. 2012;204:1–6.

Udelsman R, Lin Z, Donovan P. The superiority of minimally invasive parathyroidectomy based on 1650 consecutive patients with primary hyperparathyroidism. Ann Surg. 2011;253:585–91.

Wang TS, Ostrower ST, Heller KS. Persistently elevated parathyroid hormone levels after parathyroid surgery. Surgery. 2005;138:1130–5; discussion 1135–6.

Willatt JM, Francis IR, Novelli PM, Vellody R, Pandya A, Krishnamurthy VN. Interventional therapies for hepatocellular carcinoma. Cancer Imaging. 2012;12: 79–88.

21 The Future of Robotic Thyroid Surgery and Neck Dissection

F. Christopher Holsinger

As the preceding chapters attest, surgical robotics has moved from the realm of fantasy and science fiction to routine clinical practice. At present, the da Vinci Surgical System (Intuitive Surgical Inc., Sunnyvale, CA) is the only commercially available surgical robot. While this system is used extensively to facilitate laparoscopic minimally invasive surgery in the chest, abdomen, and pelvis, its use for surgery of the thyroid, parathyroid, and neck remains investigational. While the currently available 5- and 8-mm instruments have been appropriate for the first generation of robotic neck procedures, as technology improves, robotic systems and instruments will likely be developed whose scale and capabilities are better suited to the delicate, complex anatomy of the thyroid bed and neck.

New Robotic Systems

With robotic surgery, the surgeon and his hands are physically separate from the patient. Real surgery is performed in a virtual environment, allowing the surgeon to interact with surgical anatomy from a novel perspective, in otherwise inaccessible places and in ways that otherwise would not be possible.

F.C. Holsinger, MD, FACS
Division of Head and Neck Surgery,
Stanford University Medical Center,
Stanford, CA
e-mail: holsinger@stanford.edu

With da Vinci, a three-part robotic surgical architecture is utilized. Surgical instruments are located within a *"patient-side" cart* and are safely placed by the surgeon within the patient's body under direct and/or endoscopic guidance. A binocular 8.5- or 12-mm endoscope with dual 0° or 30° optics is used to visualize target anatomy. The three-dimensional (3-D) surgical anatomy is then recreated using the *"vision" cart,* where computer processing links the camera's image and the real-world spatial relationships of the instruments in a virtual environment. The surgeon, sitting at a *remote console cart*, can then operate within this virtual 3-D environment using "master controllers" which control and direct movements of the robotic instruments. These master controllers bear a remarkable similarity to joysticks and other handheld devices employed in video games and other virtual reality simulators. For hemostasis and energy, monopolar electrocautery and the Harmonic Scalpel® (Ethicon Endo-Surgery, Johnson & Johnson, Cincinnati, OH) are used.

Limitations of the current system include the scale of instrumentation, absence of an optimal energy source, absence of haptic feedback, and fixed angulation stereo-endoscopes. Throughout the chapters in this text, 5-mm instruments are the currently most-widely utilized for robotic neck surgery. While an improvement over 8-mm instruments, the current 5-mm instruments may still be too large for several crucial tasks, including precise and trauma-free dissection along the recurrent laryngeal nerve. The Maryland

D.J. Terris, M.C. Singer (eds.), *Minimally Invasive and Robotic Thyroid and Parathyroid Surgery*,
DOI 10.1007/978-1-4614-9011-1_21, © Springer Science+Business Media New York 2014

Dissecting Forceps have a scale resembling standard micro-Halsted dissecting forceps, though a smaller caliber, closer to the Jacobsen delicate forceps, would be preferred. Furthermore, an ideal instrument for dissection along the nerve would be fashioned with a gentle curvature that provides optimal tissue handling and traction/countertraction close to neurovascular structures. New instrumentation will likely incorporate both a smaller scale and more optimal curvature of the tip of the forceps. Although flexible at the distal end of the 5-mm instrument, the sheathed and rigid robotic arm does still limit the angle of approach to surgical anatomy. A fully flexible robotic arm throughout most of its length would allow the robotic neck surgeon to more intuitively use instruments in the thyroid bed and neck. For hemostasis, using current Intuitive Surgical instrumentation, the surgeon must choose between an 8-mm bipolar cautery Maryland Forceps and the Harmonic Scalpel (5 or 8 mm). Furthermore, in the future, a 5-mm bipolar dissecting forceps will likely be available, allowing the surgeon to manage small sites of bleeding with minimal thermal spread.

The use of the Harmonic Scalpel has been shown to be an effective surgical tool for hemostasis for thyroid and parathyroid surgery. However, ultrasonic technology requires that the surgical arm be fixed without any flexibility in the robotic arm's distal tip. This architecture may often limit the surgeon's ability to align the Harmonic Scalpel with the angle of the blood vessel or soft tissue which is being divided. Refinements in ultrasonic technology, perhaps incorporating bipolar electrocautery, may one day allow the robotic thyroid surgeon to provide better hemostasis especially along Berry's posterolateral ligament near the recurrent laryngeal nerve, without undue risk of thermal injury and the potential for either temporary or permanent neuropraxia.

Whether using remote access through either retroauricular or axillary incision, angled binocular stereo-endoscopes are a critical aspect of performing a safe robotic procedure in the neck and thyroid bed. The da Vinci provides rigid endoscopes with either 0° or 30° angulation, with an 8.5- or 12-mm diameter. The current platform offers the surgeon an unparalleled view of thyroid and neck surgical anatomy, yet in several instances, greater angulation, especially with a flexible binocular stereo-endoscope, would offer a significant clinical advantage. For instance, the use of a single ipsilateral incision to expose the anatomy of the contralateral recurrent laryngeal nerve tests the limits of the surgeon and endoscope. A variety of maneuvers described in the text provides the surgeon with a good estimation of this anatomy using the camera in the 30° down position. However, a flexible camera that would allow for 45–60° visualization would likely permit the surgeon to have better assessment of small blood vessels in the vicinity of the recurrent laryngeal nerve or alert the surgeon to unexpected patterns of branching or the presence of Zuckerkandl's tubercle.

A variety of new platforms may be coming to market in the coming years, with different configurations. These new systems will likely lead to greater integration of robotics into thyroid and parathyroid surgery.

Recommended Reading

Hockstein NG, Gourin CG, Faust RA, Terris DJ. A history of robotic surgery: from science fiction to surgical robotics. J Robot Surg. 2007;1(2):113–8.

Lee J, Chung WY. Robotic thyroidectomy and neck dissection: past, present, and future. Cancer J. 2013;19: 151–61. doi:10.1097/PPO.Ob013e31828aab61.

Mohr C. Catherine Mohr: surgery's past, present and robotic future – YouTube. http://bit.ly/15O0SHU. Accessed 21 May 2013.

Index

D.J. Terris, M.C. Singer (eds.), *Minimally Invasive and Robotic Thyroid and Parathyroid Surgery*, DOI 10.1007/978-1-4614-9011-1, © Springer Science+Business Media New York 2014

MIX
Papier aus verantwortungsvollen Quellen
Paper from responsible sources
FSC® C105338

If you have any concerns about our products,
you can contact us on
ProductSafety@springernature.com

In case Publisher is established outside the EU,
the EU authorized representative is:
Springer Nature Customer Service Center GmbH
Europaplatz 3, 69115 Heidelberg, Germany

Printed by Libri Plureos GmbH
in Hamburg, Germany